AF804417

The AHA-Syndrome and Cardiovascular Diseases

The AHA-Syndrome and Cardiovascular Diseases

Edited by
Dr. Swati Y. Bhave
Executive Director, Association of Adolescent and Child Care in India (AACCI)
Senior Visiting Consultant, Indraprastha Apollo Hospital, New Delhi
Former Senior Consultant and Postgraduate Teacher
Bombay Hospital and Medical Research Centre, Mumbai

Sunil Saini
Department of Applied Psychology
Guru Jambheshwar University of Science and Technology
Hisar - 125 001

Anshan
Tunbridge Wells, UK

CONSISTING OF KNOWLEDGE
Anamaya Publishers
New Delhi

A catalogue record for the book is available from the British Library

ISBN 978-1848290-235

Copublished by
Anshan Limited
The Control Centre
11a Little Mount Sion
Tunbridge Wells
Kent TN1 1YS
United Kingdom
Tel.: +44 (0) 1892 557767
Fax: +44 (0) 1892 530358
Email: info@anshan.co.uk
Website: www.anshan.co.uk

Sold and distributed in all the countries, except India, Pakistan, Sri Lanka, Bangladesh, Bhutan and Nepal by Anshan Limited, The Control Centre, 11a Little Mount Sion, Tunbridge Wells, Kent TN1 1YS, United Kingdom

In India, Pakistan, Sri Lanka, Bangladesh, Bhutan and Nepal by
Anamaya Publishers, F-154/2 Lado Sarai, New Delhi - 110 030, India
Email: anamayapub@vsnl.net

All rights reserved.
Copyright © 2010. Anamaya Publishers, New Delhi

No part of the material protected by this copyright notice may be reproduced or utilised in any form or by any means, electronic or mechanical, including photocopying, recording or by any information storage and retrieval system without the written permission from the copyright owner.

Printed in India.

Dedicated to

My father-in-law Mr. Shripad Bhave whose exemplary anger management in his whole life both at home and at work has resulted in his living a healthy life, even today at the age of 89 years.

Swati Y. Bhave

The loving memory of my mother, who passed away before I could present her time's most precious gift, of which she would have been very proud.

Sunil Saini

Foreword

Today's newspapers, news channels, magazines etc., are full of incidents related to anger, hostile behaviour, aggression (the AHA-Syndrome) and violence. Almost every society around the world is under the threat of war and terrorism, which is an extreme form of the AHA-Syndrome. It has been well recognised that negative emotions like the AHA-Syndrome in human beings increase the risk of hypertension, stroke and other coronary artery disease, i.e. CHD and sudden death. This is a field of active research.

The AHA-Syndrome is very common at home, office, public places and workplace at every stage of life. There is a great need to study anger, hostility and aggression in the childhood, adolescence, adulthood and older people to unfold the root cause of this growing epidemic (the AHA-Syndrome) engulfing humanity. This global issue also needs to be considered from the medical point of view.

The present volume explores the relation of psychological dimensions, particularly anger, hostility and aggression, in relation to CHD. Other dimensions such as depression, personality, stress, lifestyle behaviours, work stress, quality of life etc., have also been discussed in detail with empirical evidences.

The first section is devoted to an extensive review of the basic concept of the AHA-Syndrome. The measurement of AHA, its management and evidences regarding their consequences, especially to cardiovascular heart diseases have been discussed in detail. Early risk factors for the development of aggression and psychological well being in relation to the AHA-Syndrome with special emphasis on adolescents, gender issues have been well covered.

The second section is devoted to the relationship of the AHA-Syndrome and other emotions to cardiovascular diseases. Personality type, neuro-endocrine mechanism, marital relationships and children, emotional correlates of hypertension, hostility, depression, obesity, psychosocial factors, workplace stressors, quality of work life, self-management, early risk factors of CHD and these relationships are discussed with empirical evidences.

The third section is devoted to the management of cardiovascular diseases. Risk behaviour intervention for CHD, essential for positive cardiac health, psychological methods, nutrition and food habits, lifestyle intervention, medical management of CHD, biofeedback training and exercises in controlling cardiovascular diseases have been given full justice.

The contributors to this volume are researchers and teachers from different fields (i.e. psychology, medicine, food technology, management, physiotherapy etc.) of international and national reputation. The first editor Dr. Swati Y. Bhave is an internationally known expert on pediatrics and adolescent health. She has edited the first textbook on adolescent medicine in the country and her special interest has been in adolescent mental health. The second editor Sunil Saini, a clinical psychologist, is working on research projects on the AHA-Syndrome, development of scales and cross-cultural research on international projects.

This is a good, comprehensive volume on anger and aggression and it would be useful for students doing research in psychology and medicine for treatment of cardiovascular diseases, for practitioners at hospitals and private clinics, psychiatrists, clinical psychologists and paramedical workers.

Dr. B.K. Goyal
FAMS, FRCP, FACC (USA)
Director, Medical Education and Research
Bombay Hospital Group
Mumbai - 400 020
India

Preface

Anger, hostility and aggression (i.e. the AHA-Syndrome) and related problems are the major problems that people face today. There are increasing evidences that the AHA-Syndrome is the root cause of many of the disturbances and health problems at personal, family, workplace and societal levels. At the personal level, this may include frustration, depression, suicidal ideation, resentment, hostile attributions, school failure, school bullying, road rage, alcohol abuse, and substance abuse. At the family level, it may include marital conflict, domestic violence, parent-child discord, divorce, abuse of elders, and sexual aggression. At the workplace, the AHA-Syndrome is the leading cause of disruptions, workplace aggression, and job loss. At public places, it is the major cause of strikes, violent demonstrations, and property damage. All these emotional (anger), cognitive (hostility) and behavioural (aggression) related problems further have linkage with many physiological problems like cardiovascular heart diseases (CHD), cancer, arthritis, pain, gastrointestinal problems, respiratory diseases, irritable bowl syndrome, digestive problems, headaches etc. Thus, we see that the AHA-Syndrome affects people in almost all walks of life. In the present volume, we focus on how the AHA components develop and are effective in the progression of cardiovascular diseases. Violent crimes like terrorism and war and cardiac events like hypertension and heart attacks are the leading causes of death and disability around the world. In this volume, experienced researchers from psychology, psychiatry, medicine and other related sciences from around the world have contributed their valuable chapters with empirical evidences on how the AHA components are helpful in cardiac events. Traditional causal factors in CHD have also been discussed with more exploration.

The volume is divided into three sections. The first section is an introduction to the basic concept of the AHA-Syndrome, how it develops, and how it is experienced and expressed. Chapters 1 to 4 and Chapter 6 focus on how anger, hostility and aggression are experienced and expressed. Chapters 5 and 7 are devoted to the management of the AHA components. The second section is concerned with the relation between the AHA components and cardiovascular diseases. Chapters 8 to 12 deal with the relation between the AHA-Syndrome and CHD. Chapters 13 to 18 highlight the relation between the other dimensions of psychology and CHD. The third section covers intervention and treatment of cardiovascular diseases.

The volume is a further extension to the research literature on anger, hostility, aggression related problems and cardiovascular heart diseases in both psychology and medicine. We hope that young doctoral researchers in psychology and medicine would get benefitted from it and it would also serve as an important tool for the practitioners who are involved in the treatment of anger and aggression related problems and cardiovascular heart diseases. We thank Padma Vibhushan Dr. B.K. Goyal for agreeing to write the Foreword to this volume.

SWATI Y. BHAVE
SUNIL SAINI

Acknowledgements

We are grateful to the 34 national and international authors for their valuable contribution and helpful cooperation. We also thank M/s Anamaya Publishers, India and M/s Anshan Ltd., UK for their efforts in publishing this volume and making it available globally.

Sunil Saini is grateful to Prof. Helen Pratt, Michigan State University, USA who introduced him to Dr. Swati Y. Bhave, who encouraged and shaped his raw enthusiasm into the world of book publication. He also thanks his research assistant Ms. Neelam Goyal who has been an essential part in completing his other research assignments. He also acknowledges the support of Mr. Mukesh, In-charge, UCIC and his staff members at Guru Jambheshwar University of Science and Technology, Hisar.

SWATI Y. BHAVE
SUNIL SAINI

Contents

The AHA-Syndrome and Cardiovascular Diseases

The AHA-Syndrome and Cardiovascular Diseases
Editors: Swati Y. Bhave and Sunil Saini
Copyright © 2010 Anamaya Publishers, New Delhi, India

1. Anger, Hostility and Aggression: The AHA-Syndrome

Sunil Saini
Department of Applied Psychology, Guru Jambheshwar University of Science and Technology
Hisar - 125 001, India

Abstract: Anger, hostility and aggression – components of the AHA-Syndrome – are leading causes of today's health problems. Anger, as an emotional state, is the fundamental part of the AHA-Syndrome. It contributes to many physiological and psychological problems. Emotions and emotional style are the building blocks of a person's unique, relatively stable, and consistent pattern of personality, which dispose him/her to think, feel and behave in a particular way. Hostility, the second component, has also been found to be a major psychosocial risk factor that contributes to the etiology of coronary heart disease. Hostility involves attitudes and cognitive processes that often motivate an individual to express anger in aggressive behaviour. Aggression, the behavioural component, involves destructive or punitive behaviours that are directed towards a person or an object. Interrelations among anger, hostility and aggression, and their association with cardiovascular heart diseases (CHDs) have been identified in many empirical studies. Research findings show that the AHA-Syndrome is emerging as a major cause of cardiovascular responses and premature mortality among people at all stages of life.

Keywords: Anger, Hostility, Aggression, AHA-Syndrome.

Introduction

Human beings are one of the most blessed living creatures on this planet. However, humanity is losing its virtues day-by-day, and people are becoming more aggressive and violent. Love, kindness, compassion, caring, sharing, cooperation, and all other human values are being replaced by anger, hostility and aggression. People in everyday stressful situations respond with anger, hostility and aggression, referred to collectively as the AHA-Syndrome [1], which often results in many physiological and psychological problems.

The AHA-Syndrome is one of the leading causes of today's health problems such as, cancer and coronary heart diseases, including elevated blood pressure, hypertension and heart attacks. The experience, expression and control of anger also contributes to ulcers, respiratory and gastrointestinal problems, diabetes, eating disorders, marital conflicts and workplace aggression. Anger-related problems also result in frustration, depression and suicidal ideation, excessive drinking and food addiction, child abuse and other harrowing acts such as rape, murder, and road rage. Traffic accidents are increasing day-by-day and it is generally found that anger, hostility and aggression are the major factors behind such incidents.

History also shows that Hitler's hostility toward Jews led to mass destruction of humanity and there are still such hostile tendencies among big powers around the world, which has put our beautiful planet at risk. Hostility towards HIV/AIDS positive people is also a big hurdle in prevention and reducing this growing epidemic that endangers humanity. The September 11, 2001 terrorist attacks, the subsequent war on terrorism in Afghanistan, and the ongoing conflict between many countries around the world provide further evidence of extreme forms of the expression of anger and aggression. The continuing conflict between the Israelis and the Palestinians, India and Pakistan, and the fighting in Iraq further illustrate the unfortunate consequences relating to the expression of aggression in many parts of the world.

Experience of Anger

Anger may be experienced daily and encountered in a number of family, interpersonal and occupational situations. It is a normal reaction when circumstances are not fair or expectations are not met. Anger can be elicited by specific events, behaviours of self or others, and a combination of internal and external events. It is likely to occur when a person believes that his/her personal rights or codes have been violated. Similarly, anger can occur when a person feels powerless or threatened [2]. When anger comes from internal sources such as, when one does not get what one wants at a particular moment, a flash of anger may overwhelm one, if one does not receive acceptance or recognition when one feels this is deserved.

When anger occurs, the body goes instantly into a series of mind-body reactions involving hormones, the nervous system and muscles. This involves a release of adrenaline, which results in shortness of breath, skin flushing, muscle rigidity, and tightening in the jaw, stomach, shoulder and hands. Anger places an individual in a state of readiness, thus, one should use the energy immediately so that the body can relax and resume functioning effectively. If one maintains the state of anger for too long, it may result in considerable physical damage [3]. People with angry temperaments evoke similar response from others, thereby creating problems for themselves and others.

Anger is a fundamental part of the AHA-Syndrome [1]. It is an emotional state or feeling accompanied by arousal of the autonomic nervous system, tension in the skeletal musculature, and antagonistic thought patterns. Although everyone experiences anger on occasions, some people are clearly more prone to such experiences than others. A fiery temper may manifest itself outwardly in various forms of verbal and physical confrontations, or may be boiling for decades in a suppressed and hidden manner. According to Anderson [4], anger may be a defence to avoid painful feelings associated with failure, isolation or low self-esteem, or it may be related to anxiety about situations over which a person has no control. It can be expressed outwardly, held in, or controlled and resolved. Expressed anger may lead to negative evaluations by others, a negative self-concept and low self-esteem, family conflict and mild to severe aggression. Anger that is held in may contribute to medical conditions such as hypertension, coronary heart disease and cancer. The behavioural consequences of anger can also lead to burden for families and staff working in day and residential services, as well as to the wider community.

Emotions and emotional style are the building blocks of a person's unique, relatively stable, and consistent pattern of personality, which dispose him/her to think, feel and behave in a particular way [5, 6]. The emotion of anger may manifest itself in varying intensity from mild irritation to outbursts of fury and rage [1, 7]. According to Novaco [8], anger is a negatively toned, i.e. unpleasant emotion and internal occurrence, which is subjectively experienced as a highly aroused, agitated, and antagonistic state of mind. Novaco argues that it is an individual's appraisal of an event or situation that mediates his/her emotional arousal and behavioural response, and it determines whether or not he/she is likely to feel angry and/or behave aggressively.

In summary, anger is a frequently occurring emotion, the moderate to intense forms of which may be experienced several times a day by any individual [9]. Anger may be evoked by a variety of external stimuli – persons, objects, and situations – or internal sensations – anger-laden memories, feelings of rejection, humiliation, and anxiety – that are interpreted as provocative and wrongful [8]. Anger experienced both internally and outwardly can be harmful and lead to physiological and other psychological problems.

Expression of Anger

Anger can have both positive and negative effects, depending on how it is expressed. It is most important to learn how to express our anger in appropriate, supportive ways. How a person expresses anger in a given situation depends on past experiences, values and beliefs. Individuals learn from such experiences with their families, friends, schools, society and culture. Anger can give us energy and motivation to right a wrong and to solve a problem, but it can also be destructive, if it is not expressed appropriately. Murphy and Oberlin [10] stress that "It is sometimes okay to be angry, but it is never okay to be mean. Every angry reaction to a difficult situation has a line that separates the acceptable from the unacceptable". Anger becomes negative when people deny it, suppress it or express it inappropriately. If anger is expressed inappropriately, it can turn into other disturbing emotions such as resentment, bitterness, hostility and hate. Uncontrolled anger can also transform into destructive aggression, which has a negative impact on personal well-being, families, work environment and society.

Anger causes high levels of arousal that can last for hours or even longer, and can be expressed in many anti-social behaviours with negative consequences, including crying, yelling, sarcasm, violence, crime, rape, and murder. It can also contribute to traffic accidents, child abuse, marital conflict, divorce, job loss, increased smoking, frequent drinking, headaches, hypertension, ulcers, heart disease, stroke, diabetes, cancer, and emotional problems with anxiety and depression. Expression of anger while driving is a common phenomenon nowadays. Increasing road clashes, traffic accidents and deaths are often the result of negative thoughts while driving. Research on driving simulations has shown that angry drivers are twice as likely to become involved in accidents, especially in high stress situations [11].

Anger is expressed in three ways. It can be directed outwards against others, inwards leading to self-destructive behaviour, and towards efforts to control the experience and expression of anger itself. When anger is directed outwards, one may feel like yelling, screaming, punching someone, smashing or destroying something, or engage in other destructive expressions of anger.

When anger is directed inward or suppressed, it can also be destructive. If anger is not allowed some form of constructive external expression, it can increase the risks of high blood pressure, depression, suicidal tendencies, gastrointestinal problems, respiratory diseases, and increased smoking or drinking. The third mode is the control of anger or anger management.

Controlling anger involves calming oneself so that anger can be used constructively. Thus, anger affects us at all the four levels of our being – physical, emotional, mental and spiritual.

State and Trait Anger

Spielberger's State-Trait Anger Expression Inventory (STAXI-2) [12] distinguishes between state-anger, trait-anger, anger-out, anger-in, anger-control/out and anger-control/in. State anger is a situation specific, transitory emotional state, while trait anger refers to individual differences in a stable personality trait. Anger can be expressed physically, verbally or towards the source of irritation (anger-out), or held in and suppressed (anger-in). People who frequently experience anger arousal may also have the tendency to express their anger [1, 5]. When anger is experienced, failure to express it in assertive behaviour or overt aggression (anger-out) could reflect the voluntary inhibition of aggressive urges – i.e. repression or suppression of anger – or alternative methods of coping through other social responses, such as assertiveness [13].

Studies have shown that suppression of anger is related to elevations in cardiovascular response [14]. Also, it has been recognised for long that anger is associated with heightened levels of cardiovascular arousal that contribute to coronary heart disease. Numerous studies have tested the relationship of anger expression to resting blood pressure [15], lipid concentration [16], the severity of angiographically documented coronary stenosis [17], and all-cause mortality, including coronary heart disease (CHD) [18]. Other biological mechanisms by which anger may increase the risk of CHD include discharge of circulating catecholamines, increased myocardial oxygen demand and vasospasm [19].

Suls, Wan and Costa [20] concluded that high scores on Spielberger's STAXI Anger-In Scale, a trait measure of anger suppression, were associated with higher blood pressure levels. The STAXI Anger-Out Scale, a trait measure of the outward expression of anger, showed an inverse relationship with levels of systolic blood pressure (SBP), but not diastolic blood pressure (DBP). High anger-out individuals have also been shown to exhibit biases in their appraisals of situations, blaming others for bad events and judging that the negative behaviour was intentional [21]. Anger is also associated with increased rates of testosterone production and platelet formation, which are involved in the pathogenesis of CHD [22].

Hostility

Buss [23] defined hostility, the second component of the AHA-Syndrome, as an attitude that involves disliking others and evaluating them negatively. Eckhardt and Deffenbacher [24] regard hostility as, "A personality trait referring to appraisal and cognitive process through which the individual tends to code the other's action as harmful and unjustified acts". Schultz and Videbeck [25] defined hostility as an emotion expressed through verbal abuse, lack of cooperation, violation of rules or norms or threatening behaviour. According to Spielberger et al. [26], hostility refers to a pervasive aggressive attitude that directs an individual to express anger via aggressive behaviour.

The cognitive aspects of hostility include cynicism, mistrust, and a general belief that others are the likely sources of frustration and mistreatment [27-29]. Thus, hostility refers to an enduring trait, which involves devaluation of the worth and motives of other persons, and a relational view of being in opposition towards others [13]. Hostile people are often described as being stubborn, impatient, hot-headed, and having a cynical attitude. They frequently engage in arguments and may verbally state that they feel like hitting something or someone. Hostility shows itself in many ways that include rage, negative critical attitudes, nagging, shouting, sarcasm, gossip, resentment, hatred, slamming doors, aggressive driving, and even criminality.

Hostility manifests itself in childhood and can often be observed in children and adolescents [30]. Researchers have identified many causal contributors to the development of hostility, including genetic factors [31], family environment [32], child-rearing practices [33], Type A personality [34], life satisfaction [35], and socioeconomic status [36]. Hostility has also been associated with many mental and somatic health consequences, such as depression [37], anti-social behaviour [38], suicidal thoughts [39], and social conflict [40].

Hostility is also a major psychosocial risk factor for the etiology of CHDs [28]. Smith et al. [41] reported that highly hostile undergraduate students ascribed more conflict and less cohesion to their family life as compared to their low hostile counterparts. Smith's psychosocial vulnerability model [29] suggests that hostile people experience higher levels of stress and lower levels of social support due to their cynical nature and negative interactions with others. As increased levels of stress and low levels of social support have been consistently linked to heart disease, hostility may exert its influence on health through creating a psychosocial profile that increases the risk of heart disease.

Marital relationships are an important factor in hostile behaviour that contributes to cardiovascular disease and premature mortality [42] because negative marital interactions often evoke strong physiological responses [43]. Hostile individuals respond to provocation [44], conflict [45], and disagreement [46] with large increase in blood pressure and heart rate as compared to persons who are not hostile. Shekelle et al. [47] found that higher hostility scores predicted increases in both CHD and mortality among the 1,900 men who were followed for 20 years in the Western Electric Study. These increases in both CHD and total mortality were independent of baseline smoking status, cholesterol, blood pressure, and alcohol use. Similarly, Barefoot, Dahlstrom and Williams found a positive relation between high Multiphasic Personality Index (MMPI) hostility scores and CHD in a 25-year study of 225 physicians [48].

Aggression

Aggression is a normal part of human development. From the developmental perspective, if aggressive behaviour is manifested at an early stage, it is likely to persist and signal a risk for delinquent behaviour, which continues through adulthood. Aggressive children often become aggressive adults who, later on, serve as faulty parental models for their own children to follow. Thus, a vicious circle is formed that passes on from one generation to the other. Early aggressive behaviour consists of crying, screaming, temper tantrums, biting, kicking, throwing, and breaking objects.

Early childhood aggressive behaviour may be in response to parental authority and unrealistic expectations on the part of the parents toward their child. Later, as social interactions increase, aggression may be directed towards peers, teachers and other social authorities. During early adolescence, more serious violence develops, including gang activities, stealing, drug abuse, sex crimes and physical fights. In adulthood, aggression escalates to include assault, robbery, road rage, rape, sex crimes, murder and homicide. In cases of childhood, adolescent, and adult aggression, one common characteristic of the aggressive episode is autonomic arousal [49]. This stimulation of the autonomic nervous system is part of the fight-flight syndrome that prepares the organism for physical action.

Factors that influence the development of aggression include parental and post-natal differences, as well as physiological, psychological, social and environmental effects. Some researchers [50, 51] theorise that aggression is an innate, instinctive phenomenon, whereas others contend that aggression must be learned. Although no absolute causes for aggression have been identified, there is general agreement that both nature and nurture are important causes that interact with and influence each other [51].

Archaeological and historical evidence show that violence and aggression were prevalent among our hunter/gatherer ancestors 25,000 years ago and in the Greek, Egyptian, and Roman societies 2,000 to 3,000 years ago. Aggression is widespread in almost every society even today, and may be either appropriate, e.g. self-protective or destructive to the self and others [52]. Various psychologists and thinkers have defined aggression in different ways. The third component of the AHA-Syndrome, aggression involves potential injury to other persons [7, 50, 53-57]. Trama and Saini [58] defined aggression as behaviour directed towards any object or person with the intent to cause harm or injury directly or indirectly, physically (kicking, hitting etc.), verbally (verbal attack, sarcastic remarks, shouting etc.), psychologically (distrust, cynicism etc.), or socially (making public statements, tarnishing an individual's image, defaming a person etc.).

Most theorists consider intent as an essential element in their definitions of aggression. Historically, distinguished theorists and researchers such as Freud and Lorenz considered aggressive behaviour to be innate, but others have more recently proposed that it is a learned behaviour [59, 60]. Dollard et al. [61] defined aggression as an act whose goal is to injure another organism. An individual may strike, kick or hit various kinds of inanimate objects, but such behaviour is not viewed as aggression unless it caused harm or injury to another living organism. Spielberger et al. [26] did not include intention in defining their concept of aggression. Behavioural studies show that aggression is often associated with negative health behaviours (e.g., smoking, drug use, alcohol use, and promiscuous sex), which have the potential to compromise immune activity and increase exposure to infectious agents or carcinogens [62].

The concept of aggression has been used in many contexts, and has been applied to animal as well as human behaviour. Aggression is used to describe negative personality traits and attitudes, as well as to characterise the behaviour of both children and adults. Aggression is used in military contexts to characterise actions of one nation against another [63, 64], and in sports to denote strongly competitive behaviour. In the medical field, aggression is often linked to disorders, such as epilepsy [65]. A number of studies have demonstrated that driving under stressful traffic conditions produces physiological arousal such as elevated heart rate and blood pressure [66-69]. One of the most reliable findings in the literature has been an association between aggressive behaviour with lower resting heart rate and electrodermal activity in non-institutionalised children and adolescents [70-74].

The AHA-Syndrome

Anger, hostility and aggression are often used interchangeably to describe behaviour in the psychological and psychiatric literature. Aggressive behaviour is frequently described as being motivated by anger and hostility while hostility is often described as resulting from angry feelings that motivate aggressive behaviour. Spielberger et al. [75] refer to these overlapping concepts as the AHA-Syndrome. They have defined anger as an emotional state and hostility as a personality trait, whereas aggression refers to behaviour that involves the expression of anger. According to them, the concept of anger refers to an emotional state that consists of feelings that vary in intensity, the concept of hostility refers to attitudes that motivate behaviour, and the concept of aggression implies destructive or punitive behaviour directed towards a person or object. Interrelations among anger, hostility and aggression are as follows:

Anger and Hostility

Anger signals one's body to prepare for a fight, while hostility is being ready for a fight all the time. According to Smith [29], hostility is a system of negative beliefs about others. It is thought to have an impact on health by making a person more prone to anger. Spielberger et al. [26] have demonstrated that the T-Anger (trait-anger) scale of the STAXI is related to hostility for both males and females. Researchers have suggested that anger and hostility originate from family factors, such as attachment style and parental rearing behaviours [76].

Anger and hostility are associated with many sources of physical and psychological distress, e.g. people who remain angry and hostile much of the time indulge in less physical activity, less self-care, more smoking, more alcohol consumption and more frequent drinking and driving. Thus, hostility and anger may give rise to reckless behaviour and result in aggression. Studies have shown that hostile individuals, who experience anger more frequently, reported higher levels of conflict in their families and less marital satisfaction than those with lower hostility [41].

Anger and Aggression

Anger as an emotional state often motivates aggression, which may be described as behaviour that is planned or intended to harm, hurt or injure another person or object. However, the relationship between anger and aggression remains unclear. Aggression represents only a portion of anger-out strategies and, thus, the relationship between anger and aggression is neither simple nor straightforward [1, 5, 24, 77]. Berkowitz [78] states that anger is a perceptual experience that does not cause aggression, but often accompanies the inclination to act aggressively. He has shown that anger does not always lead to aggression but requires the presence of appropriate cues [54]. Scott [79] and Buss [80] have also demonstrated aggression in the absence of anger. Kaufmann [81] presumed anger to be neither a sufficient nor a necessary condition for the stimulation of aggressive behaviour. He stated that one problem with the relationship between anger and aggression is the lack of a unified definition of anger, as with the definition of aggression. Evidence suggests that emotional arousal may have complex facilitative effects on human aggression.

Buss [23, 80] has distinguished between two forms of aggression: (i) aggression reinforced by pain of the victim and accompanied by anger, and (ii) aggression reinforced by extrinsic reward in which anger is not involved. However, it has not been shown that injury-reinforced aggression must be accompanied by anger or any other emotion. It has also not been shown that aggression reinforced by extrinsic reward must occur in the absence of anger. Novaco considers anger to be an inherent disposition to react aggressively, which may be regarded as a causal determinant that is "neither necessary or sufficient" for aggressive behaviour to occur [82]. More specifically, the higher and more intense the arousal of anger that is experienced, the greater the risk for aggression to occur. Intense anger not only strengthens an individual's motivation to act aggressively, but also distorts his/her ability to process aggression-mitigating information.

Anger is associated with various forms of aggression, including spousal abuse [83], child abuse [84], aggressive driving [11], and murder [85]. According to Berkowitz [53, 78] and Averill [9], frustration arouses anger and provokes aggression. Anger causes high levels of arousal, which can last for hours or even longer, and may motivate aggressive behaviour. Uncontrolled anger transforms into destructive aggression, which has a negative impact on personal well-being, family relationships, work setting, and society at large. Novaco [86] has noted that hundreds of studies in experimental psychology have found that when subjects are made angry, there is an increased probability of aggression.

Hostility and Aggression

Hostility is expressed in aggressive behaviours that inflict psychological pain, e.g. insulting comments, negative gestures, undue criticism etc. This type of aggression appears in everyday life and is very common at the work place. Buss and Kaufmann distinguish between aggression and hostility. In describing a hostile person, Kaufmann [56] wrote: "We think of him as one who has a habit or propensity for disliking others, wishing them harm or aggressing against them". In a similar manner, Buss [23] suggests that hostility "involves negative evaluations of people and events and may be inferred when the attack is reinforced more by injury than by attaining the extrinsic reinforcer". From these definitions we can infer that hostility corresponds to "injury reinforced aggression". This interpretation is also consistent with the work of Bandura [57], who uses the term 'hostile aggression' to denote behaviour reinforced by injurious consequences. Buss [23] further explains that hostility typically consists "of the mulling over of past attacks on oneself, rejections and deprivations", suggesting, perhaps, that hostility is the result of punishment. Repeated punishments and suffering at the hands of others may lead to a generalised dislike of humanity, and a tendency to perceive the pain and discomfort of people as reinforcing.

According to Dodge [87], negative emotional states make aggressive boys more prone to attribute hostile intentions to other children they interact with, thereby stimulating them to behave more aggressively than they would in a neutral emotional state. Hostile behaviours are also common while driving. Negative thoughts while driving lead to anger, causing aggressive driving behaviour. In other words, these negative thoughts behind the wheel act like mental pollutants, which decrease the enjoyment of driving and result in more aggressive behaviour.

The AHA-Syndrome and Cardiovascular Disease

Cardiovascular diseases are the leading worldwide cause of death and disability, accounting for 16.7 million (29.2%) of total global deaths in 2003. An estimated 64,400,000 Americans have cardiovascular disease, which claimed 958,775 lives in the United States in 1999, or almost 40.1% of all deaths [88]. Approximately every 26 seconds, someone in the US experiences a coronary event, and someone dies every minute from one of these events. The direct and indirect costs of cardiovascular disease were estimated at US$ 133.2 billion in 2003 [89]. The World Health Organisation (WHO) estimates that 60% of the world's cardiac patients will be from India by 2010 [90]. This increase in cardiovascular disease is likely due to people becoming more sedentary in office and factory jobs, the stress associated with an urban lifestyle, people eating more processed food, and the aging of the population [91].

Most of the risk factors for cardiovascular disease that have been investigated are associated with unhealthy lifestyle factors such as, smoking, obesity, and inadequate exercise [92], lack of social support [93], various emotional disorders [94], and prolonged stressors [95]. The AHA-Syndrome has a strong relationship with cardiovascular diseases. The research literature is filled with studies of such linkage, showing that this syndrome is emerging as a major cause of cardiovascular responses and premature mortality among people at all stages of life [28]. Although the link between anger and coronary deterioration is empirically robust, research has generated mixed results as to whether it is anger expression [96, 97], or anger suppression [98] that contributes to most coronary disease. With regard to hypertension, a major risk factor for heart attacks, the preponderance of evidence indicates that the suppression of anger is most characteristic of hypertensive patients [99].

It has been known for long that anger is accompanied by heightened levels of cardiovascular arousal, which has been identified as the mechanism that translates personality and behaviour problems into cardiovascular disease [22]. Dr. John Hunter, the famous 18th century British surgeon, is often quoted as having once remarked, "My life is in the hands of any rascal that chooses to annoy me". This intuition preceded the landmark research by Barefoot et al. [48] on the association of hostility assessed in medical school with physician mortality.

Coronary heart disease caused by atherosclerotic narrowing of the coronary arteries was linked to acute psychophysiologic reactivity in a seminal review by Kranz and Manuck [100]. This relationship is facilitated by anger's link to a high-hostile disposition through several pathways. One pathway includes fat being released into the bloodstream for energy during an anger episode, but remaining unused and then converting to cholesterol. Increased cholesterol, in turn, contributes to blockage of the arteries (atherosclerotic plaque formation) that increases blood pressure and contributes to hypertension and heart disease [101]. This process contributes to the evidence linking increased anger and hostility with elevated levels of cholesterol.

Another potential pathway between anger and arterial occlusion is that arterial damage or endothelial injury results from the turbulence of blood flow associated with cardiovascular reactivity [100]. With each anger episode, blood rapidly rushes past the arterial walls, causing erosion in them. Clumps of platelets and cholesterol attach themselves to damaged spots on arteries that increase over time. As anger becomes more chronic and intense, arteriosclerotic plaque accumulates, blocking the blood's path to the coronary arteries, which can lead directly to heart failure. Thus, coronary heart diseases have a robust association with the AHA-Syndrome. There is also a strong interaction between the inter-related components of the AHA-Syndrome with many other physiological and psychological problems.

Conclusion

Evidence of strong relationships between the various components of the AHA-Syndrome (anger, hostility and aggression) and cardiovascular disorders has been summarised in this chapter. Experience and expression of anger is associated with high level of arousal leading to both psychological and physiological problems. Hostility has been shown to be an important contributor to the etiology of heart disease. Similarly, aggression has been found to be associated with negative health consequences, which compromise immune activity. Thus, the compounding effects of anger, hostility and aggression (the AHA-Syndrome) increase the risk of developing heart disease. A better understanding of the AHA-Syndrome and how it contributes to the development of cardiovascular disease is needed to help control and reduce the world's leading cause of death.

Ackowledgement

The author expresses his gratitude to Prof. Charles Spielberger for his extremely helpful comments on an earlier draft of this article.

References

1. Spielberger, C.D., Reheiser, E.C. and Sydeman, S.J., 1995a, "Measuring the Experience, Expression and Control of Anger", In *Anger Disorders: Definitions, Diagnosis, and Treatment*, H. Kassinove (Ed.), Taylor and Francis, Washington, D.C., pp. 49-67.
2. Horn, R. and Towl, G., 1997, "Anger Management for Women Prisoners", *Issues in Criminological and Legal Psychology*, 29, pp. 57-62.
3. Warren, N.C., 1990, "Make Anger Your Ally: Harnessing One of Your Most Powerful Emotions", Wolgemuth and Hyatt, Inc., Brentwood, Tennessee.
4. Anderson, L.S., 1978, "The Aggressive Child", *Pediatric Development and Behavior*, 1, Retrieved on 10 March 2002, *www.dbpeds.org/articles/article.cfm*
5. Spielberger, C.D., Ritterband, L.M., Sydeman, S.J., Reheiser, E.C. and Unger, K.K., 1995b, "Assessment of Emotional States and Personality Traits: Measuring Psychological Vital Things", In *Clinical Personality Assessment: Practical Approaches*, N.J. Butcher (Ed.), Oxford University Press, New York, pp. 42-58.
6. Tremblay, R.E. and LeMarquand, D., 2001, "Individual Risk and Protective Factors", In *Child Delinquents: Development, Intervention, and Service Needs*, R. Loeber and D.P. Farrington (Eds.), Sage Publications, Thousand Oaks, California, pp. 137-164.
7. Berkowitz, L., 1990, "On the Formation and Regulation of Anger and Aggression: A Cognitive-Neoassociationistic Analysis", *American Psychologist*, 45, pp. 494-503.
8. Novaco, R.W., 2000, "Anger", In *Encyclopaedia of Psychology*, A.E. Kazdin (Ed.), American Psychological Association and Oxford University Press, Washington, D.C., pp. 170-174.
9. Averill, J.R., 1983, "Studies on Anger and Aggression: Implications for Theories of Emotion", *American Psychologist*, 38, pp. 1145-1160.
10. Murphy, T. and Oberlin, L.H., 2001, "The Angry Child: Regaining Control When Your Child is Out of Control", Clarkson Potter, New York.
11. Deffenbacher, J.L., Lynch, R.S., Filetti, L.B., Dahlen, E.R. and Oetting, E.R., 2003, "Anger, Aggression, Risky Behavior, and Crash-related Outcomes in Three Groups of Drivers", *Behavior Research and Therapy*, 41, pp. 333-349.
12. Spielberger, C.D., 1999, "State-Trait Anger Expression-2", *Professional Manual Lutz*, Psychological Assessment Resources, Florida.
13. Smith, T.W., 1994, "Concepts and Methods in the Study of Anger, Hostility and Health", In *Anger, Hostility and the Heart*, A.W. Siegman, and T.W. Smith (Eds.), Lawrence Erlbaum Associates, Inc., Hillsdale, New Jersey, pp. 23-42.

14. Vogele, C. and Steptoe, A., 1993, "Anger Inhibition and Family History as Modulators of Cardiovascular Responses to Mental Stress in Adolescent Boys", *Journal of Psychosomatic Research*, 37, pp. 503-514.
15. Shapiro, D., Goldstein, I.B. and Jamner, L.D., 1996, "Effects of Cynical Hostility, Anger-out, Anxiety, and Defensiveness on Ambulatory Blood Pressure in Black and White College Students", *Psychosomatic Medicine*, 58, 354-364.
16. Engebretson, T.O. and Stoney, C.M., 1995, "Anger Expression and Lipid Concentrations", *International Journal of Behavioral Medicine*, 2, pp. 281-298.
17. Dembroski, T.M., MacDougall, J.M., Williams, R.B., Haney, T.L. and Blumenthal, J.A., 1985, "Components of Type A, Hostility and Anger-in: Relationship to Angiographic Findings", *Psychosomatic Medicine*, 47, pp. 219-233.
18. Eaker, E.D., Pinsky, J. and Castelli, W.P., 1992, "Myocardial Infarction and Coronary Death Among Women: Psychosocial Predictors from a 20-year Follow-up of Women in the Framingham Study", *American Journal of Epidemiology*, 135, pp. 854-864.
19. Kawachi, I., Sparrow, D., Spiro, A., Vokonas, P. and Weiss, S.T., 1996, "A Prospective Study of Anger and Coronary Heart Disease", *Circulation*, 94(9), pp. 2090-2095.
20. Suls, J., Wan, C.K. and Costa, P.T., 1995, "Relationship of Trait Anger to Resting Blood Pressure: A Meta-analysis", *Health Psychology*, 14, pp. 444-456.
21. Hazebroek, J., Howells, K. and Day, A., 2001, "Cognitive Appraisals Associated with High Trait Anger", *Personality and Individual Differences*, 30, pp. 31-45.
22. Siegman, A.W., 1994, "From Type A to Hostility to Anger: Reflections on the History of Coronary-prone Behavior", In *Anger, Hostility and the Heart*, A.W. Siegman and T.W. Smith (Eds.), Lawrence Erlbaum Associates, Inc., Hillsdale, New Jersey, pp. 1-22, 173-198.
23. Buss, A.H., 1961, *The Psychology of Aggression*, John Wiley & Sons, New York.
24. Eckhardt, C. and Deffenbacher, J., 1995, "Diagnosis of Anger Disorders", In *Anger Disorders: Definition, Diagnosis, and Treatment*, H. Kassinove (Ed.), Taylor and Francis, Washington, D.C.
25. Schultz, J.M. and Videbeck, S.L., 2005, *Lippincott's Manual of Psychiatric Nursing Care Plans*, 7th Edn., Lippincott Williams and Wilkins, Philadelphia.
26. Spielberger, C.D., Jacobs, G., Russell, S. and Crane, R., 1983, "Assessment of Anger: The State-Trait Anger Scale (STAS)", In *Advances in Personality Assessment*, Vol. 2, J.N. Butcher and C.D. Spielberger (Eds.), Lawrence Erlbaum Associates, Inc., Hillsdale, New Jersey, pp. 159-187.
27. Barefoot, J.C., 1992, "Developments in the Measurement of Hostility", In *Hostility, Coping and Health*, H.S. Friedman (Ed.), American Psychological Association, Washington, D.C., pp. 13-31.
28. Miller, T.Q., Smith, T.W., Turner, C.W., Guijarro, M.L. and Hallet, A.J., 1996, "A Meta-analytic Review of Research on Hostility and Physical Health", *Psychological Bulletin*, 119, pp. 322-348.
29. Smith, T.W., 1992, "Hostility and Health: Current Status of a Psychosomatic Hypothesis", *Health Psychology*, 11(3), pp. 139-150.
30. Woodall, K.L. and Matthews, K.A., 1993, "Changes in and Stability of Hostile Characteristics: Results from a 4-year Old Longitudinal Study of Children", *Journal of Personality and Social Psychology*, 64, pp. 491-499.
31. Rose, R.J., 1988, "Genetic and Environmental Variance in Content Dimension of MMPI", *Journal of Personality and Social Psychology*, 55, pp. 302-311.
32. Matthews, K.A., Woodall, K.L., Kenyon, K. and Jacob, T., 1996, "Negative Family Environment as a Predictor of Boys' Future Status on Measure of Hostile Attitude, Interview Behavior and Anger Expression", *Health Psychology*, 15, pp. 30-37.
33. Raikkonen, K., Katainen, S., Keskivaara, P. and Keltikangas-Jarvinen, L., 2000, "Temperament, Mothering and Hostile Attitudes: A 12-year Longitudinal Study", *Personality and Social Psychology Bulletin*, 26, pp. 3-12.

34. Thoresen, C.E. and Pattillo, J.R., 1988, "Exploring the Type A Behavior Pattern in Children and Adolescents", In *Type A Behavior Pattern: Research, Theory and Intervention*, B.K. Houston and C.R. Cynder (Eds.), John Wiley & Sons, New York, pp. 98-145.
35. Diener, E., Diener, M. and Diener, C., 1995, "Factors Predicting the Subjective Well-being of Nations", *Journal of Personality and Social Psychology*, 69, pp. 851-864.
36. Carroll, D., Smith, G.D., Sheffield, D., Shipley, M.J. and Marmot, M.G., 1997, "The Relationship Between Socioeconomic Status, Hostility, and Blood Pressure Reactions to Mental Stress in Men: Data from Whitehall II Study", *Health Psychology*, 16, pp. 131-136.
37. Barefoot, J.C., Williams, R.B., Siegler, I.C. and Schroll, M., 1995, "Depressive Effect, Hostility, and Socioeconomic Status (SES): Interrelationships and Joint Effect on Health", *Psychosomatic Medicine*, 57, p. 66.
38. Pakiz, B., Reinherz, H.Z. and Giaconia, R.M., 1997, "Early Risk Factors for Serious Antisocial Behavior at Age 21: A Longitudinal Community Study", *American Journal of Orthopsychiatry*, 67, pp. 92-101.
39. Weissman, M., Fox, K. and Klerman, G.L., 1973, "Hostility and Depression Associated with Suicide Attempts", *American Journal of Psychiatry*, 130, pp. 450-455.
40. Berkman, L. and Orth-Gomer, K., 1996, "Prevention of Cardiovascular Morbidity and Mortality: Role of Social Relations", In *Behavioral Medicine Approaches to Cardiovascular Disease Prevention*, K. Orth-Gomer and N. Schneiderman (Eds.), Earlbaum, Mahwah, NJ, pp. 51-68.
41. Smith, T.W., Pope, M.K., Sanders, J.D., Allred, K.D. and O'Keeffe, J.L., 1988, "Cynical Hostility at Home and Work: Psychosocial Vulnerability Across Domains", *J. Res. Pers.*, 22, pp. 525-548.
42. Tucker, J.S., Friedman, H.S., Wingard, D.L. and Schwartz, J.E., 1996, "Marital History at Midlife as a Predictor of Longevity: Alternative Explanations to the Protective Effect of Marriage", *Health Psychology*, 15, pp. 94-101.
43. Ewart, C.K., Taylor, L.B., Kraemer, H.C. and Agras, W.S., 1991, "High Blood Pressure and Marital Discord Not Being Nasty Matters More than Being Nice", *Health Psychology*, 10, pp. 155-163.
44. Suarez, E.C. and Williams, R.B., 1989, "Situational Determinants of Cardiovascular and Emotional Reactivity in High and Low Hostile Men", *Psychosomatic Medicine*, 51, pp. 404-418.
45. Hardy, J.D. and Smith, T.W., 1988, "Cynical Hostility and Vulnerability to Disease, Social Support, Life Stress, and Physiological Responses to Conflict", *Health Psychology*, 7, pp. 447-459.
46. Smith, T.W. and Allred, K.D., 1989, "Blood Pressure Responses During Social Interaction in High- and Low-cynically Hostile Males", *Journal of Behavioral Medicine*, 12, pp. 125-143.
47. Shekelle, R.B., Gale, N., Ostfeld, A.M. and Paul, O., 1983, "Hostility, Risk of Coronary Heart Disease and Mortality", *Psychosomatic Medicine*, 45, 109-114.
48. Barefoot, J.C., Dahlstrom, G.. and Williams, R.B., 1983, "Hostility, CHD Incidence and Total Mortality: A 25-year Follow-up Study of 255 Physicians", *Psychosomatic Medicine*, 43, pp. 59-63.
49. Raine, A., 1993, *The Psychopathology of Crime: Criminal Behavior as a Clinical Disorder*, Academic Press, San Diego.
50. Moyer, K.E., 1976, *The Psychobiology of Aggression*, Harper and Row, New York.
51. Sylwester, R., 1999, "In Search of the Roots of Adolescent Aggression", *Educational Leadership*, 57, pp. 65-70.
52. Ferris, C.F. and Grisso, T., 1996, "Understanding Aggressive Behavior in Children", *Annals of the New York Academy of Sciences*, New York, 794, pp. 426-794.
53. Berkowitz, L., 1962, *Aggression: A Social Psychological Analysis*, McGraw-Hill, New York.
54. Berkowitz, L., 1964, "Aggressive Cues in Aggressive Behavior and Hostility Catharsis", *Psychological Review*, 71, pp. 104-122.
55. Feshbach, S., 1970, "Aggression", In *Carmichael's Mannual of Child Psychology*, Vol. 2, 3rd Edn., P. Mussen (Ed.), John Wiley & Sons, New York.

56. Kaufmann, H., 1970, *Aggression and Altruism: A Social Psychological Analysis*, Holt, Rinehart and Winston, New York.
57. Bandura, A., 1973, *Aggression: A Social Learning Analysis*, Prentice-Hall, Oxford, England.
58. Trama, S. and Saini, S. (in press), "A Study of Gender Differences in Anger, Hostility, Verbal and Physical Aggression", *Indian Journal of Psychological Issues*.
59. Conger, R.D., Neppl, T., Kim, K.J. and Scaramella, L., 2003, "Angry and Aggressive Behavior Across Three Generations: A Prospective, Longitudinal Study of Parents and Children", *Journal of Abnormal Child Psychology*, 31, pp. 143-160.
60. Huesmann, L.R., Moise-Titus, J., Podolski, C.L. and Eron, L.D., 2003, "Longitudinal Relations Between Children's Exposure to TV Violence and their Aggressive and Violent Behavior in Young Adulthood: 1977-1992", *Developmental Psychology*, (Special Issue: Violent Children), 39, pp. 201-221.
61. Dollard, J., Doob, L., Miller, N., Mowrer, O.H. and Sears, R.R., 1939, *Frustration and Aggression*, Yale University Press, New Haven, Connecticut.
62. Booth, A., Johnson, D. and Granger, D.A., 1999, "Testosterone and Men's Health", *Behavioral Medicine*, 20, pp. 1-20.
63. Nordstrom, C., 1998, "Deadly Myths of Aggression, Aggressive Behavior", *Anthropological Perspectives on Aggression* (Special Issue), 24, pp. 147-159.
64. Satterfield, J.M. and Seligman, M.E.P., 1994, "Military Aggression and Risk Predicted by Explanatory Style", *Psychological Science*, 5, pp. 77-82.
65. Tebartz van Elst, L., 2002, "Aggression and Epilepsy", In *The Neuropsychiatry of Epilepsy*, M.E. Trimble and B.E. Schmitz (Eds.), Cambridge University Press, New York, pp. 81-106.
66. Taggart, P., Gibbons, D. and Somerville, W., 1969, "Some Effects of Motor Car Driving on the Normal and Abnormal Heart", *British Medical Journal*, 4, pp. 130-134.
67. Littler, W.A., Honour, A.J. and Sleight, P., 1973, "Direct Arterial Pressure and Electrocardiogram During Motor Car Driving", *British Medical Journal*, 2, pp. 273-277.
68. Stokols, D., Novaco, R.W., Stokols, J. and Campbell, J., 1978, "Traffic Congestion, Type A Behavior and Stress", *Journal of Applied Psychology*, 63, pp. 467-480.
69. Stokols, D. and Novaco, R.W., 1981, "Transportation and Well-being", In *Transportation and Well-being*, I. Altman, J.F. Wohlevill and P.B. Everett (Eds.), Plenum Press, New York, pp. 85-130.
70. Davies, J.G.V. and Maliphant, R., 1971, "Autonomic Responses of Male Adolescents Exhibiting Refractory Behavior in School", *Journal of Child Psychology and Psychiatry*, 12, pp. 115-127.
71. Schmidt, K., Solant, M.V. and Bridger, W.H., 1985, "Electrodermal Activity of Undersocialized Aggressive Children: A Pilot Study", *Journal of Child Psychology and Psychiatry*, 26, pp. 653-660.
72. Maliphant, R., Hume, F. and Furnham, A., 1990, "Autonomic Nervous System (ANS) Activity, Personality Characteristics and Disruptive Behaviors in Girls", *Journal of Child Psychology and Psychiatry*, 31, pp. 619-628.
73. Kindlon, D.J., Tremblay, R.E., Mezzacappa, E., Earls, F., Laurent, D. and Schaal, B., 1995, "Longitudinal Patterns of Heart Rate and Fighting Behaviors in 9-through 12-year Old Boys", *Journal of the American Academy of Child and Adolescent Psychiatry*, 34, pp. 371-377.
74. Raine, A., Venables, P.H. and Mednick, S.A., 1995, "Low Resting Heart Rate at Age 3 Years Predisposes to Aggression at Age 11 Years: Evidence from the Mauritius Child Health Project", *Journal of the American Academy of Child and Adolescent Psychiatry*, 36, pp. 1457-1464.
75. Spielberger, C.D., Johnson, E.H., Russel, S.F., Crane, R.J., Jacobs, G.A. and Worden, T.J., 1985, "The Experience and Expression of Anger: Construction and Validation of an Anger Expression Scale", In *Anger and Hostility in Cardiovascular and Behavioral Disorders*, M. Cheney and R. Rosenman (Eds.), McGraw-Hill, New York.

76. Grunbaum, J.A., Vernon, S.W. and Clasen, C.M., 1997, "The Association Between Anger and Hostility and Risk Factors for Coronary Heart Disease in Children and Adolescents: A Review", *Ann. Behav. Med.*, 19, pp. 179-189.
77. Kassinove, H. and Sukhodolsky, D.G., 1995, "Anger Disorders: Basic Science and Practice Issues", In *Anger Disorders: Definitions, Diagnosis and Treatment*, H. Kassinove (Ed.), Taylor and Francis, Washington, D.C., pp. 2-27.
78. Berkowitz, L., 1989, "Frustration-Aggression Hypothesis: Examination and Reformulation", *Psychological Bulletin*, 106, pp. 59-73.
79. Scott, J.P., 1958, *Aggression*, University of Chicago Press, Chicago.
80. Buss, A.H., 1971, "Aggression Pays", In *The Control of Aggression and Violence: Cognitive and Physiological Factors*, J.H. Singer (Ed.), Academic Press, New York.
81. Kaufmann, H., 1965, "Definitions and Methodology in the Study of Aggression", *Psychological Bulletin*, 64, pp. 351-364.
82. Novaco, R.W., 1994, "Anger as a Risk Factor for Violence Among the Mentally Disordered", In *Violence and Mental Disorder: Developments in Risk Assessment*, J. Monahan and H.J. Steadman (Eds.), University of Chicago Press, Chicago, pp. 21-59.
83. Boyle, D.J. and Vivian, D., 1996, "Generalized versus Spouse-specific Anger/Hostility and Men's Violence Against Intimates", *Violence and Victims*, 11, pp. 293-317.
84. Rodriguez, C.M. and Green, A.J., 1997, "Parenting Stress and Anger Expression as Predictors of Child Abuse Potential", *Child Abuse and Neglect*, 21, pp. 367-377.
85. U.S. Department of Justice, 2000, *Crime in the United States 2000: Uniform Crime Reports*, Available at *www.fbi.gov/ucr/cius_00/00crime2.pdf*
86. Novaco, R.W., 1986, "Anger as a Clinical and Social Problem", In *Advances in the Study of Aggression*, R. Blanchard and C. Blanchard (Eds.), Academic Press, New York, pp. 1-67.
87. Dodge, K.A., 1985, "Assessment and Training of Social Skills", Presented at a Symposium at the *Biennial Meeting of the Society for Research in Child Development*, Toronto.
88. AHA, 2001, *Cardiovascular Disease Costs*, American Heart Association, *www.americanheart.org*
89. AHA, 2003, *Heart Disease and Stroke Statistics: 2004 Update*, American Heart Association, Dallas, Texas.
90. Leeder, S., Raymond, S., Greenberg, H., Liu, H. and Esson, K., 2004, *A Race Against Time: The Challenge of Cardiovascular Disease in Developing Countries*, Trustees of Columbia University, New York.
91. AHA, 2006, *Heart Disease and Stroke Statistics: 2006 Update*, American Heart Association, *www.americanheart.org*
92. Siegler, I.C., 1994, "Hostility and Risk: Demographics and Lifestyle Variables", In *Anger, Hostility and the Heart*, A.W. Siegman, and T.W. Smith (Eds.), Lawrence Erlbaum Associates, Inc., Hillsdale, New Jersey, pp. 199-214.
93. Angerer, P., Siebert, U., Kothny, W., Muhlbauer, D., Mudra, H. and von Schacky, C., 2000, "Impact of Social Support, Cynical Hostility and Anger Expression on Progression of Coronary Atherosclerosis", *J. Am. Coll. Cardiol.*, 36, pp. 1781-1788.
94. Kubzansky, L.D. and Kawachi, I., 2000, "Going to the Heart of the Matter: Do Negative Emotions Cause Coronary Artery Disease", *Journal of Psychosomatic Research*, 48, pp. 323-337.
95. Kop, W.J., 1997, "Acute and Chronic Psychological Risk Factors for Coronary Syndromes: Moderating Effects of Coronary Artery Disease Severity", *Journal of Psychosomatic Research*, 43, pp. 167-181.
96. Kaplan, J.R., Botchin, M.B. and Manuck, S.B., 1994, "Animal Models of Aggression and Cardiovascular Disease", In *Anger; Hostility and the Heart*, A.W. Siegman and T.W. Smith (Eds.), Erlbaum, Hillsdale, New Jersey.

97. Siegman, A.W., Dembroski, T.M. and Ringel, N., 1987, "Components of Hostility and the Severity of Coronary Artery Disease", *Psychosomatic Medicine*, 49, pp. 127-135.
98. Haynes, S.G., Feinleib, M. and Kannel, W.B., 1980, "The Relationship of Psychosocial Factors to Coronary Heart Disease in the Framingham Study, III: Eight Year Incidence of CHD", *American Journal of Epidemiology*, 11, pp. 37-58.
99. Johnson, E.H. and Gentry, W.D., 1992, "Personality, Elevated Blood Pressure, and Essential Hypertension: A Research Agenda", In *Personality, Elevated Blood Pressure and Essential Hypertension*, E.H. Johnson, W.D. Gentry and S. Julius (Eds.), Hemisphere, Washington, D.C., pp. 319-334.
100. Krantz, D.S. and Manuck, S.B., 1984, "Acute Psychophysiological Reactivity and Risk of Cardiovascular Disease: A Review and Methodological Critique", *Psychological Bulletin*, 96, pp. 435-464.
101. Lichtenstein, M.J., Shipley, M.J. and Rose, G., 1985, "Systolic and Diastolic Blood Pressures as Predictors of Coronary Heart Disease Mortality in the Whitehall Study", *British Medical Journal*, 291, pp. 243-245.

The AHA-Syndrome and Cardiovascular Diseases
Editors: Swati Y. Bhave and Sunil Saini
Copyright © 2010 Anamaya Publishers, New Delhi, India

2. The Main Symptoms of the AHA-Syndrome: Relationships Between Anger, Hostility and Aggression in a Normal Population

J.M. Ramírez[1,2] and J.M. Andreu[1,3]
[1]Institute for Biofunctional Studies, [2]Department of Psychobiology, [3]Department of Clinical Psychology, Universidad Complutense, Madrid, Spain

Abstract: The purpose of the present study is to analyse the relationship between the main symptoms of the AHA-Syndrome – anger, hostility, and aggression – summarising the main empirical results of our research in normal people. The different definitions of aggression may be grouped according to whether the primary goal is distress or harm, focussing primarily on the objective infliction of harm, or on the subjective intention of harming. Most classifications in the literature show two kinds of aggression, even if different names are used: (i) hostile aggression – also known as reactive, impulsive, or affective – is an act, primarily oriented to hurt another individual; and (ii) instrumental aggression – also known as proactive, premeditated, or predative – is a means or tool for solving problems, or for obtaining a variety of objectives. As predicted, there was a positive correlation between the experience and expression of anger. Anger involved physiological arousal and prepared for aggression. Finally, hostility positively correlated with anger and different kinds of aggression, but not its degree of justification.

Keywords: AHA-Syndrome, Anger, Hostility, Aggression.

Introduction

The concepts of anger, hostility, and aggression, are part of a cluster often referred to as the AHA-Syndrome [1]. Anger refers to an emotion but can also be considered a personality trait. Hostility, in itself, is a multidimensional concept that can be categorised into attitudinal, emotional, and behavioural components [2]. Aggression, usually, refers to behaviours toward others; it has traditionally been classified into two distinct subtypes that, even if using many different terms, consistently follow a common dichotomy: reactive or proactive [3].

Since the design of experiments, methodologies, and therapies employed in the AHA-Syndrome are strongly influenced by the definitions adopted, it is important to start with a description of its main symptoms, in the hope that a good profile may help in a better and more comprehensive understanding of the AHA-Syndrome. This article will first present a brief theoretical consideration of the aforementioned three concepts. The aim is to present some information of how these different constructs – anger, hostility, and aggression – may be interrelated, on the understanding that a useful framework would be of fundamental importance for improving the diagnosis, prevention, and treatment of the AHA-Syndrome, which comprise emotion or affective feelings (anger), temperament or attitude (hostility) and, obviously, overt behaviour (aggression, in its strictest sense).

Even if one is obviously aware that the patients with health problems and psychiatric disorders are the closest subjects to the AHA-Syndrome, when dealing with the different symptoms and their interrelations, it may be prudent to leave aside the clinical populations and, instead, start understanding the nature and functional value, if any, of these constructs in 'normal' subjects, with a relatively homogenous environment and no significant differences in age and education. This is the main reason why undergraduate students have been chosen from a community sample for the experimental analysis, which forms the basis of the present article.

Aggression

Concept of Aggression

Before distinguishing between forms of aggression, one must be clear about the meaning of the term, because if other researchers want to replicate a research, at least there has to be a previous agreement about a precise working notion, i.e. what one is looking for, so that it allows clear operational definitions. In spite of the enormous literature available on the topic and the continuous efforts by many scholars dedicated to the scientific study of aggression, there is still considerable disagreement about its precise meaning and causes, with no singular or even preferred definition. Far from being a univocous term, aggression is often ill-defined, used with ambiguity and with a surplus of meanings. This multitude of different conceptualisations is one of the main problems in the literature. Part of the task of understanding aggression, therefore, would be to clarify its meaning.

Which definition should be chosen? Traditionally, stress has been laid on the intention to harm another living being [4], and not simply the delivery of harm, i.e. a manifest response "aimed at the injury of a target" [5-7]. This intention seems clear in some kinds of aggression but, in others, the perpetrators of the harm may be able to deny any intent to cause harm. For example, aggression would simply be the infliction of harm on others, in a behaviourist approach "that delivers noxious stimuli to another organism" [8], or as described elsewhere, "the delivery of any form of definite and observable harm-giving behaviour towards any target", without mentioning the eventual intention of the actor [9-13]. Spielberger et al. [14] did not include the intention either, when they said that the concept of aggression "implies destructive or punitive behaviour directed towards other persons or objects".

A recent analysis [15] tried to clarify these different definitions, distinguishing between proximate and ultimate goals. Intention to harm is viewed as a necessary feature in any kind of aggression, but only as a proximate goal (as in purely hostile aggression models). At the level of ultimate goal, though, there is a clear difference between different types of aggression. Thus, both robbery and physical assault are acts of aggression because both include intention to harm the victim at a proximate level. However, they typically differ in ultimate goals, with robbery serving primarily profit-based goals and assault serving primarily harm-based goals. In short, this distinction allows the discussion of the commonalities in different kinds of aggression and the distinctions between them, while including aggression with mixed motives.

Kinds of Aggression

However, difficulties inherent in defining aggression appear simple in comparison to the difficulty in establishing a classification of such an ambiguous construct. Far from being a term describing a singular dimension, aggression consists of several phenomena, which may be similar in appearance but have separate genetic and neural control mechanisms, show diverse phenomenological manifestations, have different functions and antecedents, and are instigated by different external circumstances.

Early work by Arnold Buss [8], thinking in terms of the way of doing it (how) distinguished three, not quite independent but rather overlapping dimensions [16], on which one might categorise several types of aggression: physical-verbal, active-passive, and direct-indirect. The *physical-verbal* dimension distinguishes between whether one uses physical means or words to harm another person [17, 18]. The *active-passive* dimension refers to the extent to which the aggressor actively engages in a behaviour aimed at harming someone, with passive aggression referring to causing harm by not doing something. The *direct-indirect* dimension is also relevant [8, 18-20]. Direct aggression involves face-to-face confrontation between the aggressor and the target. It is defined as any behaviour aimed at the goal of harming another living being [4]. Consistent with Buss' original formulation, this form of aggression may be either verbal or physical, e.g. direct aggression may involve screaming at another person or hitting that person. Indirect aggression is defined as any behaviour aimed at the goal of harming another living being that is delivered circuitously through another person or object, even if it must nevertheless be intended to harm someone [21]. It is a mode of aggression that avoids counterattack. It may involve both 'round about' aggression – the hated person is not attacked directly, but by devious means – and undirected aggression – there is discharge of negative affect against no one in particular [8]. Norma Feshbach [22] defined it as "responses, which result in pain to a stimulus person through rejecting and excluding him", including such actions as ignoring or denying requests. It may be either physical or verbal, e.g. indirect aggression may involve causing harm to someone's property, or talking behind someone's back.

Some researchers have also considered *non-direct* forms of aggression that cause harm by disrupting relationships [23]. Crick and Grotpeter [24] defined relational aggression as "harming others through purposeful manipulation and damage of their peer relationships", including behaviours such as exclusion and telling the target they would not be friends anymore. These forms of relationally oriented aggression include both direct and indirect behaviours. For example, telling a target they would not be friends is a direct, verbal approach, and denying a request is similarly direct. This form of aggression also involves primarily verbal aggression that causes harm by disrupting relationships.

A recent study has proposed a new typological construct of aggression, elaborated through a structural equation modelling, and assessed its statistical validity. This theoretical classification of aggression and the empirical data showed an adjusted goodness of fit index = 0.102, providing empirical support for a structural typology of aggression composed of three dimensions – biological, social, and situational. Physical and verbal aggressions were classified in a construct named *biological dimension* of aggression; indirect and critical aggression were classified in a construct called *social dimension* of aggression; and, finally, reactive and instrumental aggression were included in a construct named *situational dimension* of aggression [3].

Many other proposed classifications of human aggression, even if using different terms, consistently follow a common dichotomy – in terms of purpose (why) or goal (inferred or otherwise) – depending on whether the primary intent is distress or harm, show qualitatively different phenomenology and neurophysiology, and appear clearly distinct at the factorial level. For instance, Rosenzweig [25] delineated a specific typology of aggressive responses to frustration: a *positive/constructive* profile (need-persistence), which is adaptive as well as prosocial, and a *negative/destructive* one (ego-defence), which is maladaptive as well as antisocial. Recent studies [26, 27] suggest something similar. Loeber and Schmaling [28] applied, practically, the same criteria to antisocial conduct, proposing *overt* and *covert.*

Some researchers [29-31] distinguish between *proactive* and *reactive* aggression, whereas others [7, 32-37] prefer to talk about *instrumental* and *hostile* aggression. Some others [38, 39] prefer to call them *impulsive* and *premeditated* aggression. Among psychiatrists [40], it is usual to talk about *predatory* and *affective* aggression. Other researchers [41, 42] have also proponed to extend to humans another bimodal scheme classification originated by ethological observations in animals [43, 44]: affective *defence* and predatory *attack*. However, its application can be difficult in our species since both these components of aggression may appear together [3]. The assessment of the validity of these two constructs by factor analysis shows good internal consistency (α = 0.73). A cluster analysis confirmed this predicted dichotomy – they are independent, existing in varying degrees, with qualitatively different phenomenology and neurobiology, and appearing clearly distinct at the factorial level [30, 40, 45].

Thus, we find that aggressive behaviour has traditionally been classified into two distinct subtypes. These independent constructs, which are referred to as hostile and instrumental aggression consistently emerge in varying degrees among 'normal' persons [46]. Their more specific characteristics are as follows:

- The *hostile-impulsive-uncontrolled unplanned-reactive-hot blooded-overt-defensive-affective negative/destructive* type may be defined as an act that is primarily intended, as ultimate motive, to harm another individual. This kind of aggression has historically been conceived as being impulsive, thoughtless or thought confusion [45], emotionally charged – driven by anger and characterised by loss of behavioural control – and occurring as a reaction to some perceived provocation. Psychologically, it is associated with disruptive behaviour, hostile attribution biases, intention-cue detection deficits in interpretation, internalising problems such as, depression or somatisation, and victimisation [30]. It typically occurs with hostile facial expressions and a strong negative affect. Physiologically, it is characterised by a marked sympathetic over-arousal. Some cognitive and neurobiological deficits have been repeatedly associated with this type of people being more likely to have lower IQ [40], as well as poorer verbal skills, lower P300 amplitude [47, 48], impairment of prefrontal function [41, 49], and lower levels of CSF 5HIAA [50].
- The *instrumental-premeditated controlled-planned-proactive-cold blooded-hidden-offensive-predatory-positive/constructive* type is conceived as a non-provoked aversive act aimed at influencing others [30]. It is a premeditated means or tool for solving problems, or for

obtaining a variety of objectives other than harming the victim such as, some reward, profit, or advantage for the aggressor – power, money, control and domination, gratification with sex or drugs etc. It is purposeful and goal-oriented, thus, requiring neither provocation nor anger [51], and more likely to be acquired and reinforced [52]. Psychologically, it is associated with a positive evaluation of aggression and social gain and dominance: leadership, socialisation, reciprocal relationship and friendship with other proactive persons, aggressive models etc. Physiologically, it is marked by under-arousal. In contrast to hostile aggression, the instrumental form exhibits relatively normal psychophysiological and neuropsychological variables, with an intact control system and average IQ, similar to the ones of non-violent controls [47, 53], having relatively normal prefrontal function [41] and P300 amplitude [48]. They are not thought to be different from 'normal' people [50]. Their scores on personality measures, however, are high [53].

Distinguishing this dichotomy is an important first step in understanding the multifaceted nature of aggression, which, if forgotten, may confuse our understanding of anger and hostility [3, 54].

Anger

Understanding the role of emotions in human aggression may be helpful in illuminating its developmental origins and outcomes. Unfortunately, most investigations have been conducted independently of research on emotions. Anger refers to feelings and represents the emotional or affective component of at least of some kinds of aggressive behaviour.

State anger is defined as a psychobiological, subjective experience that, over time and across situations, "usually refers to an emotional state that involves displeasure and consists of subjective feelings that vary in intensity, from mild irritation or annoyance to intense fury and rage" [14, 55, 56]. This internal state is embedded in a specific situational context, assuming that it would fluctuate over time as a function of perceived affronts, injustice, or frustration [57]. Anger would escalate if the source is seen as being intentional, preventable, unjustified, and blamed, as well as when values are compromised, promises and expectations are broken, rules violated, personal freedom and rights abridged. It is typically accompanied by autonomic nervous system arousal such as increases in heart rate and perspiration, cognitive distortions and deficiencies, and socially constructed and reinforced scripts [58, 59].

Trait anger may be considered to be a general temperament of low threshold reactivity in which angry feelings are experienced in response to a very wide variety of relatively innocuous triggers – e.g. a short delay on a cashier's line, a slightly late mail delivery by the postal service, or noticing that a student has made unexpected spelling errors – or a more narrow pattern of reactivity to specific classes of stimuli for the person such as competition, rejection, or perceived unfairness. Anger proneness may be seen as a personality trait or characteristic conceived in terms of individual differences in the frequency over time to appraising emotional situations in an angry way (anger experience), as well as to responding in anger (readiness to act angrily) [56-58, 60-62]. Its corresponding action readiness mode is that of correcting the harm received, either in a constructive way (assertion) or in a destructive way (aggression).

Hostility

Hostility is a negative evaluation of persons and things [8], often accompanied by a clear desire to do harm or to agreed them [63]. Plutchik [64] considered it as a negative attitude that mixes anger as well as disgust, and it is accompanied by feelings of indignation, disgust, contempt and resentment towards others. On occasions, it can even become bitterness and violence. This cluster of negative feelings towards others, known as *hostile attribution* is its subjective component [65], being reflected in a disfavourable judgement on them, perceived as antagonistic and threatening [66]. According to him, hostility is expressed when we say we do not like somebody, especially if we wish him ill. A hostile person is somebody who usually does negative evaluations of and towards others, showing an overall dislike and contempt for others [14].

This attitude of resentment and suspicion can be reflected in verbal and motor responses, such as the aggressive ones [67]. Others have used the term *hostility* to describe the broad construct involving affect, cognition and behaviour, but this term has a more specific meaning involving cognitive factors [68]. The cognitive phenomenon of hostility consists of negative beliefs about and attitudes toward others, including cynicism, mistrust and denigration. Cynicism refers to the belief that others are motivated by selfish concerns and, often, mistrust is the co-occurring expectation that others are likely to be provoking and hurtful. When these cognitive factors are considered together, hostility can be seen as a general trait connoting "a devaluation of the worth and motives of others, an expectation that others are likely sources of wrongdoing, a relational view of being in opposition toward others, and a desire to inflict harm or see others harmed" [69].

Hostility in itself is a multidimensional concept that can be categorised into attitudinal, emotional and behavioural components [2]. The attitudinal component refers to negative attitudes and appraisal towards others – mistrust and cynicism. The emotional component includes emotions like anger, irritability and annoyance. The behavioural component refers to aggressive, antagonistic behaviour.

Bendig [70] reported a factor called *covert hostility*, consisting mainly of irritable acts, and *overt hostility*, consisting mainly of assault and verbal aggression. Another distinction offered more recently [68] is between the experience and expression of hostility. Experimental hostility primarily refers to subjective factors, notably the affective processes of anger and related emotions as well as the cognitive processes comprising hostility, e.g. suspicion and cynicism. In contrast, expressive or behavioural hostility refers to overt verbal or physical aggressiveness, or both.

Psychologically, hostility has a close relationship with irritability and aggression. Consequently, it is necessary to clarify in some way the complex relationship between anger, hostility and aggression. *Anger*, the easiest concept of the three, has been described earlier. *Hostility*, on the contrary, implies an attitude that usually is accompanied by feelings of anger. Both show similar physiological effects on the autonomic as well as somatic nervous systems, and in both there is a predisposition towards aggressive behaviours mainly directed at the destruction of objects, insults, or at the infliction of some harm. If anger and hostility refer to feelings and attitudes, *aggression* implies a further step, in the sense that it includes the appearance of behaviours that may be destructive, harmful or punitive when directed towards other people or objects.

Some Correlations Between the Different Constructs

This section addresses some findings to probe that there should be some correlation between the three main symptoms of the AHA-Syndrome. Specifically, the following questions are going to be addressed:

(a) Are there different types of aggression? If yes, which would be the main commonalities and distinctions between them?
(b) Is there any correlation between aggression and anger and hostility?
(c) Is there any correlation between the above-mentioned related constructs?

Hostile vs. Instrumental Aggression

Two decades of research on moral approval of aggressive acts – applying the Cuestionario de Actitudes Morales sobre Agresión (CAMA) questionnaire to urban populations of different cultures throughout the world – brought out interesting conclusions:

(1) Aggressive acts of milder intensity were more acceptable than those of stronger aggression, as expected.
(2) A factorial analysis of the principal components of CAMA and varimax rotation showed two groups of situations (> 0.35):
    (i) Those leading towards instrumental aggression, which include self-defence, defence of others, and defence of property.
    (ii) The rest of the situations with hostile responses, which include lack of communication or emotional agitation.
(3) Both kinds of aggression – instrumental and hostile – as measured by CAMA, across the studies, were significantly correlated with one another ($r = 0.34$), with a shared variance and some independence between both subscales.
(4) The level of justification of instrumental aggressive acts such as, those conducted in protection of self or other, was clearly higher than that of hostile acts with no such justification, e.g. as an expression of emotions, as a result of communication difficulties etc.
(5) Within instrumental aggression, situations defending others and in self-defence received more moral approval than did those defending property.
(6) Provoked aggression led to more approval than unprovoked aggression. For example, killing was considered more justified for altruistic reasons than as a mere expression of bad temper, whereas punishment, emotional reaction, and communication problems were seen as the least justified circumstances for aggression [3, 71-73].

In other studies [74-76] interesting differences were found analysing social representation of aggression by the Aggressive Questionnaire (AQ) [67] and the correlations between AQ and CAMA. Physical aggression obtained a significant negative correlation with hostile representation of aggression ($r = -0.48$, $p < 0.05$) but, by contrast, a high positive correlation with instrumental representation of aggression ($r = 0.44$, $p < 0.05$). Finally, justification of aggression was significantly correlated to physical aggression ($r = 0.37$, $p < 0.05$) but not to verbal aggression ($r = 0.04$, n.s.).

These findings support the contention that aggression, far from being homogeneous, shows two distinct forms, which are different from one another, and differentially related to a host of other variables. There were pronounced personality differences [53]. The observed differences suggest that the physiological aspects of behavioural control play a key role in the type of aggressive behaviour displayed. For instance, underarousal is related to hostile aggression [77, 78], while instrumental aggression shows relatively normal psychobiological variables [79] and psychophysiological functions [48].

Their moderate correlates, however, suggest that instrumental and hostile aggression are similar in some ways, as one might expect. Thus, it was predicted that those who engage in both types of aggression are less likely to be able to control their behaviour. Also, they are more likely to experience anger as well as be more impulsive and more irritable than those who do not engage in these types of aggression. Grouping aggression according to different criteria, and applying the AQ, positive and significant correlations were found between physical and verbal aggression ($r = 0.35$, $p < 0.05$) [80].

Experience of Anger vs. Expression of Anger

A careful assessment of the differences between the intensity of anger experience and the frequency with which it is expressed is not only essential for understanding problems rooted in anger, but it is also a necessary first step in treatment planning.

It was predicted that even if a certain positive correlation should be expected between subjective anger experience and objective proneness toward an angry action, its experience would be shown in greater proportion. Studies have shown a positive correlation between both, in accordance with the working hypotheses, i.e. those who experienced anger more frequently were also more likely to express anger [58, 61]. This result also matched with another previous study [81], where a significant correlation of these variables with subcortical arousal was also found. Anger involves physiological arousal and prepares for aggression.

The feelings of anger, however, were much more frequent than the readiness to commit an angry action ($r = 0.30$, $p < 00001$), even if a positive correlation might be expected between them [56]. This is, of course, reasonable as one is likely to show restraint particularly when one's actions may be harmful to others, as often happens in the expression of anger.

Though it should be added that an over-control of anger, characterised by very low levels of anger expression, in the long term may risk an inappropriate and explosive expression of anger resulting in extreme violence [82].

Anger vs. Aggression

Anger, as well as other emotions, may almost certainly be involved in some forms of aggression. Those who engage in aggression of any kind are less likely to be able to control their behaviour and more likely to experience anger. They are also likely to be more impulsive and more irritable than those who do not engage so often in aggression. Barratt [83] hypothesised that trait behavioural approach sensitivity (BAS) would be positively related to the personality traits of anger/hostility, as well as with physical aggression [84]. Anger, thus, would be a negative but approach-related emotion associated with aggression [85]. Generally speaking, people high on trait anger would be more likely to accept aggressive responses. Precisely, this was also found by comparing CAMA and AQ, i.e. there is a low, even if significant, correlation between anger and justification of aggression ($r = 0.10$, $p < 0.05$) [74].

More specifically, one would expect that trait anger would relate positively to one's measure of hostile aggression because it reflects intention of harming others, i.e. it is motivated by anger. Therefore, it would be relatively likely for irritable individuals to express hostile aggression [83]. This hypothesis was supported by a small, but significant, positive correlation between anger and the hostile representation of aggression ($r = 0.11$, $p < 0.05$), and, more specifically, between anger and communication, included within hostile situations ($r = 0.22$, $p < 0.05$), being the highest one between the AQ sub-scales verbal aggression and anger ($r = 0.60$; $p < 0.05$) [72, 76, 80].

Instrumental aggression, in contrast, may have a weaker relationship with irritability and, consequently, it would not necessarily relate positively to trait anger, because it is not directly motivated by angry feelings. Making the distinction between hostile and instrumental aggression, thus, may clarify when aggression may be maladaptive and when it may not.

Hostility vs. Aggression

A comparison between the four sub-scales of AQ showed significant positive correlation between all of them, supporting the hypothesised correlation between the personality traits anger/hostility and physical aggression, given the direct relation of both with trait BAS, as already mentioned [83, 85]. More specifically, hostility showed a higher correlation with verbal aggression ($r = 0.34$, $p < 0.05$) than with physical aggression ($r = 0.20$, $p < 0.05$) [80]. This moderate correlation between hostility and both physical and verbal aggression was mainly due to their connection with anger. For example, when anger is less, the correlations between hostility and both physical and verbal aggression would be even lower. The partial correlation with anger controlled was 0.08 between hostility and physical aggression and 0.05 between hostility and verbal aggression [7].

No correlation was found between hostility and justification of aggression ($r = 0.07$, n.s.), measured by AQ and CAMA, respectively [74]. Rather than assessing aggressive acts directly, one must remember that the CAMA questionnaire assesses attitudes and beliefs about aggression. In other words, both constructs – hostility and justification of aggression – are related to cognitive and affective facets, but not to behavioural ones, as is physical or verbal aggression. This may explain why physical aggression is moderately correlated to the justification of aggression ($r = 0.37$; $p < 0.05$) [74].

Hostility vs. Anger

It is predicted that those who engage in aggression are more likely to experience anger and be more impulsive. Consequently, some correlation between these two constructs could also be expected. In fact, an analysis of the AQ sub-scales showed the same, i.e. the highest correlation between the different sub-scales was precisely between anger and hostility ($r = 0.60$, $p < 0.05$) [80].

Conclusion

The findings reviewed in this chapter support the contention that instrumental and hostile aggression are two distinct forms of aggression, and different from one another. They are referred to being independent of one another, or as if a person does either one or the other, even if, in fact, there is also a moderate correlation with one another. Both forms of aggression share considerable variance. This significant relationship between them actually suggests that people who report using one kind of aggression also report using the other, and that aggression may be associated to a distinctive personality style, regardless of its type [77, 78].

What is the picture of both kinds of aggression that is revealed by their relationships with other aggression-related variables? Reports of engaging in hostile aggression are associated with expressing rather than controlling anger, with a more general irritability, and an inability to inhibit action. The personality traits of anger/hostility would be significantly related to aggression. An individual who uses hostile aggression might be characterised as one who is not inhibited in social interaction and is likely to experience as well as express anger. On the contrary, reports of engaging in instrumental aggression show that if one wants to be really skilful in one's pretended goal, one should control anger. An aggressive act does not have to be necessarily accompanied by anger or by the desire to hurt [86]. The traditional assumption that anger necessarily causes aggression should be questioned [66].

Finally, anger modulates aggression. First, it reduces inhibitions against being aggressive in at least two ways. Anger sometimes provides a justification for aggressive retaliation – it is part of the decision rule in the aggression script. But anger may also sometimes interfere with higher level cognitive processes, including those normally used in moral reasoning and judgement, which are part of the re-appraisal process. Second, anger allows a person to maintain an aggressive intention over time. Anger increases attention to the provoking events, increases the depth of processing of those events and, therefore, improves recall of such events.

Key Points

- The positive correlation empirically found between hostile or reactive aggression, anger, and hostility showed a high adjustment with the prototypical description and characteristics given to hostile aggression, which is also known as impulsive or affective.
- In contrast, instrumental or proactive aggression did not significantly show most of the above-mentioned characteristics.
- The use of personality measures, therefore, may help to clearly differentiate aggressive subjects from 'normal' population and, perhaps, even between them.

Acknowledgements

This work was supported by grants of the Spanish Ministry of Science and Technology (BS2001/1224), Ministry of Education and Science (SEJ2007-60303) and of Complutense University (PR1/06-14456-B) to both the authors.

References

1. Van Doornen, L.J.P., 1997, "Lipids and the Coronary Prone Personality", In *Lipids, Health and Behavior*, M. Hillbrand and R.T. Spitz (Eds.), American Psychological Association, Washington, D.C.
2. Sluyter, F., Keijser, J.N., Boomsma, D.I., van Doorne, L.J.P., van den Oord, E.J.C.G. and Snieder, H., 2000, "Genetics of Testosterone and the Aggression-Hostility-Anger Syndrome: A Study of Middle-aged Male Twins", *Twin Research*, 3, pp. 266-276.

3. Ramirez, J.M. and Andreu, J.M., 2003, "Aggression's Typologies", *International Review of Social Psychology*, 16, pp. 145-161.
4. Baron, R.A. and Richardson, D.R., 1994, *Human Aggression*, Plenum Press, New York.
5. Berkowitz, L., 1989, "Frustration-Aggression Hypothesis: Examination and Reformulation", *Psychological Bulletin*, 14, pp. 59-73.
6. Dollard, J., Doob, L.W., Miller, N.E., Mower, O.H. and Sears, R.R., 1939, *Frustration and Aggression*, Yale University Press, New Haven.
7. Feshbach, S., 1964, "The Function of Aggression and the Regulation of the Aggressive Drive", *Psychological Review*, 71, pp. 257-272.
8. Buss, A.H., 1961, *The Psychology of Aggression*, John Wiley & Sons, New York.
9. Ramírez, J.M., 1996, "Causes and Functions of Aggression", *Hiroshima Forum for Psychology*, 17, pp. 21-37.
10. Ramírez, J.M., 1998, "Aggression", In *Comparative Psychology: A Handbook*, G. Greenberg and M.M. Haraway (Eds.), Garland, New York, pp. 625-634.
11. Ramírez, J.M., 2000, *Agresión: Un Enfoque Psicobiológico*, Promolibro, Valencia.
12. Ramírez, J.M. and Rañada, A.F., 1996, *De la Agresión a la Guerra Nuclear*, Nobel, Oviedo.
13. Reynolds, M. and Andreu, J.M., 1999, "From Aggression to Nuclear War", *Aggressive Behavior*, 2, pp. 309-310.
14. Spielberger, C.D., Jacobs, G., Rusell, S.F. and Crane, R.S., 1983, "Assessment of Anger: The State-Trait Anger Scale", In *Advances in Personality Assessment*, Vol. 2, J.N. Butcher and C.D. Spielberger (Eds.), Lawrence Erlbaum Associates, Inc., Hillsdale, New Jersey.
15. Anderson, C.A. and Bushman, B.J., 2002, "Human Aggression", *Annual Review of Psychology*, 53, pp. 27-51.
16. Yudofsky, S.C., Silver, J.M., Jackson, W., Endicott, J. and Williams, D., 1986, "Overt Aggression Scale for the Objective Rating of Verbal and Physical Aggression", *American Journal of Psychiatry*, 143, pp. 35-39.
17. Berkowitz, L., 1994, "Is Something Missing? Some Observations Prompted by the Cognitive-Neoassociacionist View of Anger and Emotional Aggression", In *Aggressive Behavior: Current Perspectives*, R. Huesman (Ed.), Plenum Press, New York, pp. 35-60.
18. Björkqvist, K., 1994, "Sex Differences in Physical, Verbal and Indirect Aggression: A Review of Recent Research", *Sex Roles*, 30, pp. 177-188.
19. Björkqvist, K., Lagerspetz, K.M. and Kaukianen, A., 1992, "Do Girls Manipulate and Boys Fight? Developmental Trends in Regard to Direct and Indirect Aggression", *Aggressive Behavior*, 18, pp. 117-127.
20. Buss, A.H., 1971, "Aggression Plays", In *The Control of Aggression and Violence*, J.L. Singer (Ed.), Academic Press, New York.
21. Richardson, D.S. and Green, L.R., 2003, "Defining Direct and Indirect Aggression: The Richardson Conflict Response Questionnaire", *International Review of Social Psychology*, 16, pp. 11-30.
22. Feshbach, N., 1969, "Sex Differences in Children's Modes of Aggressive Responses Towards Outsiders", *Merrill Palmer Quarterly*, 15, pp. 249-258.
23. Richardson, D.S. and Hammock, G.S., 2003, "Defining Non-direct Aggression Raises General Questions About the Definition of Aggression", *International Review of Social Psychology*, 16, pp. 5-10.
24. Crick, N.R. and Grotpeter, J.K., 1995, "Relational Aggression, Gender and Social Psychological Adjustment", *Child Development*, 66, pp. 710-722.
25. Rosenzweig, S., 1941, "Need-persistive and Ego-defensive Reactions to Frustration as Demonstrated by an Experiment on Repression", *Psychological Review*, 48, pp. 347-349.

26. Lansford, J.E., Dodge, K.A., Bates, J.E. and Petit, G.S., 2002, "Developmental Trajectories of Reactive and Proactive Aggression", Paper Presented at the *15th World Meeting of the International Society for Research on Aggression*, Montreal, July 2002, p. 109.
27. Poulin, F., Dishion, T.J. and Boivin, M., 2002, "Proactive/reactive Aggression and Adjustment Problems in Adolescence", Paper Presented at the *15th World Meeting of the International Society for Research on Aggression*, Montreal, July 2002, p. 110.
28. Loeber, R. and Schmaling, K.B., 1985, "Empirical Evidence for Overt and Covert Antisocial Conduct Problems: A Meta-analysis", *Journal of Abnormal and Child Psychology*, 13, pp. 337-352.
29. Crick, N.R. and Dodge, K.A., 1996, "Social Information-processing Mechanisms in Reactive and Proactive Aggression", *Child Development*, 67, pp. 993-1002.
30. Dodge, K.A. and Coie, J.D., 1987, "Social Information Processing Factors in Reactive and Proactive Aggression in Children's Peer Groups", *Journal of Personality and Social Psychology*, 53, pp. 1146-1158.
31. Pitkänen-Pulkkinen, L., 1969, "A Descriptive Model of Aggression and Non-aggression and Applications to Children's Behavior", *Jyväskylä Studies in Education, Psychoplogy, and Social Research*, 19.
32. Peña, M.E., Andreu, J.M., Graña, J.L., Pahlavan, F. and Ramirez, J.M., 2008, "Moderate and Severe Aggression Justification in Instrumental and Reactive Contexts", *Social Behavior and Personality*, 36(2), pp. 229-238.
33. Aronson, E., 1992, *The Social Animal*, Freeman, New York.
34. Bandura, A., 1973, *Aggression: A Social Learning Analysis*, Prentice Hill, Englewood Cliffs.
35. Hartup, W.W., 1974, "Aggression in Childhood: Developmental Perspectives", *American Psychologist*, 29, pp. 336-341.
36. Hinde, R.A., 1970, *Animal Behaviour: A Synthesis of Ethology and Comparative Psychology*, McGraw-Hill, New York.
37. Kingsbury, S.J., Lambert, M.T. and Hendrickse, W., 1997, "A Two-factor Model of Aggression", *Psychiatry*, 60, pp. 224-232.
38. Barratt, E.S. and Slaughter, L., 1998, "Defining, Measuring and Predicting Impulsive Aggression: A Heuristic Model", *Behav. Sci. Law*, 16, pp. 285-302.
39. Houston, R.J., Stanford, M.S., Villemarette-Pittman, N.R., Conklin, S.M. and Helfritz, L.E., 2003, "Neurobiological Correlates and Clinical Implications of Aggressive Subtypes", *Journal of Forensic Neuropsychology*, 3, pp. 67-87.
40. Vitiello, B., Behar, D., Hunt, J., Stoff, D. and Ricciuti, A., 1990, "Subtyping Aggression in Children and Adolescents", *Journal of Neuropsychiatry and Clinical Neurosciences*, 2, pp. 189-192.
41. Raine, A., Meloy, J.R., Bihrle, S., Stoddard, J., LaCasse, L. and Buchsbaum, M.S., 1998, "Reduced Prefrontal and Increased Subcortical Brain Functioning Assessed Using PET in Predatory and Affective Murders", *Behavioral Sciences and the Law*, 16, pp. 319-332.
42. Weinshenker, N.J. and Siegel, A., 2002, "Bimodal Classification of Aggression: Affective Defense and Predatory Attack", *Aggression and Violent Behavior*, 7, pp. 237-250.
43. Flynn, J.P., 1976, "Neural Basis of Threat and Attack", *Biological Foundations of Psychiatry*, pp. 111-133.
44. Ramirez, J.M., 1981, "Towards a Conceptualization and Classification of Animal Aggression", *Hiroshima Forum for Psychology*, 8, pp. 11-21.
45. Barratt, E.S., Stanford, M.S., Dowdy, L., Liebman, M.J. and Kent, T.A., 1999, "Impulsive and Premeditated Aggression: A Factor Analysis of Self-reported Acts", *Psychiatric Research*, 86, pp. 163-173.
46. Bushman, B.J. and Anderson, C.A., 2001, "Is It Time to Pull the Plug on Hostile versus Instrumental Aggression Dichotomy?" *Psychological Review*, 108, pp. 273-279.

47. Barratt, E.S., Stanford, M.S., Felthous, A.R. and Kent, T.A., 1997a, "The Effects of Phenytoin on Impulsive and Premeditated Aggression: A Controlled Study", *Journal of Clinical Psychopharmacology*, 17, pp. 341-349.
48. Barratt, E.S., Stanford, M.S., Kent, T.A. and Felthous, A.R., 1997b, "Neuropsychological and Cognitive Psychophysiological Substrates of Impulsive Aggression", *Biological Psychiatry*, 41(10), pp. 1045-1061.
49. Fuster, J.M., 1997, *The Prefrontal Cortex: Anatomy, Physiology and Neuyropsychology of the Frontal Lobe*, 3rd Edn., Raven, New York.
50. Linnoila, M., Virkkunen, M., Scheinin, M., Nuuutila, R, Rimon, R. and Goodwin, F.K., 1983, "Low Cerebrospinal Fluid 5-hydroxyindoleacetic Acid Concentration Differentiates Impulsive from Non-impulsive Violent Behavior", *Life Sciences*, 33, pp. 2609-2614.
51. Berkowitz, L., 1993, *Aggression: Its Causes, Consequences and Control*, McGraw-Hill, New York.
52. Bandura, A., 1983, "Psychological Mechanisms of Aggression", In *Aggression: Theoretical and Empirical Reviews*, R.G. Geen and E.I. Donnerstein (Eds.), Academic Press, New York, pp. 39-46.
53. Stanford, M.S., Houston, R.J., Villemarette-Pittman, N.R. and Greve, K.W., 2003, "Premeditated Aggression: Clinical Assessment and Cognitive Psychophysiology", *Pers. Individ. Differ.*, 34, pp. 773-781.
54. Ramírez, J.M., "Some Dychotomous Classifications of Aggression According to its Function", *International Journal of Organisational Transformation and Social Change* (in press).
55. Spielberger, C.D., Reheiser, E.C. and Sydeman, S.J., 1995, "Measuring the Experience, Expression and Control of Anger", *Issues in Comprehensive Paediatric Nursing*, 18, pp. 207-232.
56. Van Goozen, S.H., Fridja, N.C., Kindt, M. and Van de Poll, N.E., 1994, "Anger Proneness in Women: Development and Validation of the Anger Situation Questionnaire", *Aggressive Behavior*, 20, pp. 79-100.
57. Ramirez, J.M., Fujihara, T. and Van Goozen, S.H., 2001a, "Cultural and Gender Differences in Anger and Aggression: A Comparison Between Japanese, Dutch and Spanish Students", *Journal of Social Psychology*, 141, pp. 119-121.
58. Ramirez, J.M., Fujihara, T., Van Goozen, S.H. and Santisteban, C., 2001b, "Anger Proneness in Japanese and Spanish Students", In *Cross-cultural Approaches to Aggression and Reconciliation*, J.M. Ramírez and D.R. Richardson (Eds.), NovaScience, Huntington, pp. 87-97.
59. Sukhodolsky, D.G., Kassinove, H. and Gorman, B.S., 1995, "Cognitive-behavioral Therapy for Anger in Children and Adolescents: A Meta-analysis", *Aggression and Violent Behavior*, 9(3), pp. 247-267.
60. Deffenbacher, J.L., 1992, "Trait Anger: Theory, Findings and Implications", In *Advances in Personality Assessment*, C.D. Spielberger and J.N. Bucher (Eds.), Lawrence Erlbaum Associates, Inc., Hillsdale, pp. 177-201.
61. Ramirez, J.M., Santisteban, C., Fujihara, T. and Van Goozen, S.H., 2002, "Differences Between Experiences of Anger and Readiness to Angry Action: A Study of Japanese and Spanish Students", *Aggressive Behavior*, 20, pp. 429-438.
62. Ramirez, J.M., Alvarado, J.M. and Santisteban, C., 2004, "Individual Differences in Anger Reaction to Noise", *Individual Differences Research*, 2(2), pp. 125-136.
63. Kaufmann, H., 1970, *Aggression and Altruism*, Rinehart and Winston, Holt.
64. Plutchik, R., 1980, *Emotion: A Psychoevolutionary Synthesis*, John Wiley & Sons, Inc., New York.
65. Barefoot, J.C., 1992, "Developments in the Measurement of Hostility", In *Hostility, Coping and Health*, H.S. Friedman (Ed.), American Psychological Association, Washington, D.C.
66. Berkowitz, L., 2000, "Causes and Consequences of Feelings", *Studies in Emotion and Social Interaction*, Cambridge University Press, New York.
67. Buss, A. and Perry, M., 1992, "The Aggression Questionnaire", *Journal of Personality and Social Psychology*, 63(3), pp. 452-459.

68. Miller, T., Smith, T. and Turner, C.W., 1996, "A Meta-analytic Review of Research on Hostility and Physical Health", *Psychological Bulletin*, 119(2), pp. 322-348.
69. Smith, T.W., 1994, "Concepts and Methods in the Study of Anger, Hostility and Health", In *Anger, Hostility and the Heart*, A.W. Siegman and T.W. Smith (Eds.), Lawrence Erlbaum Associates, Inc., Hillsdale, New Jersey, pp. 23-42.
70. Bendig, A.W., 1962, "Factor Analytic Scales of Covert and Overt Hostility", *Journal of Consulting Psychology*, 26, p. 200.
71. Ramírez, J.M., 2001, "Moral Approval of Aggressive Acts by Urban Students: A Cross-national Study in Four Continents", In *Cross-cultural Approaches to Aggression and Reconciliation*, J.M. Ramírez and D.R. Richardson (Eds.), NovaScience, Huntington, pp. 61-71.
72. Ramirez, J.M. and Andreu, J.M., 2006, "Aggression and Some Other Psychological Constructs (Anger, Hostility and Impulsivity): Some Comments from a Research Project", *Neurosci. Biobehav. Rev.*, 21(1), pp. 276-291.
73. Ramírez, J.M., 2007, "Justification of Aggression in Several Asian and European Countries with Different Religious and Cultural Background", *International Journal of Behavioral Development*, 31(1), Serial No. 51, pp. 9-15.
74. Andreu, J.M., Peña, M.E. and Graña, J.L., 2001, "Agresividad y Aceptabilidad de la Agresión en Jóvenes y Adolescentes de Ambos Sexos", *Clínica y Salud*, 12(2), pp. 271-284.
75. Archer, J. and Haigh, A., 1997, "Do Beliefs About Aggression Predict Self-reported Levels of Aggression?" *Journal of Social Psychology*, 38, pp. 71-84.
76. Ramirez,, J.M., Andreu, J.M. and Fujihara, T., 2001c, "Cultural and Sex Differences in Aggression: A Comparison Between Japanese and Spanish Students Using Two Different Inventories", *Aggressive Behavior*, 27, pp. 313-322.
77. Houston, R.J. and Stanford, M.S., 2005, "Electrophysiological Substrates of Impulsiveness: Potential Effects on Aggressive Behavior", *Progress in Neuro-Psychopharmacology and Biological Psychiatry*, 29(2), pp. 305-313.
78. Houston, R.J. and Stanford, M.S., 2006, "Characterisation of Aggressive Behavior and Phenytoin Response", *Aggressive Behavior*, 32, pp. 38-43.
79. Linnoila, M. and Charney, D.S., 1999, "The Neurobiology of Aggression", In *Neurobiology of Mental Illness*, D.S. Charney, E.J. Nestler and B. Bunneys (Eds.), Oxford University Press, New York, pp. 855-871.
80. Andreu, J.M., Graña, J.L. and Peña, M.L., 2002, "Adaptación Psicométrica de la Versión Española del Cuestionario de Agresión", *Psicothema*, 14(2), pp. 476-482.
81. Ramírez, J.M. and Sancho, J.L., 1995, "Influencia de la Reactivación Cortical, Subcortical y del Sexo en la Ira y el Comportamiento Agresivo", Universidad Complutense Madrid (unpublished results).
82. Allan, S. and Gilbert, P., 2002, "Anger and Anger Expression in Relation to Perceptions of Social Rank, Entrapment and Depressive Symptoms", *Personality and Individual Differences*, 32(3), pp. 551-565.
83. Barratt, E.S., 1991, "Measuring and Predicting Aggression Within the Context of a Personality Theory", *Journal of Neuropsychiatry and Clinical Neurosciences*, 3, pp. S35-S39.
84. Harmon-Jones, E. and Sigelman, J., 2001, "State Anger and Prefrontal Brain Activity: Evidence that Insult-Related Relative Left-Prefrontal Activation is Associated with Experienced Anger and Aggression", *Journal of Personality and Social Psychology*, 80(5), pp. 797-803.
85. Harmon-Jones, E., 2003, "Anger and the Behavioral Approach System", *Personality and Individual Differences*, 35(5), pp. 995-1005.
86. Averill, J.R., 1982, *Anger and Aggression: An Essay on Emotions*, Springer, New York.

The AHA-Syndrome and Cardiovascular Diseases
Editors: Swati Y. Bhave and Sunil Saini
Copyright © 2010 Anamaya Publishers, New Delhi, India

3. Measuring the Anger Components of the AHA-Syndrome

Charles D. Spielberger, Eric C. Reheiser and G. Douglas Lunsford
University of South Florida, Tampa, USA

Abstract: This article examines the concepts of anger, hostility and aggression, and reviews the evolution and development of psychometric scales for measuring the experience, expression and control of anger as components of the AHA-Syndrome. Research findings on the measurement of state and trait anger, as well as anger expression and control, which contributed to the construction and validation of the State-Trait Anger Scale (STAS), the Anger Expression (AX) Scale, and the State-Trait Anger Expression Inventory (STAXI) are described in detail. Research findings with the STAS, AX Scale and the STAXI relating to the effects of anger on health and behaviour are also briefly described.

Keywords: Anger, Hostility, Aggression, Measurement, AHA-Syndrome.

Introduction

Anger, hostility and aggression are generally recognised as important concepts in most contemporary theories of personality and psychopathology, and as important contributors to the etiology of psychoneuroses, depression, and cardiovascular disorders. However, angry feelings are frequently confounded with hostility and aggressive behaviour, and these terms are often used interchangeably in the research literature. Consequently, definitions of these constructs remain ambiguous, leading to conceptual confusion and overlapping measurement operations of questionable validity [1].

Given the substantial overlap in prevailing definitions of anger, hostility, and aggression, we have referred collectively to these constructs as the AHA-Syndrome [2], and have endeavoured to identify meaningful definitions for each concept. *Anger*, generally, refers to an emotional state, which consists of feelings that vary in intensity from mild irritation or annoyance to intense fury or rage, with associated activation or arousal of the autonomic and neuroendocrine systems [3, 4]. *Hostility*, generally, involves the experience of intensely angry feelings, but also has the connotation of complex attitudes and behaviours that include being mean, vicious, vindictive and, often, cynical. As a psychological construct, aggression describes destructive or punitive behaviours directed towards other persons or objects in the environment.

The earliest efforts to assess anger and hostility were based on clinical interviews, behavioural observations, and projective techniques such as, the Rorschach Inkblots and the Thematic Apperception Test. Physiological and behavioural correlates of anger, hostility, and various manifestations of aggression have also been investigated in numerous studies. In contrast, the phenomenology of anger, i.e. the experience of angry feelings, has been largely neglected in psychological research. Another common problem with existing measures of anger and hostility is that these scales fail to explicitly take the state-trait distinction into account. A coherent theoretical framework that distinguishes between anger, hostility and aggression as psychological concepts, and that takes the state-trait distinction into account is essential for constructing and validating psychometric measures of anger and hostility.

Although the physiological correlates of hostility and behavioural manifestations of aggression have been investigated in numerous studies, anger was largely neglected in psychological research. In her book, *Anger: The Misunderstood Emotion*, Tavris [5] identified anger as a crucial emotion that strongly impacts our daily lives, "having different consequences for our mental and physical health". As the title of the book implies, anger is still greatly misunderstood. Tavris correctly points out that "anger is not a disease, with a single cause; it is a process, a transaction, a way of communicating" [5]. She also notes that our beliefs about and interpretations of the experience of anger are important in understanding the nature of anger as an emotional reaction.

A quarter century following the publication of Tavris' book, DiGiuseppe and Tafrate noted the ubiquitous nature of anger, stating that "anger is certainly a common and universal human experience" [6]. DiGiuseppe and Tafrate also observed that "anger is the forgotten emotion", and that "our scientific knowledge concerning anger has lagged behind that of other emotional disorders". They identified some of the potential reasons that anger, as an emotional state, has received less attention than other emotions as a topic of scientific inquiry, which included the absence of a diagnostic category for anger disorders in the DSM IV, limited assessment instruments, the paucity of treatment studies on anger, and the failure of our language to discriminate between functional and dysfunctional anger.

This article endeavours to provide a coherent theoretical framework for the measurement of anger, taking into account the state-trait distinction, along with individual differences in the expression and control of anger. The construction and validation of the State-Trait Anger Expression Inventory (STAXI) for assessing the experience, expression and control of anger is also briefly described [3, 4]. It concludes with a discussion on the utilisation of the STAXI as a measure of anger in research on heart disease, depression, and disorders such as alcohol and drug abuse.

Experience, Expression and Control of Anger

Substantial evidence that anger motivates hostility in a wide range of aggressive behaviours makes clear the need to assess both anger as an emotional state, and how frequently this emotion is experienced. As a first step in developing a measure of anger, we defined *state anger* (S-Anger) as a psychobiological state or condition consisting of subjective feelings that vary in intensity, from mild irritation or annoyance to intense fury and rage, with concomitant activation or arousal of the autonomic nervous system [7]. It was further assumed that S-Anger fluctuates over time as a function of perceived affronts, injustice, or frustration. *Trait anger* (T-Anger) was defined in terms of individual differences in the frequency that S-Anger was experienced over time. Persons high in T-Anger perceive a wider range of situations as anger-provoking – annoying, irritating, frustrating – than those low in T-Anger, and more frequently experience elevations in S-Anger whenever such conditions are encountered.

DiGiuseppe and Tafrate [6] noted that Spielberger's "distinction between emotional states and traits has become one of the most important ideas in the psychology of emotions". As applied to anger, Spielberger's state/trait theory predicts the following about people high in trait anger:

- Perceive a wider range of situations as anger provoking.
- Experience state anger with greater intensity and frequency.
- Express their anger with greater negativity and less effective coping.
- Experience a higher degree of dysfunction and negative consequences.

The State-Trait Anger Scale (STAS) was constructed to assess the intensity of feelings of anger as an emotional state and individual differences in anger proneness as a personality trait [8]. In responding to the STAS S-Anger scale, examinees report their feelings of anger at a particular time by rating themselves on a four-point intensity scale, e.g. "I feel angry":

(1) Not at all.
(2) Somewhat.
(3) Moderately so.
(4) Very much so.

Examinees indicate how they generally feel in responding to the STAS T-Anger scale by rating themselves on a four-point frequency scale, e.g. "I am a hotheaded person":

(1) Almost never.
(2) Sometimes.
(3) Often.
(4) Almost always.

Alpha coefficients of 0.93 and 0.87 were found for the preliminary STAS S- and T-Anger scales administered to a large sample of university students, providing impressive evidence of the utility of the working definitions of anger that guided selection of the items for these scales [7]. The individual item-remainder correlations for the final set of 10 S-Anger and 10 T-Anger items selected for the STAS were 0.50 or higher. Factor analyses of the S-Anger items identified only a single underlying factor for both males and females, indicating that this scale measured a unitary emotional state that varied in intensity. In contrast, factor analyses of the 10 STAS T-Anger items identified two independent, substantially correlated factors, *Angry Temperament* (T-Anger/T) and *Angry Reaction* (T-Anger/R). The T-Anger/T items describe experiencing anger without specifying any provoking circumstance, e.g. "I am a hot headed person", or "I have a fiery temper". The T-Anger/R items describe reactions to situations in which anger was provoked by the negative evaluations of other persons, e.g. "It makes me furious when I am criticised in front of others".

As our research on anger has progressed, the critical importance of differentiating between the experience and expression of anger became increasingly apparent [8]. It seemed essential not only to distinguish, both conceptually and empirically, between the intensity of the experience of anger as an emotional state (S-Anger) and individual differences in anger-proneness as a personality trait (T-Anger), but also to identify and measure the characteristic ways in which people expressed their anger. Recognition of the importance of anger expression stimulated the development of scales to assess the expression and control of anger.

Measuring Anger Expression

The conceptual distinction between 'anger-in' and 'anger-out' as major modes of anger expression has long been recognised in psychophysiological research. The effects of anger expression on the cardiovascular system was a major focus of the classic studies of Funkenstein et al. [9] more than 50 years ago. They exposed healthy college students to anger-inducing laboratory conditions, and measured their pulse rate and blood pressure to determine the physiological effects of how they handled their anger. Students who became angry during the experiment and directed their anger toward an investigator or the laboratory situation were classified as anger-out; those who suppressed their anger and/or directed it at themselves were classified as anger-in. The increase in pulse rate for students classified as anger-in was three times greater than for the anger-out group.

Following the procedures used by Funkenstein et al. [9], individuals are generally classified as anger-in if they suppress their anger or direct it inward, toward the ego or self [5, 10]. When held in or suppressed, anger may be subjectively experienced as an emotional state, S-Anger, which varies in intensity. Anger directed outward generally involves both the experience of S-Anger and its manifestation in some form of aggressive behaviour. Those who express their anger in aggressive behaviour, directing it toward other persons or objects in the environment, are classified as anger-out. Anger-out may be expressed in physical acts such as slamming doors, destroying objects, and assaulting other persons, or in verbal behaviour in the form of criticism, threats, insults, or the extreme use of profanity. These physical and verbal manifestations of anger may be directed toward the source of provocation or frustration, or expressed indirectly toward persons or objects associated with or symbolic of the provoking agent.

Harburg et al. have reported impressive relationships between anger expression, elevated blood pressure and hypertension, demonstrating that anger-in and anger-out have different effects on the cardiovascular system [11, 12]. They classified individuals as anger-in or anger-out on the basis of their self-ratings of how they would express anger if treated unfairly by a supervisor, a landlord, or a police officer. Gentry [13] and his colleagues [14] have, subsequently, corroborated and extended Harburg's findings. It should be noted, however, that the procedures used by Harburg and Gentry for classifying individuals as anger-in raises important conceptual issues because individuals who do not experience anger are equated with those who experience and suppress their angry feelings. Very different personality dynamics have been attributed by Rosenzweig [15, 16] to 'impunitive' persons, who do not experience anger during anger-provoking situations, and 'intrapunitive' persons, who turn anger inward when provoked, often blaming themselves for the anger directed toward them by others.

Differentiating between how angry feelings are expressed can be accomplished by measuring the frequency that anger is suppressed (anger-in) or overtly expressed in behaviour (anger-out). The expression of anger was implicitly defined by Funkenstein et al. [9], Harburg et al. [12], and Gentry et al. [14] as comprising a single dimension, varying from extreme suppression or inhibition of anger to the expression of anger in assaultive or destructive behaviour. In keeping with this definition, Spielberger et al. [8] attempted to construct a unidimensional, bipolar measure to assess this dimension, the *Anger Expression* (AX) Scale.

As a first step in constructing the AX Scale, working definitions of anger-in and anger-out were formulated on the basis of a review of the relevant research literature. Anger-in was defined in terms of how often an individual experiences, but holds in (suppresses) angry feelings. Anger-out was defined as the frequency with which an individual expresses angry feelings in verbal or physically aggressive behaviour. However, in contrast to the procedure used by Funkenstein and Harburg of assigning subjects to dichotomous anger-in or anger-out categories, the AX Scale was designed to measure a continuum of individual differences in how often anger was held in or expressed.

Consistent with our working definitions of anger-in and anger-out, items were constructed for the AX Scale with content that ranged from strong inhibition or suppression of angry feelings (AX/In) to extreme expression of anger toward other persons or objects in the environment (AX/Out). The rating format for the AX Scale was the same as that used with the STAS T-Anger scale [17], but the instructions differed markedly from those used in assessing T-Anger. Rather than asking respondents to indicate how they generally feel, they were instructed to report "... how often you generally react or behave in the manner described when you feel angry or furious". Examples of AX Scale items are as follows:

AX/In: I keep things in; I boil inside, but I don't show it.
AX/Out: I lose my temper; I strike out at whatever infuriates me.

In responding to the AX Scale items, subjects rated themselves on the following four-point frequency scale:

(1) Almost never.
(2) Sometimes.
(3) Often.
(4) Almost always.

In a study of the relationship between anger expression and blood pressure, Johnson [18] administered a 30-item preliminary version of the AX Scale to 1,114 high school students. To verify that the AX Scale items were measuring a unitary psychological construct, students' responses to the individual items were evaluated in separate factor analyses for males and females. Although we had originally intended to develop a unidimensional, bipolar measure of anger expression, the results of the factor analyses clearly indicated that the AX items were tapping two independent dimensions, which were labelled Anger/In and Anger/Out on the basis of the content of the items with strong loadings on one of these factors and negligible loadings on the other.

Given the strength and clarity of the Anger/In and Anger/Out factors, the striking similarity (invariance) of these factors for males and females, and the large sample on which the factor analyses were based, our test-construction strategy for developing the AX Scale was modified to identify homogeneous subsets of items to comprise scales for measuring anger-in and anger-out. Based on further factor analyses [8], eight items with uniformly high loadings for both sexes on the Anger/In factor and negligible loadings on the Anger/Out factor were selected for the AX/In subscale; the median loadings of these items on Anger/In and Anger/Out were 0.665 and – 0.045, respectively. Similarly, eight items with uniformly high loadings for both sexes on the

Anger/Out factor and negligible loadings on Anger/In were selected for the AX/Out scale; the median loading of these items was 0.59 on Anger/Out, and – 0.01 on Anger/In.

Jacobs et al. [19] examined the test-retest reliability of the AX Scale over a two-week interval and found stability coefficients that ranged from 0.64 to 0.86. Johnson [18] and Pollans [20] found, essentially, zero correlations between the AX/In and AX/Out scales for both males and females in large samples of high school and college students; similar findings have also been reported for other populations [3, 21]. These findings provide strong evidence that the AX/In and AX/Out subscales are factorially orthogonal, empirically independent, and internally consistent. Clearly, these scales assess two independent anger-expression dimensions that are relatively stable over time.

Measuring the Control of Anger

The original item pool for the AX Scale consisted of several items that were included to measure the middle range of an anger-in/anger-out continuum. Three of these items – control my temper; keep my cool; and calm down faster – had substantial loadings on both the Anger/In and Anger/Out factors, and were retained in the final set of 20 AX Scale items. In subsequent research with the AX Scale, these items tended to coalesce to form the nucleus of an anger control factor [20], which stimulated the development of the AX Anger Control (AX/Con) Scale.

The first step in constructing the AX/Con scale was to assemble a pool of items with appropriate content for assessing behaviour related to the control of anger. Using the three anger control items as a guide, dictionary and thesaurus definitions of 'control' and idioms pertaining specifically to the control of anger were considered in constructing additional anger control items. The pool of AX/Con items was administered to a large sample of university students, along with the 20 AX Scale items. In separate factor analyses of the AX/Con items for males and females, a strong anger control factor and several very small factors were found for both sexes. The items with the strongest loadings on the AX/Con factor for both males and females were added to the three original AX/Con items to form an eight-item AX/Con scale.

In order to evaluate the independence of the Anger/Con factor and to determine its relation to the Anger/In and Anger/Out factors, the items comprising the eight-item AX/Con, AX/Out and AX/In scales were administered to a large sample of university students [2]. In factor analyses of responses to the 24 AX items, an anger control factor was the strongest to emerge for both males and females; all eight AX/Con items had dominant salient loadings on this factor. Well-defined Anger/In and Anger/Out factors were also found; all eight AX/In and AX/Out items had dominant salient loadings on the appropriate factor. For both sexes, the AX/Con scale correlated negatively with AX/Out ($r = -0.59$ for males, – 0.58 for females). Correlations between the AX/In and AX/Out scale were essentially zero for both sexes. The independence of the AX/In and AX/Out subscales and moderately high negative correlations of AX/Out with AX/Con have been consistently demonstrated [8, 20].

Evidence of the concurrent (convergent) and discriminant validity of the AX Scales is reflected in the correlations of these scales with other anger and personality measures [3]. Moderately high correlations of AX/Out scores with T-Anger/T scores, indicate that persons with an angry temperament are more likely to express their anger outwardly. Small but highly significant positive correlations of both AX/In and AX/Out scores with the STPI T-Anxiety scale suggested that individuals who more often suppress or express anger are likely to experience anxiety more frequently than individuals with low anger expression scores. The correlations of all three anger expression measures with the STPI T-Curiosity scale were essentially zero, providing evidence of discriminant validity.

A major reason for constructing the AX Scale was to investigate how the various components of anger contributed to the etiology of hypertension and coronary heart disease. Harburg et al. [11, 12] and Gentry et al. [14] have reported that individuals who tend to suppress anger have higher systolic and diastolic blood pressure. Williams et al. [22] found that patients with high scores on the MMPI Ho scale were more likely to develop coronary artery disease. Dembroski et al. [23] found that high ratings of potential for hostility and anger-in were positively associated with the severity of coronary atherosclerosis.

In an investigation of the relationship between anger expression and blood pressure (BP), Johnson [18] administered the AX Scale to 1,114 high school students. Measures of systolic (SBP) and diastolic (DBP) blood pressure were obtained during the same class period in which these students responded to the psychological tests. The correlations of AX/In scores with SBP and DBP were positive, curvilinear, and highly significant for both sexes. The overall pattern of correlations indicated that higher blood pressure was associated with holding anger in, and that students with very high AX/In scores had much higher BP.

Johnson [18] also examined the influence of a number of variables found to be related to BP in previous research, and found that height, weight, dietary factors (salt intake), racial differences, and family history of hypertension correlated significantly with BP. After partialing out the influence of these variables, AX/In scores were still positively and significantly associated with elevated SBP and DBP. In separate multiple regression analyses for males and females, AX/In scores were first to enter step-wise multiple discriminant equations for both sexes, and were found to be better predictors of blood pressure than any other measure.

State-Trait Anger Expression Inventory

The STAS and the AX Scale were combined to form the State-Trait Anger Expression Inventory (STAXI), which provides relatively brief, objectively-scored measures of the experience, expression and control of anger [3]. The original 44-item STAXI included 10-item S-Anger and T-Anger scales, and eight-item scales for measuring AX/Out, AX/In and AX/Con. The T-Anger scale also included factorially derived four-item subscales that assessed individual differences in T-Anger Temperament and Reaction.

Fuqua et al. [24] administered the 44-item STAXI to a large sample of college students and factor-analysed their responses to the individual items. Based on the results of their analyses, these investigators concluded that "... seven factors provided the best fit of the data to the instrument and its theoretical foundations". Almost all of the items that defined each STAXI scale and subscale had salient loadings on the appropriate factor and negligible loadings on the other factors. These findings provided strong confirmation of the factor structure of the STAXI, and evidence that the STAXI scales and subscales measured meaningful, relatively independent components of the experience, expression and control of anger.

The first six factors identified by Fuqua et al. [24] corresponded almost exactly to the five primary STAXI scales, except that items from the STAXI T-Anger scale loaded on separate T-

Anger Temperament and Reaction factors. The seventh factor identified by Fuqua et al. [24] was defined by salient secondary loadings for three of the 10 STAXI S-Anger items (Feel like... breaking things, ...banging on the table, ...hitting someone). While these items had higher loadings on Factor 1, which was defined by dominant salient loadings for all 10 S-Anger items, Fuqua et al.'s findings suggested that there might be a second S-Anger factor comprised of items with content that reflected a strong disposition to express angry feelings in aggressive behaviour. van der Ploeg [25] administered a Dutch adaptation of the 20-item STAS to male military draftees in the Netherlands. In a separate factor analysis of the 10 S-Anger items, he also found two S-Anger factors that were similar to those reported by Fuqua et al. [24].

Additional factor analyses of the 44-item STAXI provided further evidence of two distinctive, highly correlated S-Anger factors [26]. The two S-Anger factors that emerged in these analyses were labelled *Feeling Angry*, e.g. "I feel angry", and *Feel Like Expressing Anger*, e.g. "I feel like hitting someone". Further research with an expanded version of the STAXI [4] identified three S-Anger factors, the Feeling Angry factor identified in previous research and two Feel Like Expressing Anger factors that involved verbal expression, e.g. "feel like screaming", and physical expression, e.g. "feel like hitting someone". The revised and expanded 57-item STAXI-2 includes three S-Anger factors that are each assessed with five-item subscales.

The revised STAXI-2 also contains two anger control scales for measuring the control of anger-out by inhibiting the expression of anger ("keeping the lid on"), and the control of anger-in ("calming down", "cooling off") by reducing the intensity of suppressed anger. The components of anger assessed by the six STAXI scales and five subscales, as well as the number of items and the range of scores for each scale and subscale are given in Table 1, along with a brief description of what is measured by each scale.

Research with the STAXI on Anger and Health

The STAXI has proved useful for assessing the experience, expression and control of anger in normal persons and clinical patients [27-30], as well as for evaluating the effects of the components of anger on a variety of medical disorders, including hypertension, coronary heart disease and cancer [4]. Comparing the STAXI test scores with appropriate scale norms is an important first step in test interpretation. Norms for the STAXI scales are reported in the Test Manual for male and female high school and college students and working adults [3, 4]. In addition, there are norms for the following special interest groups – general medical and surgical patients, prison inmates and military recruits.

The STAS, AX Scales and the STAXI have been used extensively in research on the relationship between anger and health [31-37]. Suppressed anger has been consistently identified as an important factor in elevated BP and hypertension [38-44]. High AX/In scores, especially when associated with low AX/Out scores and high levels of anxiety, have been found to be associated with elevated blood pressure [18, 45] and hypertension [46]. Very high scores on both the AX/In and AX/Out scales may place an individual at risk for coronary artery disease and heart attacks, especially for persons who are high in anger control.

The effects of anger expression on cardiovascular disease, as measured by the STAXI AX/Out scale, were investigated for a very large sample of male health professionals (N = 23,522), aged 50 to 85 years with no previous history of coronary heart disease (CHD) [47]. The

Table 1. Brief description of the STAXI-2 scales and subscale

STAXI-2 Scale/Subscale	No. of items	Scale/ range	Description of scale/subscale
State Anger *(S-Ang)*	15	15-60	Measures the intensity of angry feelings at a particular time, and the extent to which a person feels like expressing anger verbally or physically
Feeling Angry *(S-Ang/F)*	5	5-20	Measures the intensity of the angry feelings the person is currently experiencing
Feel Like Expressing Anger Verbally *(S-Ang/V)*	5	5-20	Measures the intensity of current feelings related to the verbal expression of anger
Feel Like Expressing Anger Physically *(S-Ang/P)*	5	5-20	Measures the intensity of current feelings related to the physical expression of anger
Trait Anger *(T-Ang)*	10	10-40	Measures individual differences in anger as a personality trait in terms of how often angry feelings are experienced over time
Angry Temperament *(T-Ang/T)*	4	4-16	Measures the disposition to experience anger without specific provocation
Angry Reaction *(T-Ang/R)*	4	4-16	Measures the frequency that angry feelings are experienced in situations that involve negative evaluations, e.g. being attacked, or treated badly
Anger Expression-Out *(AX-O)*	8	8-32	Measures how often angry feelings are expressed in aggressive behaviour directed toward other persons or objects in the environment
Anger Expression-In *(AX-I)*	8	8-32	Measures how often angry feelings are experienced and suppressed, but not expressed
Anger Control-Out *(AC-O)*	8	8-32	Measures how often a person endeavours to prevent and control the expression of angry feelings by "keeping the lid on"
Anger Control-In *(AC-I)*	8	8-32	Measures how often a person attempts to reduce and control angry feelings by calming down or cooling off

participants in this study responded to a mail questionnaire and were followed for two years (1996-98). Men with higher AX/Out scores had a reduced risk for myocardial infarction, as compared with those with lower anger expression scores. Anger expression was also inversely associated with risk of stroke. It would be important to determine if the men with low AX/Out scores who developed CHD were also very high in anger control.

The STAXI scales have been used extensively to investigate the role of anger in Type-A behaviour [48-55]. McMillan [56] used the STAXI scales to assess the anger experienced by patients undergoing treatment for Hodgkins disease and lung cancer. Kinder et al. [57, 58] used the STAXI scales in a series of studies of psychological factors that contributed to chronic pain. Stoner [59] investigated the effects of marijuana use on the experience and expression of anger.

The STAXI scales have also been used in a number of studies to evaluate the effects of anger on alcohol and drug abuse. Giancola [60] found that higher trait anger was associated with alcohol-related aggression in 204 healthy social drinkers (111 men, 93 women) between 21 and 35 years of age, particularly for men. Williamson [61] evaluated the anger of male and female alcoholics admitted to a detoxification centre. Men had significantly higher scores on the STAXI, State Anger, Anger-In and AX scales, and significantly lower scores on Anger Control. Females had significantly higher scores only on the State Anger scale. In a study of cannabis, cocaine, and opiate abusers, only the cocaine abusers had higher scores on several of the STAXI scales [62].

Conclusion

Conceptual ambiguity and confusion in theoretical interpretations of anger, hostility and aggression were briefly reviewed. Recent advances in the conceptualisation of anger, which have stimulated the development of improved instruments for the measurement of the experience, expression and control of anger were also examined. The procedures employed in developing and validating new psychometric instruments for measuring the experience, expression, and control of anger were described in detail. Research findings utilising the STAS, AX Scales and the STAXI to assess the relationship of anger with hypertension, CHD, and other medical disorders were briefly examined.

In a comprehensive evaluation and critique of the STAXI, James Moses [28] concluded that the STAXI is a "specific, sensitive, psychometric instrument", and that "there is a great potential for its use to significantly further our understanding of important stress-based and stress-influenced syndromes, and to help in identifying effective means by which such disorders may be reversed and prevented" [28]. The utilisation of the STAXI in research in a number of countries with different languages will greatly help to clarify and validate the concepts on which this inventory was based, and will identify cultural similarities and differences in the effects of anger on health, behaviour and medical problems.

References

1. Biaggio, M.K., Supplee, K. and Curtis, N., 1981, "Reliability and Validity of Four Anger Scales", *Journal of Personality Assessment*, 45, pp. 639-648.
2. Spielberger, C.D., Krasner, S.S. and Solomon, E.P., 1988, "The Experience, Expression and Control of Anger", In *Health Psychology: Individual Differences and Stress*, M.P. Janisse (Ed.), Springer Verlag, New York, pp. 89-108.
3. Spielberger, C.D., 1988, *Manual for the State-Trait Anger Expression Inventory (STAXI)*, Psychological Assessment Resources, Inc., Odessa, Florida.
4. Spielberger, C.D., 1999, *Professional Manual for the State-Trait Anger Expression Inventory-2 (STAXI-2)*, Psychological Assessment Resources, Inc., Odessa, Florida.
5. Tavris, C., 1982, *Anger: The Misunderstood Emotion*, Touchstone, New York.
6. DiGiuseppe, R. and Tafrate, R.C., 2007, *Understanding Anger Disorders*, Oxford University Press, New York.
7. Spielberger, C.D., Jacobs, G., Russell, S. and Crane, R., 1983, "Assessment of Anger: The State-Trait Anger Scale", In *Advances in Personality Assessment*, Vol. 2, J.N. Butcher and C.D. Spielberger (Eds.), Lawrence Erlbaum Associates, Inc., Hillsdale, New Jersey, pp. 159-187.

8. Spielberger, C.D., Johnson, E.H., Russell, S.F., Crane, R.J., Jacobs, G.A. and Worden, T.J., 1985, "The Experience and Expression of Anger: Construction and Validation of an Anger Expression Scale", In *Anger and Hostility in Cardiovascular and Behavioral Disorders*, M.A. Chesney and R.H. Rosenman (Eds.), Hemisphere/McGraw-Hill, New York, pp. 5-30.
9. Funkenstein, D.H., King, S.H. and Drolette, M.E., 1954, "The Direction of Anger During a Laboratory Stress-inducing Situation", *Psychosomatic Medicine*, 16, pp. 404-413.
10. Averill, J.R., 1982, *Anger and Aggression: An Essay on Emotion*, Spring-Verlag, New York.
11. Harburg, E., Blakelock, E.H. and Roeper, P.J., 1979, "Resentful and Reflective Coping with Arbitrary Authority and Blood Pressure: Detroit", *Psychosomatic Medicine*, 3, pp. 189-202.
12. Harburg, E., Erfurt, J.C., Hauenstein, L.S., Chape, C., Schull, W.J. and Schork, M.A., 1973, "Socio-ecological Stress, Suppressed Hostility, Skin Color and Black-White Male Blood Pressure: Detroit", *Psychosomatic Medicine*, 35, pp. 276-296.
13. Gentry, W.D., 1972, "Biracial Aggression: I. Effect of Verbal Attack and Sex of Victim", *The Journal of Social Psychology*, 88, pp. 75-82.
14. Gentry, W.D., Chesney, A.P., Gary, H.G., Hall, R.P. and Harburg, E., 1982, "Habitual Anger-coping Styles: I. Effect on Mean Blood Pressure and Risk for Essential Hypertension", *Psychosomatic Medicine*, 44, pp. 195-202.
15. Rosenzweig, S., 1976, "Aggressive Behavior and the Rosenzweig Picture Frustration Study", *Journal of Clinical Psychology*, 32, pp. 885-891.
16. Rosenzweig, S., 1978, *The Rosenzweig Picture Frustration (P-F) Study Basic Manual and Adult Form Supplement*, Rana, St. Louis.
17. Spielberger, C.D., 1983, *Manual for the State-Trait Anxiety Inventory: STAI(Form Y)*, Consulting Psychologists Press, Palo Alto.
18. Johnson, E.H., 1984, "Anger and Anxiety as Determinants of Elevated Blood Pressure in Adolescents", *Ph.D. Dissertation* (Unpublished), University of South Florida, Tampa, USA.
19. Jacobs, G.A., Latham, L.E. and Brown, M.S., 1988, "Test-retest Reliability of the State-Trait Personality Inventory and the Anger Expression Scale", *Anxiety Research*, 1, pp. 263-265.
20. Pollans, C.H., 1983, "The Psychometric Properties and Factor Structure of the Anger Expression (AX) Scale", *Master's Thesis* (Unpublished), University of South Florida, Tampa, USA.
21. Knight, R.G., Chisholm, B.J., Paulin, J.M. and Waal-Manning, H.J., 1988, "The Spielberger Anger Expression Scale: Some Psychometric Data", *Journal of Clinical Psychology*, 27, pp. 279-281.
22. Williams, R.B., Haney, T.L., Lee, K.L., Kong, Y., Blumenthal, J. and Whalen, R.E., 1980, "Type A Behavior, Hostility and Coronary Atherosclerosis", *Psychosomatic Medicine*, 42, pp. 539-549.
23. Dembroski, T.M., MacDougall, J.M., Williams, R.B., Haney, T.L. and Blumenthal, J.A., 1985, "Components of Type A, Hostility, and Anger-in: Relationship to Angiographic Findings", *Psychosomatic Medicine*, 47, pp. 219-233.
24. Fuqua, D.R., Leonard, E., Masters, M.A., Smith, R.J., Campbell, J.L. and Fischer, P.C., 1991, "A Structural Analysis of the State-Trait Anger Expression Inventory (STAXI)", *Educational and Psychological Measurement*, 51, pp. 439-446.
25. van der Ploeg, H.M., 1988, "The Factor Structure of the State-Trait Anger Scale", *Psychological Reports*, 63, p. 978.
26. Forgays, D.G., Forgays, D.K. and Spielberger, C.D., 1997, "Factor Structure of the State-Trait Anger Expression Inventory", *Journal of Personality Assessment*, 69, pp. 497-507.
27. Deffenbacher, J.L., 1992, "Trait Anger: Theory, Findings and Implications", In *Advances in Personality Assessment*, Vol. 9. C.D. Spielberger and J.N. Butcher (Eds.), Lawrence Erlbaum Associates, Inc., Hillsdale, New Jersey, pp. 177-201.
28. Moses, J.A., 1992, "State-Trait Anger Expression Inventory", In *Test Critiques*, D.J. Keyser and R.C. Sweetland (Eds.), Vol. IX, Research Edition, PRO-ED, Inc., Austin, Texas, pp. 510-525.

29. Spielberger, C.D., Reheiser, E.C. and Sydeman, S.J., 1995, "Measuring the Experience, Expression, and Control of Anger", In *Anger Disorders: Definitions, Diagnosis and Treatment*, H. Kassinove (Ed.), Taylor & Francis, Washington, D.C., pp. 49-76.
30. Spielberger, C.D., Ritterband, L.M., Sydeman, S.J., Reheiser, E.C. and Unger, K.K., 1995, "Assessment of Emotional States and Personality Traits: Measuring Psychological Vital Signs", In *Clinical Personality Assessment: Practical Approaches*, J.N. Butcher (Ed.), Oxford University Press, New York, pp. 42-58.
31. Brooks, M.L., Walfish, S., Stenmark, D.E. and Canger, J.M., 1981, "Personality Variables in Alcohol Abuse in College Students", *Journal of Drug Education*, 11, pp. 185-189.
32. Cavanaugh, D.J., Kanonchoff, A.D. and Bartels, R.L., 1987, "Menstrual Irregularities in Athletic Women May be Predictable Base on Pre-training Menses", Department of Work Psychology, Ohio State University, Columbus (Unpublished).
33. Johnson, E.H. and Broman, C.L., 1987, "The Relationship of Anger Expression to Health Problems Among Black Americans in a National Survey", *Journal of Behavioral Medicine*, 10, pp. 103-169.
34. Johnson-Saylor, M.T., 1984, "Relationships Among Anger Expression, Hostility, Hardiness, Social Support, and Health Risk", *Ph.D. Dissertation* (Unpublished), University of Michigan, Ann Arbor.
35. Schlosser, M.B., 1986, "Anger, Crying and Health Among Females", *Paper Presented at the 94th Annual Convention of the American Psychological Association*, Washington, D.C.
36. Vitaliano, P.P., 1984, "Identification and Intervention with Students at High Risk for Distress in Medical School", *Ph.D. Dissertation* (Unpublished), University of Washington, Seattle, USA.
37. Vitaliano, P.P., Maiuro, R.D., Russo, J., Mitchell, E.S., Carr, J.E. and van Citters, R.L., 1986, "A Biopsychosocial Model to Explain Personal Sources of Medical Student Distress", *Proceedings of the 26th Annual Conference on Research in Medical Education*, 26, pp. 228-234.
38. Deshields, T.L., 1986, "Anger and Assertiveness in Essential Hypertension", University Microfilms No. 85-24, 330, *Dissertations Abstracts International*, 46, p. 3212B.
39. Gorkin, L., Appel, M., Holroyd, K.A., Saab, P.G. and Stauder, L., 1986, "Anger Management Style and Family History Status as Risk Factors for Essential Hypertension", Ohio University, Athens (Unpublished).
40. Hartfield, M.T., 1985, "Appraisals of Anger Situations and Subsequent Coping Response in Hypertensive and Normotensive Adults: A Comparison", *Ph.D. Dissertation*, University of California, *Dissertation Abstracts International*, 46, p. 4452B.
41. Johnson, E., Spielberger, C., Worden, T. and Jacobs, G., 1987, "Emotional and Familial Determinants of Elevated Blood Pressure in Black and White Adolescent Males", *Journal of Psychosomatic Research*, 31, pp. 287-300.
42. Kearns, W.D., 1985, "A Laboratory Study of the Relationship of Mode of Anger Expression to Blood Pressure", *Master's Thesis* (Unpublished), University of South Florida, Tampa, USA.
43. Schneider, R.H., Egan, B. and Johnson, E.H., 1986, "Anger and Anxiety in Borderline Hypertension", *Psychosomatic Medicine*, 48, pp. 242-248.
44. van der Ploeg, H.M., van Buuren, E.T. and van Brummelen, P., 1988, "The Role of Anger in Hypertension", *Psychotherapy and Psychosomatics*, 43, pp. 186-193.
45. Bongard, S. and al'Absi, M., 2005, "Domain-specific Anger Expression and Blood Pressure in an Occupational Setting", *Journal of Psychosomatic Research*, 58(1), pp. 43-49.
46. Crane, R.S., 1981, "The Role of Anger, Hostility and Aggression in Essential Hypertension", *Ph.D. Dissertation*, University of South Florida, Tampa, USA, *Dissertation Abstracts International*, 42, p. 2982B.
47. Eng, P.M., Fitzmaurice, G., Kubzansky, L.D., Rimm, E.B. and Kawachi, I., 2003, "Anger Expression and Risk of Stroke and Coronary Heart Disease Among Male Health Professionals", *Psychosomatic Medicine*, 65(1), pp. 100-110.

48. Booth-Kewley, S. and Friedman, H.S., 1987, "Psychological Predictors of Heart Disease: A Quantitative Review", *Psychological Bulletin*, 101, pp. 343-362.
49. Croyle, R.T., Jemmott, J.B. III and Carpenter, B.D., 1988, "Relations Between Four Individual Difference Measures Associated with Cardiovascular Dysfunction and Anger Coping Style", *Psychological Reports*, 63, pp. 779-786.
50. Goffaux, J., Wallston, B.S., Heim, C.R. and Shields, S.L., 1987, "Type A Behaviors, Hostility, Anger and Exercise Adherence", *Paper Presented at the 8th Annual Session of the Society of Behavioral Medicine*, Washington, D.C., March.
51. Herschberger, P., 1985, "Type A Behavior in Non-intensive and Intensive Care Nurses", *Master's Thesis* (Unpublished), University of South Florida, Tampa, USA.
52. Janisse, M.P., Edguer, N. and Dyck, D.G., 1986, "Type A Behavior, Anger Expression and Reactions to Anger Imagery", *Motivation and Emotion*, 10, pp. 371-385.
53. Krasner, S.S., 1986, "Anger, Anger Control and the Coronary Prone Behavior Pattern", *Master's Thesis* (Unpublished), University of South Florida, Tampa, USA.
54. Matthews, K.A., Glass, D.C., Rosenman, R.H. and Bortner, R.W., 1977, "Competitive Drive, Pattern A, and Coronary Heart Disease: A Further Analysis of Some Data from the Western Collaborative Group Study", *Journal of Chronic Diseases*, 30, pp. 489-498.
55. Spielberger, C.D. and London, P., 1982, "Rage Boomerangs: Lethal Type-A Anger", *American Health*, 1, pp. 52-56.
56. McMillan, S.C., 1984, "A Comparison of Levels of Anxiety and Anger Experienced by Two Groups of Cancer Patients During Therapy for Hodgkin's Disease and Small Cell Lung Cancer", *Master's Thesis* (Unpublished), University of South Florida, Tampa, USA.
57. Curtiss, G., Kinder, B., Kalichman, S. and Spana, R., 1988, "Affective Differences Among Subgroups of Chronic Pain Patients", *Anxiety Research: An International Journal*, 1, pp. 65-73.
58. Kinder, B., Curtiss, G. and Kalichman, S., 1986, "Anxiety and Anger as Predictors of MMPI Elevations in Chronic Pain Patients", *Journal of Personality Assessment*, 50, pp. 651-661.
59. Stoner, S.B., 1988, "Undergraduate Marijuana Use and Anger", *Journal of Psychology*, 122, pp. 343-347.
60. Giancola, P.R., 2002, "The Influence of Trait Anger on the Anger-Aggression Relation in Men and Women", *Alcoholism: Clinical and Experimental Research*, 26(9), pp. 1350-1358.
61. Williamson, J.D.M., 2001, "Anger and Anger Control Among Recovering Alcoholics", *Dissertation Abstracts International – Section B: The Sciences and Engineering*, 62(5-B), p. 2508.
62. Aharonovich, E., Hueco, T., Nguyen, M.S., Edward, V. and Nunes, E.V., 2001, "Anger and Depressive States Among Treatment-seeking Drug Abusers: Testing the Psychopharmacological Specificity Hypothesis", *The American Journal on Addictions*, 10, pp. 327-334.

The AHA-Syndrome and Cardiovascular Diseases
Editors: Swati Y. Bhave and Sunil Saini
Copyright © 2010 Anamaya Publishers, New Delhi, India

4. Displaced Aggression in Children and Adolescents

Thomas F. Denson
School of Psychology, University of New South Wales, Sydney, NSW 2052, Australia

Abstract: Nearly all research on displaced aggression has been conducted with adult participants. Thus, very little is known about displaced aggression in children and adolescents. This article reviews the limited empirical work available on the subject and proposes a theoretical framework for understanding displaced aggression in children. Finally, it concludes with suggestions for future research.

Keywords: Displaced aggression, Aggression, Children, Adolescents, Aggression model.

Introduction

Displaced aggression occurs when a person is provoked, is unwilling or unable to retaliate against the original provocateur and, subsequently, aggresses against an innocent target. The phenomenon is robust in adults [1]. However, very little is known about displaced aggression in children and adolescents. This article reviews the experimental research on displaced aggression in children and adolescents. Although far from being established as a robust phenomenon, there is some evidence that children and adolescents do engage in displaced aggression and also that five-year-old children demonstrate a sophisticated understanding of this phenomenon. The article also introduces a theoretical framework for understanding displaced aggression in this age range. The framework focusses on exposure to displaced aggression, the development of social information processing related to displaced aggression, and variables that may moderate reactions to provocation, as well as the occurrence and intensity of displaced aggression. Finally, some suggestions are given regarding future avenues for research with children and adolescents including bullying, mass school violence, culture, and the development of individual differences in displaced aggression.

Case Scenario of Displaced Aggression in Children

Nine-year-old Nick is chasing his dog around the house with his favourite toy water gun. Despite repeated admonitions from his father to stop running fast, Nick crashes into the coffee table and breaks an expensive flower vase. As punishment, his father takes away his toy and sends him to his room. On his way down the hallway to his room, Nick stops to push his little brother to the floor.

This anecdote illustrates the behavioural phenomena of displaced aggression, which occurs when a person is frustrated or provoked, is unwilling or unable to retaliate against the original provocateur and, subsequently, aggresses against a seemingly innocent target [2, 3]. In adults, the phenomenon is robust. A meta-analysis of 49 articles reporting on laboratory experiments revealed that the construct has a moderate effect size (d = + 0.54) [1]. Although interest in displaced aggression declined toward the end of the 1970s, recent research reflects rejuvenated awareness of the construct [4-8]. This phenomenon also occurs in animals including fish, rats and non-human primates, suggesting an evolutionary contribution [9-12].

Existing Research

Early work examined displaced aggression from the drive-reduction perspective espoused by Dollard et al. and was rooted in Freudian tradition [2]. This 'hydraulic' perspective emphasised the need to aggress following a frustration or provocation. It posits that if the aggressive drive is not directed toward the original source of displeasure, one might aggress against an innocent target as a means to satiate one's aggressive urges.

In an early investigation of 24 children (4 to 6 years old), Jegard and Walters [13] manipulated frustration by having the experimenter arbitrarily take away either a lot of candy (high frustration condition) or a little candy (low frustration condition) from the children. There was no control condition. Following the frustration manipulation, participants were placed in a room with both a stuffed dog and an inflated Bobo doll with a child's face. They were allowed to hit either or both of these objects. Displaced aggression was operationalised as hitting the stuffed dog only. The only significant result was that boys hit the Bobo doll more than girls, but boys and girls did not differ in frequency of hitting the dog. The lack of a no frustration control condition and the assumption that hitting the stuffed dog (but not the inflated doll) indicated displaced aggression precludes firm conclusions about the occurrence of displaced aggression in this experiment.

In a second early experiment, 108 middle-class children (4 to 6 years old) played a card game that served as the context for a frustration manipulation [14]. In the high and low frustration conditions, participants learned to associate losses with cards depicting a child and wins with a blank card. In the control condition, losses were associated with a blank card and wins were associated with a child figure. The children were then given the opportunity to shoot cards that depicted similar or dissimilar children to the child figures from the previous card game. When boys lost to the child in the card game, they shot similar targets more than dissimilar targets, suggesting that similarity of the target may be an important moderator of displaced aggression. In contrast, girls tended to shoot at dissimilar targets more than similar targets after losing.

Foss and Fouts [15] set out to examine the catharsis hypothesis in the context of displaced aggression in children. The catharsis hypothesis states that releasing angry feelings following provocation or frustration will improve one's mood [16]. In addition to an affective improvement, the catharsis hypothesis also posits that subsequent aggressive behaviour will be lessened. In this experiment, 44 middle-class children (8 to 11 years old) were either interrupted twice during a counting task (frustration condition) or not (no frustration condition). They were then either given the opportunity to 'take out' their aggressive urges by tearing up cardboard boxes (catharsis condition) or not (no catharsis condition). Finally, the children were asked to play a board game by themselves. The researchers assessed displaced aggression as the extent to which the children knocked over game pieces. Consistent with the catharsis hypothesis, those children who were frustrated and not allowed to engage in the cathartic box tearing demonstrated the most destructive behaviour during the board game task. No gender effects were reported.

The only experiment to date on displaced aggression with adolescents reported on 160 male and female Indian high school students (14 to 17 years old) who were frustrated by an experimental confederate during a cognitive task (frustration condition) or not (control condition) [17]. Participants were allowed to deliver electric shocks within the context of a teacher-learner task to either the provocateur (direct aggression) or to an innocent confederate (displaced aggression). Those participants who were frustrated delivered significantly more shocks to the provocateur and the innocent confederate than participants in the control condition. Moreover, they shocked the innocent confederate with intensity equal to the provocateur, suggesting a strong displaced aggression response. The study is notable for its large sample, inclusion of a control condition, and use of a physical measure of displaced aggression. No gender effects were reported.

Additional experimental work moved away from the Dollard et al. model [2] and emphasised social-cognitive perspectives on displaced aggression in children. Two experiments within this framework assessed the children's understanding of the causes of displaced aggression, but did not assess actual behavioural displaced aggression [18, 19]. Social-cognitive approaches could have important implications for the development of individual differences in displaced aggression. In the first of these experiments, 3 to 5 years old children viewed videotapes of older children engaging in either moderate or extreme acts of displaced aggression [19]. Although the 3-year-olds demonstrated some fundamental understanding of the concept, only the 5-year-olds demonstrated a complex understanding of displaced aggression. More specifically, the 5-year-old children were able to identify anger as the cause of the behaviour of the child in the video and could explain that the initial provocation ultimately led to the act of displaced aggression. Interestingly, the older children also identified that the child in the video may ruminate about the provocation.

The second of these studies showed the same videotaped episodes of displaced aggression [19] to 5-, 7-, and 9-year-old children [18]. The purpose of the study was to determine which broader social cognitive abilities co-vary with children's ability to understand displaced aggression. Understanding of displaced aggression in the 5-year-olds was related to an ability to describe others in psychological terms rather than physical terms. In 7- and 9-year-old children, their understanding was associated with the ability to infer mental states in others. The authors suggested that "...children's growing awareness of psychological characteristics such as, motives, intentions, frustration and aggressive tendencies surely contribute to the concept of displaced aggression". It should also be noted that children's understanding of displaced aggression may be dependent on the use of short, easily digestible videos, as other studies that have investigated this same area using verbal narratives failed to find an understanding of displaced aggression in children until they reached grade school [20].

Suggestions

Based on the present review of the existing literature on displaced aggression in children and adolescents, few firm answers are available. The following two important questions readily surface:

(i) Do children and adolescents engage in displaced aggression when provoked or frustrated? Only two experiments in children and one experiment with adolescents support this notion

[14, 15, 17]. Thus, although this evidence suggests that children as young as 4-years-old engage in acts of displaced aggression, the basic phenomenon is not well-established.

(ii) Do children understand the causes of displaced aggression? It appears that even very young children can demonstrate an understanding of the phenomena when it is presented in easily digestible video format [18, 19]. As children become older, their understanding of the causes of displaced aggression becomes quite complex, even to the extent of inferring mental states and moods in others. Not surprisingly, this more complex understanding is linked to the development of advanced social cognitive abilities in children [18].

Because of the expense, practical difficulty and ethical concerns of conducting aggression research in children, perhaps, it is not surprising that little research exists in this area. Nonetheless, the following are three specific issues that need to be addressed in future research:

(i) Complete designs are necessary to infer displaced aggression. Thus, a no provocation control condition should be included in studies of displaced aggression.

(ii) Attempts should be made to operationalise displaced aggression as consistent with the commonly adopted definition of aggression as "intent to cause harm" [21]. For instance, in some of the studies, children aggressed against inanimate objects. Although surely destructive and a valid dependent measure in its own right, it is doubtful if this would qualify as displaced aggression according to modern definitions, i.e. inanimate objects cannot feel and as such cannot be 'harmed'. Perhaps displaced aggression directed against animate objects may be more informative about real-world displaced aggression than destructive acts against inanimate objects.

(iii) Future work on displaced aggression should incorporate modern models of aggressive behaviour such as, Huesmann's developmental model [22], or the more recent General Aggression Model [21].

Much progress has been made in understanding aggression in the past few years. Extending these advances in aggression research to the domain of displaced aggression in youth may greatly increase our understanding of this important phenomenon.

A Theoretical Framework

Figure 1 presents a theoretical framework for understanding the development and occurrence of displaced aggression in children and adolescents. This framework relies heavily on prior models of aggression and represents an extension of principles found in these models into the specific domain of displaced aggression in young people [21-25]. It is intended as a starting point for future empirical work.

A central assumption of the model is that engaging in acts of displaced aggression begins with exposure to such behaviour while young. Such exposure biases social information processing, which, in turn, affects how the child reacts to provocations. This reaction is moderated by both person (e.g., genes, personality) and situational (e.g., social roles, norms) variables. Negative reactions to the provocation then increase the likelihood that displaced aggression will occur. Certain situational variables moderate this effect such that they influence the degree of displaced aggression and likelihood of its occurrence.

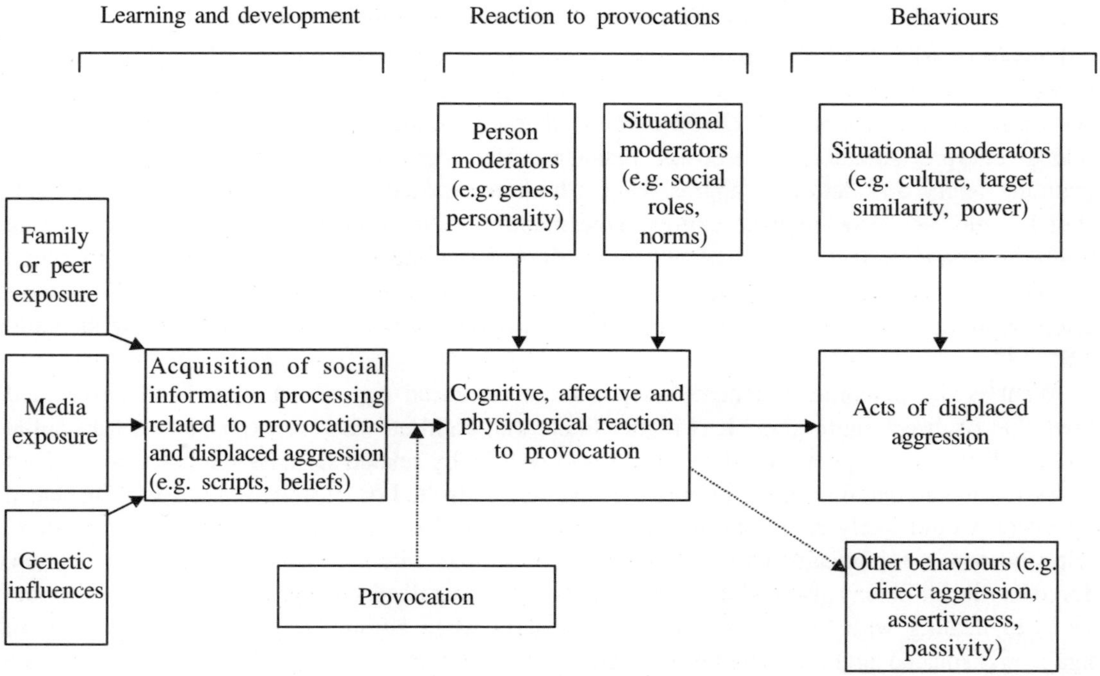

Fig. 1. A theoretical framework for understanding displaced aggression in children and adolescents.

Learning and Development

It is well-known that aggressive children come from aggressive homes [26]. Thus, children's first exposure to displaced aggression is likely to occur within the home. For instance, a child may observe that when a parent returns home complaining about a frustrating day at work, the parent may behave aggressively toward others in the household – including the child. This notion has recently been empirically validated. The degree of abuse that workers received from their supervisors was associated with increased displaced aggression in the workers' homes, as reported by family members [6]. Over time, the child may learn to pair the angered parent with the acts of displaced aggression. The ultimate effect of this pairing is that, eventually, the child 'learns' that harming undeserving others may be an appropriate and effective method of behaving when one is confronted with a provocation. Such a social learning perspective [23] may help explain why adults who were abused as children are at increased risk of abusing their own children relative to those who were not abused as children [27, 28].

Another source of exposure to acts of displaced aggression may be violent media, which has been meta-analytically linked with the development of aggressive behaviour in children [29, 30]. While acts of displaced aggression are presumably less common than acts of direct aggression in the media, violent media may still contain a significant amount of displaced aggression. Finally, genetic influences may predispose children to acquire aggressive social information processing. Indeed, in studies that have been able to statistically separate the two types of influences, both genes and socialisation experiences are powerful determinants of aggressive behaviour in children [31].

Acquisition of Social Information Processing Related to Displaced Aggression

Building on earlier social learning perspectives, cognitive models of individual differences in aggressive development postulate that repeated exposure to aggression results in changes in social information processing [22, 32]. These changes in social information processing lead a child to interpret situations in a hostile manner, which then increases the likelihood of his/her becoming angry and behaving aggressively. Children exposed to aggression adopt aggression-related cognitive knowledge structures. Huesmann [22] mentioned two types of knowledge structures – *scripts* and *normative beliefs*. Scripts determine how one should react to social interactions, what cues one should pay attention to and how one should behave. Normative beliefs about aggression describe how appropriate this type of behaviour is perceived by the child [22].

What is the outcome of repeated exposure to displaced aggression, specifically, over and above that of direct aggression? It is highly likely that children who are exposed to a substantial amount of displaced aggression develop scripts specifically related to it. While a script of direct aggression would entail harming the provocateur when insulted or frustrated, a script of displaced aggression would likely entail harming innocent others following a provocation. Over time these scripts become automatically activated in memory when the child is confronted with a provocation. Moreover, the child may also endorse normative beliefs about displaced aggression as an appropriate means of dealing with life's provocations, especially when admired role models, e.g. a parent engage in displaced aggression themselves. Given that children as young as 5-year-old demonstrate a sophisticated understanding of displaced aggression, even exposure at this early age may lead to the development of altered social information processing [18, 19].

Reaction to Provocations

The General Aggression Model [21] posits three mediating internal states that are involved in exacerbating responses to provocations – *cognition* (e.g. the accessibility of aggressive constructs, scripts); *affect* (e.g. anger); and *physiological arousal* (e.g. cardiovascular reactivity). Although not specific to displaced aggression *per se*, it is likely that children and adolescents, who have developed hostile social information processing, will perceive provocations as highly aversive and, therefore, react with increased cognitive, affective and physiological reactivity relative to those with less hostile cognitive biases. For instance, aggressive boys display better recognition memory for aggressive stimuli than non-aggressive stimuli [33], and respond with more anger and retaliation to ambiguous provocations [34].

Additional person moderators may explain how children and adolescents react to provocations. In adults, individual differences in displaced aggression have been linked to tendencies to ruminate about provocations, as well as behavioural inhibition [35]. Rumination is important because it maintains angry affect and the cognitive accessibility of aggressive constructs [36]. Moreover, in adults, angry rumination delays cardiovascular recovery to provocations [37]. Behavioural inhibition is important because it implies that individuals high in this trait do not respond immediately and directly to life's provocations. Rather, they may feel a complex emotional response consisting of a conflict between approach motivation (anger) and avoidance motivation (anxiety). For example, one item on the Behavioural Inhibition Scale [38] – "I feel pretty worried or upset when I think or know somebody is angry at me" – illustrates this point. In addition to personality variables, gender, genes and other biological differences between individuals may increase the negativity of the reaction to the provocation. Examples include genetic deficiencies in monoamine oxidase A (MAOA) gene, which has been linked to aggression [39, 40], and hormone levels such as testosterone [41].

Situational variables are also capable of influencing reactions to provocations. These may include social roles and context-dependent norms, among others. If the source of a provocation or frustration is seen as legitimate due to the social role they occupy, it is likely that the child will not respond as intensely to the provocation as to an illegitimate source of provocation. For example, if a child is told by his/her parent or teacher to cease a certain behaviour, then he/she is likely to exhibit less reactivity than if issued the same ultimatum by a bossy peer. In one experiment, adults directed less displaced aggression toward high status targets than low status targets, presumably due to lower levels of anger [42]. Group norms may also play a role in moderating responses to provocations, to an extent that some families or groups of children and adolescents condone displays of anger and aggression in response to provocations. Extreme reactions may be more likely among these group members.

Acts of Displaced Aggression

Once a sufficient degree of aggressive cognition, angry affect and/or physiological arousal is elicited by a provocation, various behaviours may follow suit. Displaced aggression is just one such behaviour. Others include, but are not limited to, direct aggression toward the provocateur, dealing assertively, yet non-aggressively with the provocateur, or behaving passively. Several situational factors make displaced aggression more or less likely:

(i) If the original source of provocation or frustration is no longer available, direct aggression is obviously not an option for the child.

(ii) If a second minor annoyance or 'trigger' to aggress follows the initial provocation, children may respond with an excessive amount of aggression that exceeds "tit-for-tat" matching rules [43, 44]. This hypothesis is based on experimental evidence in adults within the triggered displaced aggression paradigm [8].

(iii) If the degree of similarity between the original provocateur and the target of aggression is high, this may also increase displaced aggression. Moore [14] reported that, at least for boys, target similarity increased displaced aggression toward an inanimate object. This is consistent with meta-analytic findings, which suggest that the degree of similarity between the provocateur and target increases displaced aggression in adults [1]. Further work with children and adolescents could explore this issue.

(iv) Another situational variable that may moderate the degree of displaced aggression is the power of the target. If the only available target of displaced aggression is high in status or power, e.g. a teacher or parent, displaced aggression is likely to be inhibited under these circumstances. As stated earlier, adults directed less displaced aggression toward high status targets than low status targets [42], but this variable has yet to be investigated in children and adolescents.

New Directions

Now, I consider a broader conceptualisation of displaced aggression among children and adolescents. Specifically, recent theoretical advances in displaced aggression may lead to a greater understanding of some forms of violent and aggressive behaviour that affect young people. For instance, person and situational determinants of displaced aggression may explain important social problems such as bullying and school shootings. These issues are discussed along with the role of culture and the development of individual differences in displaced aggression.

Bullying

Although displaced aggression may not explain all instances of bullying, it is possible that this type of aggression is frequently an instantiation of displaced aggression. As mentioned earlier, children who are exposed to displaced aggression in the home are likely to develop scripts and normative beliefs related to this behaviour [22]. Thus, when angered, bullies may likely aggress against innocent schoolmates. Interpreting some instances of bullying as displaced aggression may be advantageous from a research perspective. As an instantiation of displaced aggression, bullying is susceptible to the same person and situation moderators that affect other types of displaced aggression. Eventually, examining bullying from a displaced aggression perspective may lead to the development of interventions that reduce bullying. Nonetheless, this may prove difficult as habitual bullies are likely to be locked into a cycle of displaced aggression whereby they receive punishment from authority figures because they are aggressive, which further increases the likelihood of engaging in subsequent displaced aggression toward safer targets such as fellow school children.

Mass School Violence

Although mass violence in schools is rare, it has nonetheless received much media and scientific attention in recent years. School violence is an interesting case because it is often a mix of direct aggression (attacking those perceived to be the source of torment), displaced aggression (attacking innocents), and sometimes suicide (attacking the self). Many of these instances involve some type of social rejection. Although in real world settings, it is difficult to determine whether social rejection is a consequence of aggression or a cause, we know from laboratory experiments that social rejection is a powerful elicitor of displaced aggression in adults [45]. In a review of 15 school shootings that occurred from 1995 to 2001, researchers concluded that social rejection was present in all but two of the cases [46]. Although some of these cases represented direct aggression, mass killings may often represent specific instances of displaced aggression because innocents are often harmed. Gaertner and Iuzzini [47] have suggested that the perceived entitativity of groups of students may moderate the degree of violence, suggesting that groups that are perceived as cohesive units may elicit more displaced aggression. Among adults, perceived entitativity is associated with the extent to which all group members are perceived as being responsible for the negative actions of a single member [35].

Culture

With the exception of one experiment [17], all of the work on displaced aggression in children and adolescents has been conducted with middle-class American children. Based on one experiment conducted with adults from the United Kingdom and Hong Kong, there is good reason to expect that culture may be an important moderator of displaced aggression. Redford [48] found that participants from Hong Kong were more likely to report displaced aggression action tendencies

– operationalised as wanting to harm inanimate objects – than participants from the UK. Conversely, participants from the UK were more likely to report more direct aggression action tendencies than participants from Hong Kong. The author speculated that collectivistic cultures might emphasise more displaced aggression in the purpose of maintaining group harmony, whereas individualistic cultures emphasise direct confrontation. Although it remains to be seen whether these findings generalise to displaced aggression against humans, culture may prove a powerful moderating force in determining the relative degree of displaced versus displaced aggression that is displayed.

Development of Individual Differences

We know that adults vary in the extent to which they tend to harm innocent others when in a bad mood [35]. Denson et al. have named this trait displaced aggression and it is related to, yet distinct from, general AHA. Among adults, individual differences in displaced aggression explained a substantial proportion of the variance in domestic abuse over and above general AHA [35]. Thus, identifying childhood influences that may affect the development of this personality dimension is of societal importance.

Those high in trait displaced aggression tend to ruminate following provocations and harm those closest to them [35]. Thus, the combination of rumination and exposure to displaced aggression in the home may increase the likelihood that children will grow up to be displaced aggressors. Early identification of children who ruminate and have abusive parents may circumvent this developmental trajectory. In addition, because individual differences in general AHA stabilise around 8-years old [49], the preschool and early grade school years may be an especially sensitive period for the development of individual differences in displaced aggression.

Conclusions

Although far from being established as a robust phenomenon, there is some evidence that children and adolescents do engage in displaced aggression and that by about 5 years of age, children demonstrate a sophisticated understanding of this phenomenon. In the present work, an initial theoretical framework for understanding displaced aggression has been introduced. The framework focusses on exposure to displaced aggression in early childhood, the development of social information processing related to displaced aggression, and variables that may moderate reactions to provocations, as well as the occurrence and intensity of displaced aggression. In addition, by exploring displaced aggression within the context of bullying, mass school violence, and culture, we may increase our understanding of these important social problems. Furthermore, understanding how some individuals develop into adults who tend to engage in frequent acts of displaced aggression may eventually benefit society.

Key Points

- ❑ Although far from being established as a robust phenomenon, there is some evidence that children and adolescents engage in displaced aggression.
- ❑ By age five, children demonstrate a sophisticated understanding of displaced aggression.
- ❑ A theoretical framework for understanding displaced aggression in children and adolescents is proposed.

- Suggestions for future research, including bullying and mass school violence as forms of displaced aggression, cultural influences and the development of individual differences in displaced aggression are discussed.

References

1. Marcus-Newhall, A., Pedersen, W.C., Carlson, M. and Miller, N., 2000, "Displaced Aggression: A Meta-analytic Review", *Journal of Personality and Social Psychology*, 78, pp. 670-689.
2. Dollard, J., Doob, L.W., Miller, N.E., Mowrer, O.H. and Sears, R.R., 1939, "Frustration and Aggression", Yale University Press, Oxford, UK.
3. Hovland, C. and Sears, R., 1940, "Minor Studies in Aggression – VI: Correlation of Lynchings with Economic Indices", *Journal of Psychology*, 9, pp. 301-310.
4. Bushman, B.J., Bonacci, A.M., Pedersen, W.C., Vasquez, E.A. and Miller, N., 2005, "Chewing on It Can Chew You Up: Effects of Rumination on Triggered Displaced Aggression", *Journal of Personality and Social Psychology*, 88, pp. 969-983.
5. Denson, T.F., Pedersen, W.C. and Miller, N., 2006, "The Displaced Aggression Questionnaire", *Journal of Personality and Social Psychology*, 90, pp. 1032-1051.
6. Hoobler, J.M. and Brass, D.J., 2006, "Abusive Supervision and Family Undermining as Displaced Aggression", *Journal of Applied Psychology*, 91.
7. Pedersen, W.C., Gonzales, C. and Miller, N., 2000, "The Moderating Effect of Trivial Triggering Provocation on Displaced Aggression", *Journal of Personality and Social Psychology*, 78, pp. 913-927.
8. Vasquez, E.A., Denson, T.F., Pedersen, W.C., Stenstrom, D.A. and Miller, N., 2005, "The Moderating Effect of Trigger Intensity on Triggered Displaced Aggression", *Journal of Experimental Social Psychology*, 41, pp. 61-67.
9. Clement, T.S., Parikh, V., Schrumpf, M. and Fernald, R.D., 2005, "Behavioral Coping Strategies in a Cichlid Fish: The Role of Social Status and Acute Stress Response in Direct and Displaced Aggression", *Hormones and Behavior*, 47, pp. 336-342.
10. Hoffmann, P., Thorén, P. and Ely, D., 1987, "Effect of Voluntary Exercise on Open-field Behavior and on Aggression in the Spontaneously Hypertensive Rat (SHR)", *Behavioral and Neural Biology*, 47, pp. 346-355.
11. Overli, O., Korzan, W.J., Larson, E.T., Winberg, S., Lepage, O., Pottinger, T.G. et al., 2004, "Behavioral and Neuroendocrine Correlates of Displaced Aggression in Trout", *Hormones and Behavior*, 45, pp. 324-329.
12. White, B.C., Dew, S.E., Prather, J.R., Stearns, M., Schneider, E. and Taylor, S., 2000, "Chest-rubbing in Captive Wooly Monkeys (*Lagothrix lagotricha*)", *Primates*, 41, pp. 185-188.
13. Jegard, S. and Walters, R.H., 1960, "A Study of Some Determinants of Aggression in Young Children", *Child Development*, 31, pp. 739-747.
14. Moore, S., 1964, "Displaced Aggression in Young Children", *Journal of Abnormal and Social Psychology*, 68, pp. 200-204.
15. Foss, L. and Fouts, G., 1977, "Effects of Frustration and Cathartic Opportunity on Aggression", *Psychological Reports*, 41, pp. 319-326.
16. Bushman, B.J., Baumeister, R.F. and Phillips, C.M., 2001, "Do People Aggress to Improve their Mood? Catharsis Beliefs, Affect Regulation Opportunity, and Aggressive Responding", *Journal of Personality and Social Psychology*, 81, pp. 17-32.
17. Sulthana, P., 1987, "The Effect of Frustration and Inequity on the Displacement of Aggression", *Asian Journal of Psychology and Education*, 19, pp. 26-33.

18. Miller, P.H. and DeMarie-Dreblow, D., 1990, "Social-cognitive Correlates of Children's Understanding of Displaced Aggression", *Journal of Experimental Child Psychology*, 49, pp. 488-504.
19. Weiss, M.G. and Miller, P.H., 1983, "Young Children's Understanding of Displaced Aggression", *Journal of Experimental Child Psychology*, 35, pp. 529-539.
20. Dollinger, S.J. and McGuire, B., 1981, "The Development of Psychological-mindedness: Children's Understanding of Defense Mechanisms", *Journal of Clinical Child Psychology*, 10, pp. 117-121.
21. Anderson, C.A. and Bushman, B.J., 2002, "Human Aggression", *Annual Review of Psychology*, 53, pp. 27-51.
22. Huesmann, L.R., 1998, "The Role of Social Information Processing and Cognitive Schema in the Acquisition and Maintenance of Habitual Aggressive Behavior", In *Human Aggression: Theories, Research and Implications for Social Policy*, R.G. Geen and E. Donnerstein (Eds.), pp. 73-109.
23. Bandura, A., 1979/1986, "The Social Learning Perspective: Mechanisms of Aggression", In *Psychology of Crime and Criminal Justice*, H. Toch (Ed.), Waveland Press, Prospect Heights, USA, pp. 198-236.
24. Berkowitz, L., 1993, *Aggression: Its Causes, Consequences and Control*, McGraw-Hill, New York.
25. Miller, N., Pedersen, W.C., Earleywine, M. and Pollock, V.E., 2003, "A Theoretical Model of Triggered Displaced Aggression", *Personality and Social Psychology Review*, 7, pp. 75-97.
26. Eron, L.D., 1987, "The Development of Aggressive Behavior from the Perspective of a Developing Behaviorism", *American Psychologist*, 42, pp. 435-442.
27. Kaufman, J. and Zigler, E., 1987, "Do Abuse Children Become Abusive Parents?" *American Journal of Orthopsychiatry*, 57, pp. 186-192.
28. Widom, C.S., 1989, "Does Violence Beget Violence? A Critical Examination of the Literature", *Psychological Bulletin*, 106, pp. 3-28.
29. Anderson, C.A. and Bushman, B.J., 2001, "Effects of Violent Video Games on Aggressive Behavior, Aggressive Cognition, Aggressive Affect, Physiological Arousal and Prosocial Behavior: A Meta-analytic Review of the Scientific Literature", *Psychological Science*, 12, pp. 353-359.
30. Hogben, M., 1998, "Factors Moderating the Effect of Televised Aggression on Viewer Behavior", *Communication Research*, 25, pp. 220-247.
31. Brendgren, M., Vitaro, F., Boivin, M., Dionne, G. and Pérusse, D., 2006, "Examining Genetic and Environmental Effects on Reactive versus Proactive Aggression", *Developmental Psychology*, 42, pp. 1299-1312.
32. Crick, N.R. and Dodge, K.A., 1994, "A Review and Reformulation of Social Information-processing Mechanisms in Children's Social Adjustment", *Psychological Bulletin*, 115, pp. 74-101.
33. Coleman, J.M. and Kardash, C.M., 1999, "Encoding and Retrieval of Ambiguous and Unambiguous Information by Aggressive and Non-aggressive Elementary Boys", *Child Study Journal*, 29, pp. 133-151.
34. Camodeca, M., Goossens, F.A., Schuengel, C. and Terwogt, M.M., 2003, "Links between Social Informative Processing in Middle Childhood and Involvement in Bullying", *Aggressive Behavior*, 29, pp. 116-127.
35. Denson, T.F., Lickel, B., Curtis, M., Stenstrom, D.M. and Ames, D., 2006, "The Roles of Entitativity and Essentiality in Judgments of Collective Responsibility", *Group Processes and Intergroup Relations*, 9, pp. 43-61.
36. Pedersen, W.C., Denson, T.F., Goss, R.J., Vasquez, E.A. and Miller, N., 2006, "The Impact of Rumination on Aggressive Thoughts, Feelings, Behavior and Arousal", *Unpublished Manuscript*.
37. Suchday, S., Carter, M.M., Ewart, C.K., Larkin, K.T. and Desiderato, O., 2004, "Anger Cognitions and Cardiovascular Recovery Following Provocation", *Journal of Behavioral Medicine*, 27, pp. 319-341.

38. Carver, C.S. and White, T.L., 1994, "Behavioral Inhibition, Behavioral Activation and Affective Responses to Impending Reward and Punishment: The BIS/BAS Scales", *Journal of Personality and Social Psychology*, 67, pp. 319-333.
39. Eisenberger, N.I., Way, B.M., Taylor, S.E., Welch, W.T. and Lieberman, M.D. (in press), "Understanding Genetic Risk for Aggression: Clues from the Brain's Response to Social Exclusion", *Biological Psychiatry*.
40. Shih, J.C., Chen, K. and Ridd, M.J., 1999, "Monoamine Oxidase: From Genes to Behavior", *Annual Review of Neuroscience*, 22, pp. 197-217.
41. Ramirez, J.M., 2003, "Hormones and Aggression in Childhood and Adolescence", *Aggression and Violent Behavior*, 8, pp. 621-644.
42. Epstein, R., 1965, "Authoritarianism, Displaced Aggression and Social Status of the Target", *Journal of Personality and Social Psychology*, 2, pp. 585-589.
43. Axelrod, R., 1984, *The Evolution of Cooperation*, Basic Books, New York.
44. Gouldner, A.W., 1960, "The Norm of Reciprocity", *American Sociological Review*, 25, pp. 161-178.
45. Twenge, J.M., Baumeister, R.F., Tice, D.M. and Stucke, T.S., 2001, "If You Can't Join Them, Beat Them: Effects of Social Exclusion on Aggressive Behavior", *Journal of Personality and Social Psychology*, 81, pp. 1058-1069.
46. Leary, M.R., Kowalski, R.M., Smith, L. and Phillips, S., 2003, "Teasing, Rejection and Violence: Case Studies of the School Shootings", *Aggressive Behavior*, 29, pp. 202-214.
47. Gaertner, L. and Iuzzini, J., 2005, "Rejection and Entitativity: A Synergistic Model of Mass Violence", In *The Social Outcast*, K.D. Williams, J.P. Forgas and W. von Hippel (Eds.), Psychology Press, New York, USA, pp. 307-320.
48. Redford, P., 1999, "Self-construal and Action Tendencies in Hong Kong and the United Kingdom", In *Merging Past, Present and Future in Cross-cultural Psychology*, W.J. Lonner, D.J. Dinnel, D.K. Forgays and S.A. Hayes (Eds.), Swets and Zeitlinger, Lisse, The Netherlands, pp. 367-386.
49. Eron, L.D. and Huesmann, L.R., 1990, "The Stability of Aggressive Behavior: Even into the Third Generation", In *Handbook of Developmental Psychopathology*, M. Lewis and S.M. Miller (Eds.), Plenum, New York, USA, pp. 147-156.

The AHA-Syndrome and Cardiovascular Diseases
Editors: Swati Y. Bhave and Sunil Saini
Copyright © 2010 Anamaya Publishers, New Delhi, India

5. How Can We Reduce Anger?

Usha Ram
University of Pune, Pune - 411 007, India

Abstract: This article discusses anger and techniques for its reduction, as presented in ancient Indian text, namely, the *Bhagwadgita*. Firstly, anger is defined; its origin and etiology are explained according to the *Bhagwadgita*. The processes in which the cognitions and the emotion of anger develop are explained. This is followed by an explanation of the four ways to reduce anger. The article will aid in the understanding of anger according to the Indian psychological perspective. Once anger is understood the techniques that help to reduce it may be mastered.

Keywords: Roots of anger, Cognitive basis, *Triguna*, Reduction techniques.

Introduction

Several thinkers from ancient times have defined anger. It is one of the primary or basic emotions mentioned in both Western and Eastern thought and theories formulated to study and discuss emotion [1, 2]. The importance of anger can be seen in human experience across the world when one reflects on the universality of emotional expressions studied by Ekman and O'Sullivan [3], and Philippot, Feldman and Coats [4], all cited in Feldman [5].

Considering that anger is common to human experience, several psychologists have embarked on the study of anger, looking into its arousal, maintenance, duration, frequency, consequences or effects on health, other emotions like pride, guilt and distress [6-11].

By the simplest of definitions and agreements, "anger occurs toward an object/person which/who is an obstacle to fulfilling one's desired goal" [12]. The ancient Indian book of wisdom, the *Bhagwadgita* describes anger as "all-devouring.... enemy here", meaning in this world [13].

Since anger has disastrous consequences on us, the angry person and the target of the anger, handling an emotion, which leads to hostility, vengeance, aggression and destruction to the one experiencing these states and to the recipients of the angry behaviour, is important. If we understand the roots of anger, handling or reducing this emotion will become that much simpler.

Where Does Anger Come From?

Anger reduction has at its root the cognitive approach. Cognising (knowing) this emotion may in itself be called "taking the bull by its horns". In other words, knowledge will provide us with the power to rule this emotion than it ruling us.

In our efforts to understand or knowing anger, I refer to the *Bhagwadgita*. Through its 18 chapters, this splendid ancient book has provided us information – which, when used appropriately, becomes wisdom for us – that desire is the root cause of anger. Indeed, Chapter II Verses 62-63 describe the source or root of all our problems, whether anger, stress, pain or sorrow. These two verses read:

> *When a man thinks of objects 'attachments' for them arise;*
> *From attachment 'desire' is born; from desire arises 'anger';*
>
> II-62 [14]
>
> *From anger comes 'delusion'; from delusion 'loss of memory';*
> *From loss of memory the 'destruction of discrimination';*
> *From destruction of discrimination he 'perishes'...*
>
> II-63 [14]

These two verses specifically show how repeatedly thinking of any object(s) leads to attachment to them and to desires to have or possess them. The objects of the world are experienced through our five senses of hearing, smell, sight, taste and touch. These objects may have provided us pleasure (or pain) in the past and the desire for them to be present (or absent) is our attachment. Since these are sense-experiences, the objects are called sense-objects [e.g. see II-58-62 [14]]. There is a desire (*kama*) to repeat the experience of pleasure.

Anger (*krodh*) is the result of unfulfilled desire. Greed (*trisna*) is the consequence of fulfillment of desire, causing further desire for the same pleasure. Suppressed anger (*kshobh*) is experienced when one is annoyed or angry with a person who is senior or superior to one or in situations where one cannot express the anger.

Bhagwadgita has talked about the relation between *kama* and *krodha*, thus:

> "*It is desire, it is anger, born of the guna called rajas, consumer of much, very evil; know it to be your enemy here in this world*"
>
> III-37 [15, p. 160]

This verse indicates that *kama-krodha* (desire-anger) are at the root of human pain for it is under the sway of *kama-krodha* that we commit errors or what we call 'wrong doings'. When in anger, rationality has no room to operate, delusion sets in, discrimination ability drops, leading one to perform wrong or undesirable acts.

Desire, the root of our anger, arises only when there is an awareness of one's being, i.e. of 'I am' (*aham asmi*), a prerequisite of *kama* arousal. This awareness is pleasurable and activates desire for repetition of this pleasure in various ways.

Kama operates at three levels viz., body (*deha*), mind (*manas*) and intellect (*buddhi*). The *kama* at the body (*deha*) level is through the five senses and the five sense organs, e.g. desire for food, sleep and sex. At the psychological or *manas* level, pleasure-pain, joy-sorrow and such bipolar emotions and feelings are accordingly desired to be present or absent. We find human desires for love, feelings of security, self-esteem, recognition etc. It may be noted here that needs and desires are to be distinguished. Needs are to be met for sustenance and they subside when gratified while desires are for pleasure. Fulfillment of one desire leads to the emerging desire for the same or similar pleasure. A need becomes a desire when one gets pleasure from need-gratification and gets attached to this pleasure [13]. Thus, the *kama* is born, followed, in time, by frustration, anger and its consequences.

The third kind of *kama* is at the intellectual level. This is a desire for thoughts and ideas, which gives satisfaction or pleasure to one. The person is driven to seek stimulation and gratification at an intellectual level. It provides pleasure, and an attachment develops for the repeated pleasure. Obstacles in reaching intellectual goals may be many, causing the arousal of ire. Thus, we have physical desires (*dehavasana*), psycho-social desires (*lokavasana*) and intellectual desires (*sastravasana*). These are called desires for the non-soul (*anatmavasana*) as against the desires for the self/soul (*atmavasana*). The desires for the self emerge only when attachment to the worldly objects (non-soul) are transcended.

As long as our identity is limited to our body, mind and intellect (BMI) the non-self desires hound us and we experience related emotions. The identity is limited to the 'I', 'me' and 'mine', i.e. ego (*aham*). The restricted identity causes obstructions in growth experiences to transcend the world of emotional experiences. Human desires when frustrated cause distress because these desires have selfish motives and are fulfilled at the cost of others' discomfort or suffering [13]. These selfish desires are called *kamana* (II-71).

Desires appear first at the cognitive level in the form of an idea or thought. The instrument of the intellect (*buddhi*) is mind (*manas*) that gets activated by the emergence of the thought/idea and pursues the idea by the activation of related memories of pleasure. Next, the body gets the momentum toward gratification of the desire. The individual's awareness of 'being' is important here when s/he becomes aware of "I want/desire". The awareness of 'being' is cognitive. The desire is, thus, cognitive – an activating force born of an activating force *rajas* (III-57), one of the *triguna* (three properties/qualities) in all creation.

The combination of matter (*prakriti*) and spirit (*atma*) produces *triguna* (XIV-5). *Satwa* (goodness, knowledge XIV-6), *rajas* (activity, passion XIV-7), and *tamas* (ignorance, inactivity XIV-8) are the three *gunas*, which determine one's personality and behaviour.

People dominated by *rajas* are "given to lust and anger, strive to obtain by unlawful means hoards of wealth for sensual enjoyments" (XVI-12) [16]. Such people are egoistic, power-crazy, lusty, angry, malicious, hateful and move toward destruction than happiness, aiming at vengeance through hostile actions, which do not bring any long-term peace and satisfaction to the self or others. The strength of this state aroused by *rajas* gets acted through the body by *tamas* (e.g. ignorance) "without any consideration of consequences waste injury to others or one's own ability" (XVIII-25) [14].

It is quite evident from the above that high *rajasic* egoism blinds the person who is now angry (because of obstacles to his/her goals or frustration of desires). The individual cannot rein anger, which is not understood. Controlling anger is not acquired through suppression but by bringing to oneself the clarity regarding the role of egoism in the arousal, maintenance and non-gratification of one's desires (demands). Briefly speaking, incorporating the full meaning of II-62, 63 verses is perhaps the beginning of anger reduction.

Persistent indulging in thoughts related to the event that activated the anger leads a person to hostility, aggression and violence. This indulgence at the thought level develops attachment to the event to resolve it and not to reduce it. It paves the way to hostility. The feelings of hostility harbour feelings of hatred and desires for settling scores through vengeance, which is again a form of aggression and violence. What degree of peace – mental and physical – can there be where a person contemplates and works on planning to avenge his/her frustration-based anger! Filled with such feelings which stem from anger, there is no room for knowledge or reason or for love that soothes distress. Thus, knowledge makes way for wisdom regarding human emotions of love and devotion, as well as appropriate actions carried out in an appropriate manner. In all the wars waged between nations in our world the realisation of the folly of the act of war emerges later. The peoples of two nations have had no time to understand that the cause for the war-behaviour was anger arising out of frustration of desires, which had blinded them. Aggression and violence govern the leadership of warring nations and they are found lacking wisdom at the said time. Hindsight emerges after colossal damage has been done. What happens at an interpersonal level is seen occurring at an international level!

Can anything be done to stop us from our self-destructive self-ruinous behaviour? Reduce anger!

How Do We Reduce Anger?

People often talk of anger management. It is a cliché like stress-management. Management would mean effective functioning of anger with the goal in view. Perhaps we may want to reduce the frequent and/or prolonged experiences of anger and its consequences. This does not mean 'controlling' anger. Anger-control distinctly would end in anger-suppression, leading to bottling the emotion and allowing its effects on health.

We hear people say "I am hot-tempered... I want to do something about this...". In fact, one of my earliest clients in 1979 was a 22-year-old student who said these words in a loud voice and talked about how he kept getting angry and later feeling sorry. (In his case, I had used the cognitive approach then called RET).

To reduce anger or overcome the frequency, duration, and intensity of anger one first needs to understand that one is interested in this activity, as it requires an intense effort to work on this consciously. The oft-cited advice is to count from one to ten when one is angry so that the anger is not expressed either verbally or in action. Counting may help temporarily but it does not reduce anger in the individual's personality.

There are four ways to work on anger reduction: Cognitive (*jnana*), affective (*bhakti*, devotion)), behavioural (*karma*), i.e. action or deed, and meditation (*dhyana*). Now, we take a look at each of these ways.

Cognitive (*Jnana*)

This deals with knowing/obtaining information on anger to understand it fully. Once anger is understood, as discussed earlier, one can move to reduce it through knowing the ideas or thoughts about the obstacles to achieving one's goals. This helps to again understand what one's expectations and/or demands are about people and events in one's path to reach one's goal. Once the expectations and demands regarding others and oneself are identified, one can take a look at its realistic component: "is my expectation realistic?" An intense desire (*kamana*) operates when the idea contains, e.g. "I must have it and only in this way", or "she ought to have waited for me". Both the statements carry imperatives as an insistent component making the desire for fulfillment intense. Such intensity in the thought is indicative of high egoism. Fulfillment of these demands inflates the ego and *kamana* persists. *Kamana* is related to the sense-objects that provide pleasure-displeasure through the five senses, as well as the intellect and mind, as mentioned earlier. The body and the senses are perishable. Therefore, *kamana* pertaining to the body, mind and intellect are transient.

> *"The contacts with sense objects, O' son of Kunti, which caused*
> *heat and cold, pleasure and pain, have a beginning and end;*
> *they are impermanent: endure them bravely O' descendent of Bharata*"
>
> II-14 [16]

"A desire in itself cannot and does not bring about disturbances in the mind as our longing after those very same desires does." [16] Overcoming the cravings or *kamana* for the pleasures of the sense-objects can be achieved through "discrimination and proper intellectual evaluation of the sense-objects" [16].

This is the cognitive process that Ellis has presented in his rational-emotive therapy about five decades ago. He said that there is an event/happening (A), which activates the emotion of anger perceived and reported by the experiencer as the consequence (C) of A. On perceiving the event, in fact, the perceiver's beliefs, thoughts, or ideas get activated based on which the perceiver enters into a self-talk (B). This self-talk involves making imperative statements using words like 'must', 'should', and 'ought'. These statements are demands, evaluations and expectations regarding the event, which may (or may not) include a person. These statements require to be reconstructed after debating (D) with oneself about the realistic aspect of the demand. For example, "she should have waited for me. She ought not to have left without me...". Here no amount of insistence changes the event. Instead, reconstructing the self-talk to, "it would have been so convenient had she waited for me", or "I would have preferred her to have waited for me than going away", would change the feeling from anger to maybe just a slight disappointment. Beliefs such as, "I must have no difficulty in life", "everything must happen just the way I want", "people must appreciate all that I do" etc., lead to anger among other distressing feelings. Thus, replacing these irrational ideas by rational non-demanding ones will contribute to reducing the intensity of our desires. The rational approach helps in changing our beliefs and in reducing our selfness (egoism). With the decrease in egoism the *rajasic ahamkar* becomes weaker, thus, reducing anger.

Besides this rising above the *kamana* is the realisation regarding one's identity or ego. Our belief is that "I am the doer" because our "mind is deluded by our egoism" (III-27). If we realise that our identity is not limited to our BMI and to their connections with the world of objects with limited experiences of 'I' and 'mine', but that 'I' is expansive, then the transience of our experiences will be realised and will no longer be desirable.

These realisations and understandings help reduce the *kamana* to have the functional *kama* for subsistence and, thus, anger, hostility, vengeance, and aggression would be at abeyance.

Affective (*Bhakti*)

This is the second way and also second stage in the basic psychological process that all humans possess. Affect is an important aspect of the psychological composition of all humans. This method helps to get freedom from anger and its consequences at the physical and psychosocial levels. Devotion (*bhakti*) arises out of the cognitive component of trust and faith. Trust and faith are the outcome of knowledge. Knowledge here is not only of what anger (or for that matter any emotion) is and how it occurs, but of transcending this knowledge to reach wisdom regarding all of creation, not only of oneself and one's world consisting of humans and nature on the planet Earth. Once we know the source of all creation, we, according to the *Bhagwadgita*, would come to experience love/devotion for the 'form' of this source. The source, the creator, is manifest or unmanifest. Devotion (*bhakti*) for the manifest is easier to experience than for the unmanifest, which may be at the conceptual, abstract level only. To love a concept is difficult for us! Thus, said *Krishna*:

> "*Greater is their trouble whose minds are set on the 'Unmanifest';*
> *For the goal, 'Unmanifest' is very hard for the embodied to reach.*"
>
> (XII-5) [16]

The above stanza indicates that as long as we are attached to the body that we are in, it is very difficult to focus our attention on and devotion for the unmanifest or formless source of creation of the universe that includes us. Attachment to the body involves a life of sensuality and satisfying cravings of the body through the five senses, satisfying emotional and intellectual cravings through the vehicle of the body. Thus, once devotion is awakened for the creator of our world, if we progressively rise above the limited transient bodily or physically activated desires, our devotion will lead to the surrender to the creator, enabling us to gain freedom from the bindings of BMI.

The devotion makes one realise who one is. This realisation brings an end to egoism (*ahamkar*) and, thus, to anger and other such emotions. Only the supreme love prevails in one and for all from one! *Bhakti* frees the person from wants and the person

> "*... is pure, efficient, detached, ready to meet every demand I make on him as a humble instrument of my work.*"
>
> (XII-16) [14]

Such devotion enables a person to be in equilibrium, to rise above the bipolar emotions and

> "*... he does not rejoice, nor hates, nor grieves, nor desires, renouncing good and evil, full of devotion, is dear to Me.*"
>
> (XII-17) [16]

The devoted person treats all alike – friend and foe – and is free from attachment (XII-18). For him, censure and praise are equal; he is silent, content with anything, is not attached to any home, is steady-minded and filled with devotion (XII-19).

The last (20th) stanza of Chapter XII speaks for the profundity of the effect of *bhakti*. Making *bhakti* as one's way of life, being endowed with unshaken faith in the Supreme, with the "capacity to assimilate spiritual ideas into ourselves through subjective personal experience" [16], enables one to rise above *kamana*. One becomes free of it and its related emotional experiences and psychosocial and physical (health) consequences. Rising above enables one to know the transience of *kamana* and the futility of indulging in and remaining at these levels of emotion.

Behavioural (*Karma*)

In the basic psychological process it was noted that behaviour is related to our feelings. We recall that our desires are fulfilled or satisfied only through some action or behaviour. The body carries out the behaviour with all its organs active. In this respect, *Bhagwadgita* says:

> *"The right is to work only, but never to its fruits; let not the fruit-of-action be thy motive, nor let the attachment be to action."*
>
> (II-47) [16]

There is a purpose in one's acts and behaviour – a goal to be reached. Achieving the goal is a desire. Working, striving, doing something to satisfy the desire is *karma.* The *karma* is carried out with the sole purpose set before oneself. But the counsel in the above-mentioned stanza is the secret of one's real achievements.

When one embarks on an activity to achieve a set goal, in most cases, one finds oneself considering the goal not being achieved. In the event one does not reach the goal, what then is the anxiety about? Our attention is on the goal than on the act to reach it. The fear or anxiety is because one is attached to it and, later, one even justifies the means used. There may be an ego-involvement in both the means and the end, believing that one did all to get the goal.

In being involved with the fruits of the actions, one loses sight of what one is doing. The rewards/fruits of one's action – future is the focus of attention – are in one's actions in the present. Worrying about possible failure ruins the present focus, too. Therefore, be in the present – the action (*karma*) – since the future (reward/fruit/outcome) will soon be the present. So do not attach yourself to the outcome, but heed the action at hand and perform it to the best of your knowledge and let the future take care of the rest. Do not work with your mind on the reward but on the task at hand. We may then note what this stanza has to say: a person who follows this stanza:

1. Understands that his/her concern is only with his/her action.
2. Is not involved with the results of the action (fruit).
3. Is not concerned with getting a specific outcome of her/his action.
4. Understands that these ideas do not indicate being active [16].

Thus, one has a right to action but never to the outcome/fruit of that action. The result of the action is not really in one's hands as there are several variables operating at a given point in time, which may influence the action, thus, bringing about an outcome far different from the desired one. This can then become a cause for irritation, annoyance, anger, hostility and aggression or violence. All these then may affect one's mental and physical health, and social relations.

Meditation (*Dhyana*)

Late Ma Indiradevi, a spiritually evolved lady in Pune, India said in one of her discourses that in prayer we speak to the Creator and in meditation He speaks to us! This 'speaking' is enlightening us, giving us knowledge, wisdom, not necessarily the way we talk to Him.

Meditation is a process where there is an effort to withdraw one's attention from sense objects to which one's desires are attached. In desiring, one's attention is on the sense-objects, which provide pleasure or reduce, remove pain. In the world of sense-objects, one is controlled by desires, while in meditation that provides knowledge, one is the master of the desires.

Having withdrawn one's mind from the transient world, one can focus on the Self, or universal consciousness, *Atman*, God, Creator. By and by this steady focus emerges and the transience and futility of the indulgence in desiring the world of sense-objects dawns.

> "*Let the yogi try constantly to keep the mind steady, remaining in solitude, alone with the mind and body controlled, free from hope and greed.*"
>
> (VI-10) [16]

> "*Abandoning without reserve all desires born of Sankalpa, and completely restraining the whole group of senses by the mind from all sides.*"
>
> (VI-24) [16]

Gradually, quietness is attained, the mind is focussed on the Self (Creator) and no thoughts prevail (VI-25). Having achieved this state of focussing and free from distraction or disturbance from any thought

> "*Supreme bliss verily comes to this Yogi (person) whose mind is quite peaceful, whose passion is quietened, who is free from sin, and who has become BRAHMAN.*"
>
> (VI-27) [16]

It is this serenity that many want in this world, free from all types of thoughts that arise in the intellect *(buddhi)* because of the *rajas* being influential, cause agitation in the mind (*manas*) and bring forth related behaviour (*karma*), which descends on the meditator when s/he persists at it.

Conclusion

The four ways of reducing anger are very intimately interconnected. In fact, even as we start understanding anger, the process of reduction has begun, because we have begun to understand the very creation, leading us to know the source of creation upon which the devotion, dormant in all, is awakened. This devotion enables us to do our *karma* appropriately; meditating also becoming a part of this *karma*. In effect, all these processes become one as we are guided by the source of creation. This is the way to reduce not only anger but all negative feelings and rise above the gates to self-destruction.

> "*These are three gates of hell, destructive of the Self – lust, anger, and greed; therefore, one should renounce these three.*"
>
> (XVI-212) [16]

There is, thus, liberation through renunciation!

Key Points

- ❑ Anger, its origin and etiology has been explained according to the *Bhagwadgita*.
- ❑ According to the *Bhagwadgita*, attachment and desire are the root causes of anger.
- ❑ The four ways of anger reduction have been emphasised viz., cognitive (*jnana*), affective (devotion (*bhakti*)), behavioural (*karma*), i.e. action/deed, and meditation (*dhyana*).

References

1. Ekman, P., 1992, "Are There Basic Emotions?" *Psychological Review*, 99(3), pp. 550-553.
2. Izard, C.E., 1992, "Basic Emotions, Relations Among Emotions and Emotion-cognition Relations", *Psychological Review*, 99(3), pp. 561-565.
3. Ekman, P. and O'Sullivan, M., 1991, "Facial Expressions: Methods, Means and Moves", In *Fundamentals of Nonverbal Behavior*, R.S. Feldman and B. Rime (Eds.), Cambridge University Press, Cambridge, UK.
4. Philippot, P., Feldman, R.S. and Coats, E.J., 1999, *Social Determinants of Nonverbal Behavior*, Cambridge University Press, Cambridge, UK.
5. Feldman, R.S., 2001, *Social Psychology*, 3rd Edn., Prentice-Hall, Upper Saddle River, New Jersey.
6. Bishop, G.D. and Quah, S.H., 1998, "Reliability and Validity of Measures of Anger/hostility in Singapore: Cook and Medley Ho Scale, STAXI, and Buss-Durkee Hostility Inventory", *Personality and Individual Differences*, 24, pp. 867-878.
7. Chon, K.K. and Kang, H.J., 2000, "Toward an Improved Understanding of Anger: A Control Theory Approach", *Korean Journal of Health Psychology*, 5(2), pp. 146-170.
8. Crane, R.S., 1981, "The Role of Anger, Hostility and Aggression in Essential Hypertension", Doctoral Dissertation, University of South Florida, *Dissertation Abstracts International*, 42, p. 2982B.
9. Ghosh, S.N. and Sharma, S., 1998, "Trait Anxiety and Anger Expression in Patients with Essential Hypertension", *Journal of the Indian Academy of Applied Psychology*, 24, pp. 9-14.
10. Mendes de Leon, C.F., 1992, "Anger and Impatience/irritability in Patients of Low Socio-economic Status with Acute Coronary Heart Disease", *Journal of Behavioral Medicine*, 15, pp. 273-284.
11. Sharma, S., 2003, "Life Events Stress, Emotional Vital Signs and Hypertension", *Psychological Studies*, 48, pp. 53-65.
12. Ram, U., 2000, "Roots of Anger and Aggression: Indian Wisdom from the Bhagawad Gita", *Korean Journal of Health Psychology*, 5(2), pp. 171-180.
13. Ramsukhdas, 1996, *Srimad Bhagwadgita*, Gita Press, Gorakhpur.
14. Easwaran, E., 1997, *The Bhagawad Gita: For Daily Living*, Vols. 1-3, Jaico, Delhi.
15. Rama, 1985, *Perennial Psychology of the Bhagwad Gita*, The Himalayan International Institute of Yoga, Science and Philosophy of the USA, Honesdale.
16. Chinmayananda, 1976, *The Holy Geeta*, Central Chinmaya Mission Trust, Bombay.

The AHA-Syndrome and Cardiovascular Diseases
Editors: Swati Y. Bhave and Sunil Saini
Copyright © 2010 Anamaya Publishers, New Delhi, India

6. Youth Aggression and At-Risk Behaviour Interventions

Sheila Royo Maxwell and Christopher D. Maxwell
School of Criminal Justice, Michigan State University, East Lansing, Michigan, USA

Abstract: The present chapter reviews aggression and violence by kids and youth. Aggression is discussed in terms of the range of its definitions for such behaviour. The etiology and epidemiology of aggression and violence are framed within the public health ecological model. Specifically, the chapter examines the multiple definitions of aggression and violence, discusses the etiology of youth aggression and violence, and discusses prevention/intervention models and techniques. It enables the reader to understand the multi-faceted characteristic of aggression, the response mechanisms generally employed and the challenges presented in these responses, as well as the necessity for a multi-faceted, multi-level approach to understanding and preventing aggression.

Keywords: Youth aggression, Youth violence, Anti-social behaviour, Prevention techniques, Intervention techniques.

Introduction

Serious aggression and violence by youth garner media attention worldwide, and has been a cause for alarm in many societies [1]. Reports of youth violence and maladaptive aggression in schools, at sporting events, on the streets, and at home have become frequent occurrences globally. Many societies, particularly those in the West, have channelled considerable resources into understanding the etiology of such behaviours and finding reasonable preventative solutions.

Since the late 1970s, scholars have produced substantial literature to help understand and prevent youth violence and aggression. It is now clear that aggression and violence is a persistent problem that has profound personal and societal ramifications. Also, this problem and its etiology is multi-faceted and, thus, requires a multi-pronged response [1-4].

This chapter examines some of the responses and interventions to youth aggression, particularly the challenges inherent in creating and implementing workable programmes. To begin, some discussion of definitions is necessary, given the multi-faceted views and approaches to aggression.

Definitions

Inherent in the multi-disciplinary nature of aggressive and violent behaviours, the definitions and explanations for these behaviours have also varied. For example, what is often referred to as *instrumental* aggression, i.e. aggression committed to obtain some gain, e.g. in robberies, gang assaults, and other predatory acts [3], may come under the category of *adaptive* aggression if such acts were committed for the purpose of survival and self-preservation. But they may also be categorised as *maladaptive* or *hostile* aggression if such acts were committed without any provocation or under an entirely predatory context [2]. For those working in the field of criminal justice or the law where the primary goal is to establish criminality, distinctions across the contexts or precursors of these behaviours may not be as important as determining whether the elements of a criminal act can be established. However, for those working in clinical settings, the developmental and environmental contexts of these behaviours are important elements in understanding and developing workable interventions.

So what is aggression? A commonly, but by no means totally accepted definition by social scientists defines aggression as "any form of behaviour directed toward the goal of harming or injuring another living being who is motivated to avoid such treatment" [2]. This definition avoids *intentionality*, i.e. the purpose as conceived by the actor for committing the act – which can often be hard to determine and is fraught with challenges of definitions. It also considers aggression as a form of *behaviour* and not merely an attitude or a belief. Therefore, anger or frustration towards another but without the consequent behaviour (such as punching, screaming, or insulting) is not classified as aggression. If the anger or frustration turns to verbally insulting or shoving another, then it is classified as *aggression*. This definition also calls for harm or injury to another, where harm is not limited to physical injury but can include any type of aversive consequence, e.g. fear, distress, or embarrassment [2]. Moreover, self-inflicted harm, e.g. suicides, are also incorporated even though the 'other' is essentially the same person inflicting the harm. While this definition is functional in that it provides some boundaries as to what behaviours are categorised as aggressive, other anti-social symptoms like hyperactivity, deceitfulness, or defiance can also be lumped into this definition. These behaviours, often referred to as *conduct disorders* (CDs), have been closely linked to aggression. Studies have linked aggression with other anti-social symptoms showing that CDs and aggression most often ensue from similar source stressors such as mental health disorders [3]. To clarify forms and types of aggression, a functional categorisation is adopted in this chapter, which enables a better categorisation of the complexity and varied facets of aggression, its explanations, and appropriate interventions.

This commonly used categorisation dichotomizes aggressive behaviour into the bipolar continuum of *overt* and *covert aggression* [5]. Covert aggression covers internalising behaviours (self-harming) such as running away, truancy, or alcohol and drug use while overt aggression covers externalising behaviours (other-harming or other-disruptive) such as threats, temper tantrums, and other openly confrontational acts of aggression like hitting, kicking, punching or even fatal aggression. Research and psychometric evidence have provided support for this bipolar continuum of aggressive behaviours [3, 5, 6], making this a functional characterisation for researchers and clinicians.

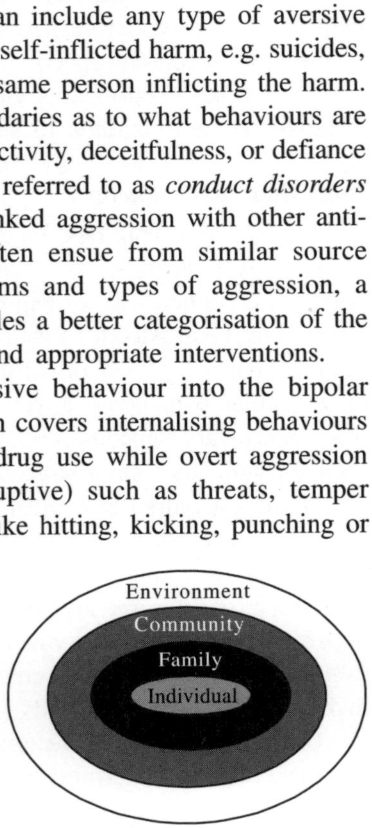

Fig. 1. The ecological model.

With this categorisation in mind, still another useful tool employed by public health professionals and researchers that is currently widely used is the framing of aggression and violence into an ecological model (Fig. 1). The model is based upon the public health approach of preventing disease or injury by considering not just the individual who is affected or at risk, but the individual's relationship to his/her surroundings such as the family, schools, peer groups, community etc. [7]. This framework, therefore, provides a more holistic approach to the understanding and prevention of aggression and violence.

Etiology and Epidemiology

Presumed causes of aggression are as varied as the disciplines that study the behaviour. These range from explanations emanating from social and economic structures (e.g. familial structures, parental rearing, parent-child interaction, peer dynamics etc.), to biological explanations (e.g. genes, brain functioning, hormones, activities of the central nervous system etc.), predisposing conditions (e.g. hyperactivity) and many others. The ecological framework assists in organising this multitude of potential predisposing and causative factors for aggression and violence. Within each level of the ecological framework, a plethora of research has been completed that outlines many factors highly correlated with aggression and violence. None of each factor by itself, however, can sufficiently explain the variability in participation, seriousness, or the frequency of aggression and violence across populations. Only when a number of factors converge are determinations plausible on who may or may not act aggressively at some point. Western literature attests that virtually all criminal offenders display disturbed behaviours at some point well before their crime commences [8-11]. This makes it possible to provide intervention that reduces aggression before it develops into criminality. Following the ecological framework, we now highlight certain aspects that have been substantiated in the literature as often co-occurring with youth aggression and violence. These aspects have been used in many preventative programmes and continue to stimulate innovative programming endeavours.

Individual Risk Factors

A host of individual risk factors have been identified as co-occurring with aggression and violence. Among these are *acquired* biological deficits such as a low birthweight, prenatal and postnatal complications, or exposure to neurotoxins, e.g. lead [12, 13], alcohol (particularly those affected by Fetal Alcohol Syndrome (FAS)) [14], cocaine [15, 16] etc. Studies are mixed on the definitiveness of the effects of these acquired biological deficits on behavioural problems. Often, no particular pathogenic effect is consistently observed across all affected individuals. Effects most likely vary depending upon the level and point of exposure, as well as associated familial, societal, and other environmental risks that may interact with these deficits.

Besides acquired biological deficits, inherited biological characteristics such as temperament or hormonal levels have also been associated with aggression and violence. Children who show fearlessness and impulsiveness very early in life have been shown to have higher levels of aggression, early onset into anti-social activities, and crime and violence later in life [17]. This is particularly pronounced when temperament is combined with other familial and environmental dysfunctions such as familial conflict, poverty, academic underachievement or failure, or upbringing in high-crime neighbourhoods [18].

Other individual risk factors comprise biases and deficits in cognitive processing that may include biases in interpreting social events [19-21]; consistently attributing hostile intent to ambiguous cues; limitations in the sequential processing of information, or endorsing beliefs that aggression is a legitimate response to a host of social challenges. Studies have found that highly aggressive children often incorrectly attribute hostile intentions to peers on matters that are generally ambiguous such as accidentally getting hit by a ball in the playground. This hostile attribution then leads to aggressive retaliation, and if consistently repeated, 'marks' the child as generally hostile. This evokes hostility among peers and leads to isolation and a more hostile environment where the child must now interact [19]. Studies have also found that an early and consistent rejection by peers also poses aggression risk [22] and victimisation of the aggressive child [23]. In turn, the rejection and victimisation appear to be associated with increased anti-social behaviour and aggression by such children.

Familial Risk Factors

Besides individual risk factors, a host of factors categorised as 'familial' have also been shown as highly correlated with aggression and violence. The family, generally considered as an institution that holds society together, has long been considered an important mediator or facilitator of anti-social behaviours, aggression and violence. Research on youth aggression certainly bears out the significance of familial factors in youth behaviours. Among important familial factors often correlated with aggression are: parental rejection and neglect, a history of criminal activity by a parent/parents, anti-social personality by a parent/parents, endorsement of aggressive conduct, failure to teach non-violent and effective methods of solving interpersonal problems, low emotional cohesion, and a high frequency of negative over positive communication [24]. In addition, the lack of parental supervision and inconsistent disciplinary practices have been shown to be among the best predictors of conduct disorders and delinquency among youth [25, 26].

Research also shows that harsh and continued physical punishment by parents on children may elicit short-term obedience, but it tends to increase aggression in the long run. Moreover, violence and aggression between parents that are witnessed by children have also been shown as highly related to both covert and overt aggression [13, 27, 28].

Community/Environmental Factors

The factors related to community/environment are not always found in the home but are those that youth may come in contact with in the course of their social activities and lifestyles. Among the ones listed here are those that have been found to be consistently linked with aggression and violence such as access to firearms [29], involvement with alcohol and other drugs, involvement with anti-social groups or deviant peers who share the same norms regarding the appropriateness of aggression, and the early and consistent exposure to violence in the mass media [30] and around one's neighbourhood [31]. Many studies conducted on each of these factors show consistently strong correlations with aggression and violence. However, none of these factors consistently show the same effect across all exposed individuals. Variations are often observed depending upon interactions between or among many risk factors.

Besides the individual, familial and community/environmental risk factors outlined here, other neighbourhood characteristics have also been shown, at least in Western literature, as correlated with youth aggression. Worth noting among these are levels of education, with higher educated neighbourhoods showing lower rates of aggression and officially recorded violence [32, 33]. Likewise, a large percentage of female-headed households, i.e. households where a divorced or widowed mother is the sole head of the family unit, has often also been shown as highly correlated with youth aggression [34]. Unlike other explanations of aggression, however, these factors have not been examined across nations and cultures. Generalisability across cultural milieus, therefore, still needs to be examined and verified. Conversely, a factor that may be important in other countries but perhaps not so much in Western societies is the presence of prolonged societal conflicts or war, where violence may increasingly become socially acceptable.

Prevention and Interventions

The vast array of studies on youth anti-social, aggressive, and violent behaviours have led to numerous preventative and intervention techniques to address this multi-faceted, persistent and, in many cases, growing social problem. Just as there are varied definitions of aggression, prevention and intervention techniques have also varied across disciplines, ranging from criminalisation to cognitive restructuring or familial and community-based interventions [3, 19, 35, 36]. Primarily, a society's response to aggression and violence is the enactment of laws and sanctions to protect the general public. Michael Tonry and David Farrington [37], two distinguished criminologists, have argued that governments in most countries make public safety among their core responsibilities. This includes the imposition of sanctions for those who are legally found to criminally aggress or commit violence. Increasingly, however, the use of law enforcement as the primary tool to advance public safety shows only modest effects on the rates of serious crimes [38].

In European countries and in the United States (US), prevention and intervention efforts for various types of anti-social behaviours have become significant complements to the enforcement approach. Particularly, the conglomeration of research on aggression and violence provided the impetus for developing prevention and intervention techniques. This body of research shows that the factors that put a youth at risk for aggression and violence are generally tractable and measurable. As such, efforts can be made to prevent aggression before it begins.

Prevention efforts generally characterise programmes that address the risks for problem behaviours 'before' they even emerge, while intervention efforts are programmes designed to address already exhibited and observable problem behaviours. Many programmes have both prevention and intervention components, while some focus specifically on either prevention or intervention strategies. In the following sections, some of the major programming strategies (involving both preventative and intervention techniques) are discussed, followed by a discussion of several programme types tested in the US, and a discussion of the effects of these programmes that can be determined from evaluation studies.

Although there is a broad array of approaches for the prevention of aggression and violence, the following three emerge as among the major approaches:

Law Enforcement Approaches

Law enforcement strategies comprise the enactment of new laws or the changing of existing laws, enforcement techniques, or sentencing and correctional policies and practices to prevent crime through deterrence, incapacitation, rehabilitation, and indirectly through socialisation and the restructuring of normative contexts. These programmes and techniques are most often administered through the institutions that comprise the criminal justice system – principally, the police, the courts and corrections – or in collaboration with these institutions. A number of strategies to curb youth aggression, violence and the opportunities that precipitate them had been attempted under this 'law enforcement' umbrella, with mixed results.

A common strategy is the prohibition or criminalisation of certain behaviours through the enactment of laws or regulations proscribing such behaviours. For example, the rush of awareness on school violence across the US since the early 1990s triggered by well-publicised shootings, ushered changes across the nation on laws regarding the carrying of concealed weapons and, particularly, the carrying of weapons (knives, cutters, handguns, etc.) on school grounds. Since the mid-1990s, many states have disallowed the carrying of weapons in schools, with provisions for expulsion among those violating these regulations, and/or provisions for criminal prosecution [39]. Indeed, aggression carries the potential for fatality or serious harm when weapons are available. Thus, the prohibition of carrying weapons, particularly handguns in schools seems like a reasonable response. This policy is bolstered by data that indicate a decrease in the prevalence of carrying weapons in schools and, more importantly, decrease in the occurrences of violence across schools in the US since the mid-1990s [36].

Another common strategy is in augmenting punishments for proscribed behaviours. Since the mid-1980s in the US, punishments for the felonious use and selling of illicit substances had been increasingly augmented to such degrees that by the late-1990s, it became clear among policymakers that this was the primary reason for dramatic increases in prison populations [40]. For the youth, perhaps one of the most common and oft-debated topic across the nation is the transfer of the prosecution of youthful offenders from juvenile courts (a more informal court proceeding) to adult trial courts [36]. Many states across the US have increasingly allowed the prosecution of young offenders (typically less than age 18 years, the age of majority in the US) in adult courts where they would often face more severe sanctions, instead of the juvenile courts. The juvenile courts are characterised by more informal proceedings where rehabilitation and not punishments are typically stressed. The general effects of these transferred prosecutions are yet to be determined, but law and justice scholars have lamented that this loss of focus on young offenders in favour of punishment severity is detrimental to the treatment of young offenders in the justice system.

A similar strategy called 'boot camps' has also been attempted and continues to be used for young offenders in many states. Boot camps are prison sanctions that take on the characteristic of a military boot-camp training where physical labour, calisthenics, and physical exertion are emphasised over typical prison routines [41]. These sanctions became popular in the early-1990s as a form of punishment that is both swift and severe [42]. Support for these modalities had been spearheaded by politicians and advocates of tough criminal sanctions, and momentum for its use was evident in the early- to mid-1990s when many states began adopting some form of boot-camp prisons for juveniles [42]. However, support for such modalities began to wane when a preponderance of evaluation results showed nil to negative effects on recidivism [41].

Regardless of the prevention technique or type of intervention, the goal of most law enforcement and punishment strategies is ultimately deterrence. It could be deterrence by those who are being punished so that they do not recommit offences (specific deterrence) or those who have not committed but have the capacity to commit crimes (general deterrence) so that they are discouraged from committing crimes for the fear of sanctions [43]. Across multiple studies on the effectiveness of deterrence, however, support for such measures is mixed. Nevertheless, nations and governments continue to rely heavily on law enforcement and punishment measures to curb criminal behaviour, including youth aggression and violence. Perhaps because this procedure is the most accessible and manipulable for many governments, one can expect continued reliance on law enforcement measures and punishments as the primary response to crime, violence and aggression. However, a nation attempting to begin law enforcement or punishment measures needs to be conscious of the extant and past practices in other nations to avoid repeating the errors committed by these nations.

Community/Situational Approaches

Based upon the premise that behaviours, particularly criminal activities are contextual and opportunistic, situational initiatives are typically designed to alter social contexts so as to prevent the occurrence of specific types of anti-social activities. This is done by reducing the opportunities, benefits and rewards, and increasing the risks for such activities. Situational prevention strategies range from simple 'target hardening' to the more sophisticated methods of deflecting offenders and reducing inducements for anti-social behaviours. Aggression in schools, for example, might be prevented by the presence of appropriate guardians who can provide supervision and monitor the activities of children in school settings that are typically ripe for intensive interactions and displays of emotion, e.g. classrooms, hallways, playgrounds, mess halls during lunches, breaks etc. Situational approaches also call for altering physical structures that promote or enhance opportunities for aggression. For example, to lessen opportunities for serious harm when confrontations within schools erupt, a small percentage of public schools in the US began using metal detectors or instituted random metal detector checks to discourage carrying of concealed weapons in schools [39].

The mobilisation of community organisations to build awareness and promote consolidated responses to violence and aggression is another integral part of the community/situational approach. This is particularly demonstrated in many domestic violence responses in the US, where community units such as hospitals, the police, neighbourhood and other civic organisations or schools are made aware of tell-tale signs of abuse (for children and adults) and the appropriate responses to suspected or even witnessed abusive events.

Developmental Approaches

Developmental approaches are designed to prevent the 'root causes' of aggression and violence in individuals by reducing risk factors associated with aggression, and increasing the protective factors. The latter are those that potentially decrease an individual's likelihood of engaging in a risk behaviour by either decreasing the level of risk experiences or moderating the relationship between risk and behaviour. These programmes are based upon numerous research evidence showing that risk factors experienced by individuals throughout their life course affect their beliefs, attitudes and, ultimately, behaviours. Early experiences, therefore, determine later behaviours. Developmental theories suggest that not only are some individuals more prone than others to engage in anti-social activities given similar situations, but that they are also more prone than others to place themselves in situations that favour anti-social activities. Research has consistently shown a strong correlation between aggression and early childhood behaviours like hyperactivity, restlessness, or mental health problems [17, 19]. Aggressive behaviour during childhood (6-13 year age group) has also been shown to consistently predict later violence among males, though research results for aggressive females are less consistent [44]. An early onset of aggression and delinquency is also associated with later acts of serious and chronic violence, as is the involvement in other forms of anti-social behaviours like substance use, stealing, the destruction of property etc. [17]. The developmental approach, therefore, examines the pathways for and progression of anti-social behaviours, as well as the appropriate behaviour for children at certain ages. This avoids inappropriately diagnosing or labelling children who display certain characteristics or display a particular profile as more aggressive or more prone than others for continued anti-social behaviours – a potentially detrimental label.

Developmental approaches generally attempt to prevent aggression and anti-social behaviours by working with children before problem behaviours manifest themselves. Three levels of approaches are often employed: primary and secondary prevention efforts, and the tertiary intervention level. Often, distinctions between primary and secondary efforts, as well as secondary and tertiary efforts can be fuzzy.

Primary prevention is the implementation of a programme that does not target any one person or place but is more population based. It is designed to address general problem behaviours before any of these behaviours take hold. For example, the Drug Abuse Resistance Education (DARE) is a primary prevention effort in the US. DARE does not target one particular person or school but is an education programme given to school children from fifth grade in both private and public schools throughout the country. DARE's basic objective is to raise awareness about the negative effects of illicit substance use, and to raise pro-social attitudes, coping skills and behaviours.

Secondary prevention programmes typically target particular people or places that have displayed certain risk factors or low levels of a given problem. Programmes in this area are designed to reduce the severity of the risk or prevent the risk from progressing to more serious forms or to anti-social behaviour patterns. Examples are programmes that target children of incarcerated parents, or of parents who are domestic combatants, or parenting training for low-income, single parents.

Tertiary interventions are programmes designed to address a particular problem that has already taken hold. These are usually conducted in clinics or residential facilities, such as in counselling and intensive residential treatments for substance abusers, or treatment for perpetrators of domestic violence.

Although a number of primary, secondary, and tertiary programmes have been implemented across the US and other countries, evaluations of many programmes show mixed results. Often, there are many limitations in terms of the target population, sufficient funding, getting cooperation and help across a number of stakeholders and entities that are centrally or marginally affected by the programme, the lack of sufficient follow-up period for research evaluations to detect significant changes in the behaviours of participants, and others. Practitioners and researchers agree, however, that multi-level and multi-faceted responses to aggression and violence are key to successful programmes.

Example Programmes

One programme each at the primary, secondary and tertiary level that has shown some promise in the US is outlined here. Descriptions of these programmes are excerpted from the Center for the Study and Prevention of Violence at the University of Colorado [45].

Primary Prevention: The PATHS Programme

The Promoting Alternative THinking Strategies (PATHS) curriculum is a comprehensive programme developed for use in the classroom setting for elementary school children. This curriculum is ideally initiated at the beginning of school and should continue through Grade 5. It is designed to promote emotional and social competencies to reduce aggression and other behaviour problems among the children, as well as enhance the educational process in the classroom [46]. Information and activities are also included for use by parents. PATHS lessons include labelling, expressing, assessing and managing feelings, controlling impulses, delayed gratification, and other lessons about self-awareness, communication, problem-solving and decision-making [46]. Teachers receive training in a two-to-three-day workshop and in bi-weekly meetings with a curriculum consultant [46]. The curriculum has been shown to reduce behavioural risk and improve protective factors such as improved self-control, thinking and planning skills, use of more effective conflict-resolution strategies, and other positive behaviours [46].

Secondary Prevention: Big Brothers Big Sisters of America

The Big Brothers Big Sisters of America (BBBSA) has been around for almost a century. The programme provides adult support and friendship to at-risk youth, typically from ages 6 to 18 years who belong to single parent homes. BBBSA adopts a case management approach, where service is delivered by volunteers but case managers screen applicants and create a match between applicants and volunteers. The volunteers interact and develop a one-on-one relationship with their matched youth. The relationship is terminated by case managers when eligibility requirements for either party are no longer met, or when either party can no longer fully participate in the relationship. Rigorous standards for screening applicants and volunteers are followed. Evaluation of the programme (after an 18 month period) showed that BBBSA youth were 46% less likely than a control group (non-participants) to initiate illicit drug use during the study period. The BBBSA youth were also 27% less likely to initiate alcohol use than the control group. Academic performance was also better for the participants, and they displayed higher quality relationships with their guardians/parents and peers [47].

Tertiary Intervention: Functional Family Therapy

Functional family therapy (FFT) is an outcome-driven prevention/intervention programme for youth of age 11 to 18 years who have demonstrated a range of maladaptive behaviours such as delinquency, violence, substance use, and a host of conduct disorders [48]. FFT emphasises factors that reduce risk and build protective mechanisms such as communication training, conflict-resolution strategies, building individual, family, and larger system relationships, technical aids for drug and alcohol use etc. To accomplish behavioural changes, FFT utilises a phasic approach, with each phase of the programme building upon the other [48]. A wide range of interventionists are utilised including mental health technicians, degreed mental health professionals, probation officers, and other para-professionals under supervision.

Clinical trials have demonstrated promising results. Among these, FFT has shown effective treatments of adolescents with a host of conduct disorders and drug abuse disorders, prevention of further occurrences of the problem, prevention of adolescent involvement with the criminal justice system, and built protection for younger children in the same families from a host of conduct disorders [48].

Conclusion

Drawing from existing research on youth aggression and violence, this chapter traces the multi-faceted definitions of and responses to youth aggression, a global phenomenon. Clearly, a holistic understanding of aggression encompasses individual, familial and community/environmental factors. Effective responses are those that seek to address the many facets of this behaviour. Biological, neurobiological and psychological sources of aggression are often insufficient explanations in and of themselves. Combined with social and community/environmental stressors, a more complete profile of consistently aggressive youth can be drawn. Consequently, prevention and intervention techniques can be outlined. The insufficiency of purely punitive measures in curbing youth aggression and violence has also been outlined. Several primary and secondary prevention efforts, as well as tertiary intervention strategies have returned positive outcomes.

Key Points

- Aggression and violence are common but are not inevitable parts of human life. Aggression by youth is tractable and techniques can be employed to prevent aggression and violence, or reduce their occurrence.
- Aggression does not often manifest as a singular behaviour problem, but is linked to multiple problem behaviours with multi-faceted source stressors.
- Individual risk factors interact with broader social, cultural and economic contexts. Thus, addressing aggression and violence across levels of the ecological model will have more sustained, widespread effects than any narrow, singular approach.

References

1. Krug, E.G., Dahlberg, L.L., Mercy, J.A., Zwi, A.B. and Lozano, R., 2002, *World Report on Violence and Health*, World Health Organisation, Geneva, Switzerland.
2. Baron, R.A. and Richardson, D.R., 1994, *Human Aggression*, Plenum Press (A division of Plenum Publishing Corporation), New York.
3. Connor, D.F., 2002, *Aggression and Antisocial Behavior in Children and Adolescents*, Guilford Press, New York.
4. Eron, L.D., Gentry, J.H. and Schlegel, P., 1994, *Reason to Hope: A Psychosocial Perspective on Violence and Youth*, American Psychological Association, Washington, D.C.
5. Loeber, R. and Schmaling, K., 1985, "Empirical Evidence for Overt and Covert Patterns of Antisocial Conduct Problems: A Meta-analysis", *Journal of Abnormal Child Psychology*, 13, pp. 337-352.
6. Achenbach, T.M., Conners, C., Quay, H., Verhulst, F. and Howell, C., 1989, "Replications of Empirically Derived Syndromes as a Basis for Taxonomy of Child/Adolescent Psycopathology", *Journal of Abnormal Child Psychology*, 17, pp. 299-323.

7. Fraser, M.W., 1996, "Aggressive Behavior in Childhood and Early Adolescence: An Ecological-developmental Perspective on Youth Violence", *Social Work*, 41(4), pp. 347-361.
8. Farrington, D. and Hawkins, J.D., 1991, "Predicting Participation, Early Onset and Later Persistence in Officially Recorded Offending", *Criminal Behavior and Mental Health*, 1(1), pp. 1-33.
9. Loeber, R. and Farrington, D.P., 2000, "Young Children Who Commit Crime: Epidemiology, Developmental Origins, Risk Factors, Early Interventions and Policy Implications", *Development and Psychopathology*, December, 12(4), pp. 737-762.
10. Moffitt, T.E., 1993, "Adolescent-limited and Life-course-persistent Antisocial Behavior: A Developmental Perspective", *Psychological Review*, 100, pp. 674-701.
11. Synder, J., Pichard, J., Schrepferman, L., Patrick, M.R. and Stoolmiler, M., 2004, "Child Impulsiveness-inattention, Early Peer Experiences, and the Development of Early Onset Conduct Problems", *Journal of Abnormal Child Psychology*, December, 32(6), pp. 579-594.
12. Bellinger, D., Leviton, A., Allred, E. and Rabinowitz, M., 1994, "Pre- and Post-natal Lead Exposure and Behavior Problems in School-aged Children", *Environmental Research*, 66, pp. 12-30.
13. Wasserman, G., Staghezza-Jaramillo, B., Shrout, P., Popovac, D. and Graziano, J., 1998, "The Effect of Lead Exposure on Behavior Problems in Preschool Children", *American Journal of Public Health*, 88, pp. 481-486.
14. Olson, H.C., Streissguth, A., Sampson, P. and Brookstein, F., 1998, "Neuropsychological Deficits in Adolescents with Fetal Alcohol Syndrome: Clinical Findings", *Alcoholism: Clinical and Experimental Research*, 22, pp. 1998-2012.
15. Chasnoff, I., Anson, A., Hatcher, R., Stenson, H., Iaukea, K. and Randolph, L., 1998, "Prenatal Exposure to Cocaine and Other Drugs: Outcome at Four to Six Years", *Annals of the New York Academy of Sciences*, 846, pp. 314-328.
16. Richardson, G., 1998, "Prenatal Cocaine Exposure: A Longitudinal Study of Development", *Annals of the New York Academy of Sciences*, 846, pp. 144-152.
17. Caspi, A. and Silva, P.A., 1995, "Temperamental Qualities at Age Three Predict Personality Traits in Young Adulthood: Longitudinal Evidence from a Birth Cohort", *Child Development*, 66, pp. 486-498.
18. Maziade, M., Caron, C., Cote, R., Merette, C., Bernier, H., Laplante, B. et al., 1990, "Psychiatric Status of Adolescents Who Had Extreme Temperaments at Age 7", *American Journal of Psychiatry*, 147, pp. 1531, 1536.
19. Hudley, C., Britsch, B., Wakefield, W.D., Smith, T., Demorat, M., Cho, S.-J., 1998, "An Attribution Retraining Program to Reduce Aggression in Elementary School Students", *Psychology in the Schools*, 35(3), p. 271.
20. Hudley, C. and Graham, S., 1993, "An Attributional Intervention to Reduce Peer-directed Aggression Among African-American Boys", *Child Development*, 64, pp. 124-138.
21. Crick, N. and Dodge, K., 1994, "A Review and Reformulation of Social Information-processing Mechanisms in Children's Social Adjustment", *Psychological Bulletin*, 115, pp. 74-101.
22. Coie, J., Dodge, K. and Kupersmidt, J., 1990, "Peer Group Behavior and Social Status", In *Peer Rejection in Childhood*, S. Asher and J. Coie (Eds.), Cambridge University Press, Cambridge, UK, pp. 17-59.
23. Schwartz, D., McFadyen-Ketchum, S., Dige, K., PEttit, G. and Bates, J., 1998, "Peer Group Victimisation as a Predictor of Children's Behavior Problems at Home and in School", *Developmental Psychopathology*, 10, pp. 87-99.
24. Rothbaum, F. and Weisz, J., 1994, "Parental Caregiving and Child Externalising Behavior in Nonclinical Samples: A Meta-analysis", *Psychological Bulletin*, 116, pp. 55-74.
25. Loeber, R. and Stouthamer-Loeber, M., 1986, "Family Factors as Correlates and Predictors of Juvenile Conduct Problems and Delinquency", In *Crime and Justice: A Review of the Research*, M. Tonry and N. Morris (Eds.), Vol. 7, The University of Chicago Press, Chicago, pp. 29-150.

26. Patterson, G., Reid, J. and Dishion, T., 1992, *Antisocial Boys*, Castalia, Eugene.
27. Maxfield, M.G. and Widom, C.S., 1996, "The Cycle of Violence: Revisited 6 Years Later", *Archives of Pediatrics and Adolescent Medicine*, April, 150, pp. 390-395.
28. Maxwell, C.D. and Maxwell, S.R., 2003, "Experiencing and Witnessing Familial Aggression and their Relationship to Aggressive Behaviors of Filipino Adolescents", *Journal of Interpersonal Violence*, December, 18(2), pp. 1432-1451.
29. Berkowitz, L., 1994, "Guns and Youth", In *Reason to Hope: A Psychosocial Perspective on Violence and Youth*, L.D. Eron, J.H. Gentry and P. Schlegal (Eds.), American Psychological Association, Washington, D.C., pp. 251-279.
30. Huesmann, L.R., Moise-Titus, J., Podolski, C.-L. and Eron, L., 2003, "Longitudinal Relations Between Children's Exposure to TV Violence and their Aggressive and Violent Behavior in Young Adulthood: 1977-1992", *Developmental Psychology*, 39(2), 201-221.
31. Cantor, J., 2000, "Media Violence", *Journal of Adolescent Health*, 27, pp. 30-34.
32. Attar, B.K., Guerra, N.G., Tolan, P.H., 1994, "Neighborhood Disadvantage, Stressful Life Events and Adjustments in Urban Elementary School Children", *Journal of Clinical Child Psychology*, 23, pp. 391-400.
33. Sampson, R.J., Morenoff, J.D., Gannon-Rowley, T., 2002, "Assessing "Neighborhood Effects": Social Processes and New Directions in Research", *Annual Review of Sociology*, Vol. 28, Annual Reviews, Palo Alto, pp. 443-478.
34. Hoffman, J.P., 2006, "Family Structure, Community Context and Adolescent Problem Behaviors", *Journal of Youth and Adolescence*, 35(6), p. 867.
35. Huesmann, L.R., Maxwell, C.D., Eron, L.D., Dahlberg, L.L., Guerra, N., Tolan, P. et al., 1996, "Evaluating a Cognitive/Ecological Program for the Prevention of Aggressive", *American Journal of Preventive Medicine*, 12(2 (Suppl.)), pp. 120-128.
36. Snyder, H.N. and Sickmund, M., 2006, *Juvenile Offenders and Victims: 2006 National Report*, U.S. Department of Justice, Office of Justice Programs, Office of Juvenile Justice and Delinquency Prevention, Washington, D.C.
37. Tonry, M. and Farrington, D.P., 1995, "Strategic Approaches to Crime Prevention", In *Building a Safer Society: Strategic Approaches to Crime Prevention*", M. Tonry and D.P. Farrington (Eds.), *Crime and Justice: A Review of Research*, The University of Chicago Press, Chicago, Vol. 19, pp. 1-20.
38. Sherman, L.W., Gottfredson, D., MacKenzie, D., Eck, J., Reuter, P., Bushway, S., 1997, "Preventing Crime: What Works, What Doesn't, What's Promising", *A Report to the United States Congress*, Prepared for the National Institute of Justice by Department of Criminology and Criminal Justice, University of Maryland, p. 416.
39. OJJDP, 1998a, *Annual Report on School Safety*, U.S. Department of Justice, Office of Justice Programs, Office of Juvenile Justice and Delinquency Prevention, Washington, D.C., NCJ 173934.
40. Woolredge, J., 1996, "A State-level Analysis of Sentencing Policies and Inmate Crowding in State Prisons: Research Note", *Crime and Delinquency*, July, 42(3), pp. 456-466.
41. MacKenzie, D.L., Brame, R., McDowall, D. and Souryal, C., 1995, "Boot Camp Prisons and Recidivism in Eight States", *Criminology*, August, 33(3), pp. 327-357.
42. Morash, M. and Rucker, L., 1990, "A Critical Look at the Idea of Boot Camp as a Correctional Reform", *Crime and Delinquency*, 36(2), pp. 204-224.
43. Antunes, G. and Hunt, A.L., 1978, "Certainty and Severity of Punishment", In *Justice and Corrections*, N.B. Johnston and L.D. Savitz (Eds.), John Wiley and Sons, New York, pp. 381-389. Reprinted from: 1973, "The Impact of Certainty and Severity of Punishment on Levels of Crime in American States: An Extended Analysis", *Journal of Criminal Law and Criminology*, Vol. 64, pp. 486-493.

44. Hawkins, D.J., Herrenkohl, T.I., Farrington, D.P., Brewer, D., Catalano, R.F., Harachi, T.W. et al., 2000, *Predictors of Youth Violence*, U.S. Department of Justice, Office of Justice Programs, Office of Juvenile Justice and Delinquency Prevention, Washington, D.C.
45. CSPV, 2006, *Blueprints of Violence Prevention*, www.colorado.edu/cspv/blueprints/model/overview.html
46. Greenberg, M., Kusche, C. and Mihalic, S., 1998, "Promoting Alternative Thinking Strategies (PATHS)", In *Blueprints for Violence Prevention Series*, D. Elliott (Ed.), Book Ten, Center for the Study and Prevention of Violence, Institute of Behavioral Science, University of Colorado, Colorado.
47. McGill, D., Mihalic, S. and Grotpeter, J., "Big Brothers Big Sisters of America", In *Blueprints for Violence Prevention Series*, D. Elliott (Ed.), Book Ten, Center for the Study and Prevention of Violence, Institute of Behavioral Science, University of Colorado, Colorado.
48. Alexander, J., Barton, C., Gordon, D., Grotpeter, J., Hansson, K., Harrison, R. et al., 1998, "Functional Family Therapy", In *Blueprints for Violence Prevention Series*, D. Elliott (Ed.), Book Three, Center for the Study and Prevention of Violence, Institute of Behavioral Science, University of Colorado, Colorado.

The AHA-Syndrome and Cardiovascular Diseases
Editors: Swati Y. Bhave and Sunil Saini
Copyright © 2010 Anamaya Publishers, New Delhi, India

7. Management of the AHA-Syndrome

Sunil Saini[1] and Sangeeta Trama[2]
[1]Department of Applied Psychology, Guru Jambheshwar University of Science and Technology Hisar - 125 001, India
[2]Department of Psychology, Punjabi University, Patiala - 147 002, India

Abstract: Anger, hostility and aggression are emerging as the major risk factors in many physiological and psychological problems. This article examines the various ways of dealing with components of the AHA-Syndrome, i.e. anger, hostility and aggression. The ill-effects of anger and aggressive feelings are cited. Intervention strategies on the part of family, teachers and individuals have been emphasised with empirical evidences.

Keywords: Anger, Hostility, Aggression management.

Introduction

Anger, hostility and aggression (AHA)-Syndrome is one of the major evils that people face today almost everywhere. There is increasing evidence that the AHA-Syndrome is the root cause of many health problems like marital conflict, family discord, divorce, abuse of elders, failure at school, workplace disruptions, job loss, traffic accidents, alcoholism, drug abuse, sexual aggression, rape, murder, terrorism and other physiological problems like blood pressure, hypertension, brain stroke, heart attacks, diabetes, respiratory problems, cancer etc. Day-by-day increasing incidences of robbery, kidnapping, assault, road rage, sexual crimes, war and terrorist activities all around the world, particularly among adolescents has put parents, school teachers and other social thinkers in a dilemma. Hence, it has become necessary to unfold the root causes of this growing epidemic and to manage it effectively. There are many AHA-Syndrome management techniques for a variety of situations, including family, school, public places, workplace etc. In this article, we focus on the management of the AHA-Syndrome at individual, family and school level.

Anger is a type of emotion that has specific characteristics like feelings of extreme displeasure, rage, frustration and hostility directed towards oneself or others. According to Spielberger [1] anger is "an emotional state that varies in intensity from mild irritation to intense fury and rage". Anger is expressed in different ways, i.e. directed inward, outward or controlling. The control of anger is the most effective way of anger expression. This article focusses on how anger and its associates, hostility and aggression, are managed in everyday life. Some people express anger by *displacing* it, i.e. taking it out on something/someone other than the one they are angry at, by kicking doors, blaming their spouses/children. Anger is probably the most poorly handled emotion in our society. Some common causes of anger are frustration, hurt, disappointment, harassment, annoyance and threats. Anger has been found to be related to frustration [2], driving anger [3], hostility [4], aggression [5], and crime [6]. Non-expressed anger can disrupt relationships, affect thinking patterns and cause various biological problems like heart disease, high blood pressure, digestive problems, etc. Anger is generally found to be at the core of aggression. Uncontrolled anger can cause various emotional and behavioural problems. It triggers aggression and violence. Due to the strong relation between the two, it is necessary to curb anger in order to control aggression.

Hostility is defined as an attitude that involves disliking others and evaluating them negatively [7]. Negative thoughts and feelings result in hostility. According to Spielberger et al. [4], hostility refers to a pervasive aggressive attitude that directs an individual to express anger through aggressive behaviour. Hostility shows itself in many ways, which include rage, negative and critical attitude, nagging, shouting, sarcasm, gossip, resentment, hatred, slamming doors, aggressive driving, and even criminality. Hostility results in anger and aggression if not controlled. Therefore, we see that hostility is the major factor behind anger and aggression. Thus, hostility management is of utmost importance to control anger and aggression.

Aggression is the intentional harming of another – characterised by verbal or physical attack. It may be driven by emotional arousal or it may be instrumental in securing a goal action intended to harm someone. It is a form of behaviour directed towards the goal of harming or injuring another living being who is motivated to avoid such treatment [8]. One needs to look around to understand the seriousness of the problem of aggression in today's society and also how it is affecting human potential in various fields. There is conflict all around us: at the family level (between parents, children, husband and wife, etc.); at the school level (between teachers and students, among teachers, among students, etc.); at the society level (among different groups) on various issues such as caste, religion, etc.; at the national level on various issues (between states like Haryana and Punjab, and Andhra Pradesh and Karnataka on water-related issues); at the international level (between countries like India and Pakistan, the United States and Iraq, Israel and Palestine etc.). All forms of conflict are causing a great loss of time, effort, money, as well as loss of life/property to humanity. All this has a common cause, i.e. aggression.

Anger, hostility and aggression hamper one's effectiveness in almost every situation. Some of the ill effects are ineffectiveness, loss of self-control, loss of peace of mind, disturbance of sense of equilibrium, inattentiveness, inability to concentrate, reduction in ability to think and reason, emotional outburst, hampering of communication, inadequate/inappropriate human relation skills, wastage of strength, loss of time, effort and energy, decreased output, inability to focus on the problem, job loss and disturbed relationships.

Due to these costs associated with the AHA-Syndrome, researchers have tried to identify various risk factors that increase the likelihood of anger, hostility and aggression among children and adults, i.e. individual characteristics, home environment, relations with peers, school failure, exposure to violence shown on media, community and societal factors. Hyperactivity, restlessness, risk-taking, poor social skills and certain beliefs and attitudes (e.g. the necessity of revenge) appear to favour the development of delinquent behaviour. Low income, inadequate education, high family stress, single parenthood, marital discord, maternal depression, and parental drug abuse are all factors that place children at particularly high risk of developing the AHA-Syndrome.

Inconsistent, critical, abusive, and disengaged parenting or teaching behaviour are also important risk factors for the development and maintenance of aggressive behaviour of children at home and in the classroom.

Therefore, it is necessary for the family members, school teachers, behavioural scientists and social workers to come forward and eradicate the root causes of the AHA-Syndrome, so that human potential may be enhanced for the betterment of society. Most importantly, there is a need to identify the level/context, which gives rise to the development of anger, hostility and aggression, and then delineate the ways in which these can be curbed, and healthy behavioural patterns can be encouraged. There are many factors that affect the development and progression of anger, hostility and aggression among children. This article discusses some important techniques of the AHA-Syndrome management at the family and school level and also for the individual.

Management of the AHA-Syndrome at the Family Level

Families are one of the most prominent groups in our culture. Parents can provide a marvelous environment of love and encouragement as well as arenas for anger, hostility and aggression. Nowadays, with the changing social practices, families are shrinking. More and more dual-income and nuclear families are coming up. Due to increased professional responsibilities and other problems such as differing views of parents, marital discord etc., and inappropriate communication between elders and children, families are becoming more disturbed. Anger experts are of the view that anger develops more often in the family in marital as well as parent-child relationships. Therefore, adequate parental training is very much required for healthy development of the child. Some important ways of managing the AHA-Syndrome at the family level are as follows:

Do Not Put Excessive Demand

Parents should not impose excessive demands on children. Children, especially elder ones, should have a say in decision making. Excessive demands can ruin their independence and capabilities, as well as make them more depressed and irritated, which can result in aggression. Goals set by an individual are more likely to be achieved instead of ones that have been imposed upon her/him. Therefore, children should be encouraged to think and take decisions according to their interests and capabilities.

Proper Parental Attention

Children of working parents are also likely to develop some deviant behaviours, including anger, hostility and aggression, because they may not get proper parental attention and guidance in everyday problems. Therefore, parents should exercise time management so that their work conditions do not cause them to ignore their child's well-being.

Do Not Argue/Conflict in Front of Children

Domestic violence is very common in families nowadays and directly affects youngsters. Children who are exposed to marital conflicts are more likely to exhibit anger, hostility and aggression. Hence, parents should not engage in quarrels/confrontation in front of their kids to prevent hampering the latter's emotional, cognitive, behavioural and overall development.

Public Awareness Programmes

In urban societies children face abuse and illtreatment, which adversely affects their personality development. Later on, it results in development of the AHA-Syndrome. Public awareness activities, advertisement and home visit programmes can help in reducing child abuse and other related maladies. Children should be encouraged to join community organisations/institutions to do social work and develop the habit of caring for others.

Respond to Initial Sign of Deviance

Children express their angry feelings by kicking, screaming, swearing, hitting or throwing things. They do not know other ways to express such feelings to attract parental attention. So parents must learn to respond to initial signs of deviance that a child shows, before the irritation worsens and relatively permanent inadequate behavioural patterns are formed.

Avoid Gender Discrimination

Family members must ensure that sons and daughters are praised equally for equal achievement. Children must be encouraged to voice their opinion sensibly and logically rather than resorting to temper tantrums, hitting etc. Do not expect your children to be reasonable at all times.

Develop Loving Relationships

Parents play an important role in reducing anger and aggression by raising children in a safe and loving domestic environment. Every child needs a strong, loving relationship with a parent/another adult to feel safe, secure and to develop a sense of trust. Those children whose parents are involved in their life are less likely to develop emotional (i.e. anger), cognitive (i.e. hostility) and behavioural problems (i.e. aggression). Warm and affectionate relationships with parents have been associated with children forming the ability to develop and maintain successful marriages, social friendships and relationships with their own children [9]. Thus, positive, warm and affectionate relationships should be fostered in parent-children relations for a healthy and prosperous life later on. Children should be taught the values of kindness, love, care, honesty and responsibility so that these values are inculcated right from childhood. These characteristics help in developing self-confidence, courage and inner strength that may later help in solving conflicting situations.

Do Not Encourage Anti-social Behaviour

At times, it is found that parents of anti-social children and youth do not discourage their behaviour. They consider it appropriate and normal. In this way, such children are given permission to be aggressive by their parents [10, 11]. Parents of such children should not be careless in this regard. They should talk to or admonish their kids when the initial anti-social behaviour is seen so that the children refrain from developing such behaviours.

Peer Relations

Peer relations play a very important role in young people's lives. Peers typically replace the family as the centre of a young person's socialising and leisure activities. Peers may influence each other to engage in anti-social behaviour [12]. Teenagers have multiple peer relationships and they confront multiple 'peer' cultures. Most often, peers reinforce family values, but they also have the potential to encourage negative behaviours. Peer pressure may encourage aggression, drug use, violence, delinquency, gangs, and failure at school. Therefore, adolescents require proper guidance. Parents (as well as teachers) should encourage healthy self-development of concept of self-worth in teenagers, and how they can resist peer pressure for indulging in maladaptive or risk behaviours (anger, hostility and aggression).

Accept Shortcomings in Children

Parents should teach children to live in the present and accept themselves as they are. When children accept their shortcomings, there may not be intense internal conflicts, which are the major causes of several problems.

Avoid Criticism

Pre-school children eagerly engage in new projects and activities. Failure and criticism can lead to feelings of guilt and frustration, which result in anger, hostility and aggression. Therefore, instead of criticism, positive enthusiasm and appreciation should be encouraged.

Management of the AHA-Syndrome at the School Level

The problem of the AHA-Syndrome is found to be very common in children. Anger, hostility and aggression are the most difficult feelings, attitudes and behaviours to manage for students. Teachers can help children in dealing with all the components of this syndrome constructively. Therefore, teachers' training is very important in implementing effective classroom management strategies in managing the AHA-Syndrome, and enhancing social and academic competence. Students often have trouble in accurately perceiving social situations, have misperception and misinterpretation, which provoke anger. The most important thing is how students feel, think and behave in a particular situation. Various strategies on the part of teachers are given as follows:

Behaviour Modification

Aggression is a learned behaviour. Theories of learning can be helpful in shaping appropriate behaviour in children. Behaviour modification techniques based on operant conditioning can be used to deal with aggression and its related behavioural problems like delinquency, smoking, drug abuse, alcoholism etc., which are commonly found predictors of aggression.

Develop Creativity

Healthy reading material should be encouraged during leisure time for the development of creativity and other cognitive abilities in children. Both parents and teachers can help in developing such habits in children.

Moral Education

Moral education should be part of the school curriculum. Early school experiences provide the base for the moral development of children. Therefore, sincere efforts should be made on the all-round development of children.

Develop More Recess Activities

Recess in school encourages all areas of development as children interact, use verbal and non-verbal communication, make decisions, solve problems, and deal with the emotional trials and tribulations of their interactions [13]. Hence, recess – now almost absent or rare – should be encouraged in schools to promote healthy social development in children.

Reward

Activities like best student for a noble cause/social work should be awarded and praised in schools so that other students could adopt such behaviour. Such programmes can boost positive attitudes among children.

Social Participation

Youth who belong to a socially appropriate group, which is sponsored and supported by the school (e.g. academic club or social organisation), are less likely to demonstrate aggression and violence [14]. Thus, children should be encouraged to join such groups/organisations.

Vocational Training

Vocational training that can provide job prospects to children in future should be encouraged. It can also lead to decrease in unemployment, which can otherwise turn children aggressive and resort to unlawful ways of earning money.

Programme for Poor Academic Performance

School failure often leads to aggression. Therefore, programmes should be made to handle problems faced by children due to poor academic performance and under-achievement. Children should be trained if they are not doing well academically. They can divert their potential to some other useful activities and in other fields where their potential can be effectively utilised.

School Environment

Unfavourable school environment, like cramped personal space for children, congested rooms, unplanned design of school layout, dark and/or dirty rooms, lack of play facilities etc., may also lead to the development of the AHA-Syndrome in children. It may lead to the development of frustration. So children should be sent to a properly organised school environment that provides adequate arrangements for diverse activities. Students often become the target of teacher politics. Therefore, a healthy inter-personal environment must be fostered in the educational institutions. Moreover, teachers must not carry their internal politics, vices and prejudices to the classrooms.

Teachers may use behaviour techniques, such as satiation, time-out and over-correction for adequately dealing with a student's aggressive behaviour. Teachers are also targets of hostility and aggression at school. Between 1995 and 1999, in the US, teachers were victims of 342,000 non-fatal crimes per year. In 1994, 12% of all elementary and secondary school teachers were threatened with injury by a student from their school [15]. Such acts should be punished strongly or such students may be debarred to set an example in the school so that others are afraid of following suit. Teachers must maintain a high profile in terms of behavioural expectations from the student and a message should be sent to the families that violence will not be tolerated.

Professional Health

A counselor or school psychologist should be present in every school to help children resolve their conflicts and counsel them to reduce their inclination toward the development of the AHA-Syndrome.

Finally, the programme for managing the AHA components should be a part of the curriculum. Goldstein's PREPARE curriculum is one of the best known packaged anger management programmes [16]. The first part of PREPARE lays emphasis on teaching skills and behaviours that are more appropriate than angry or aggressive response. The PREPARE curriculum outlines a number of steps that students can use to understand how they perceive the situation that made them angry and how to remind themselves to think through alternative ways to perceive that situation and control their anger.

Intervention Strategies for Extreme Forms of Anger, Hostility and Aggression

Extreme forms of aggression are a threat to humanity. These must be punished immediately so that it gets established in the mind of everyone that if one flouts norms and indulges in anti-social behaviour then punishment and even externment is unavoidable. Capital punishment too must be given in extreme cases when the offender repeatedly indulges in anti-social activities that may harm the victim physically/psychologically.

Government and social institutions must provide economically supporting programmes such as vocational training so that law offenders are able to support themselves in life later on. Proper counselling services along with health services must be provided to jail inmates and juvenile delinquents. Rehabilitation centres are required for offenders convicted for violent acts so that repetition of crimes does not take place [17]. The various intervention strategies are as follows:

Discipline Style

Meaning of life should be taught to children so that life's experiences become more meaningful to them. Inadequate discipline like lack of control, controversial demands, authoritarian attitude and over-possessiveness lead to behavioural problems in children, which is linked to aggression. These should be avoided.

Be Non-judgemental

Assess the situation before assuming that the "bad individual is at fault". Do not label individuals as good or bad since it affects their self-concept development. There may be subtle instigators that promote aggressive behaviour. Keep explanations as simple as possible. Cognitively impaired individuals may have problems with lengthy, complex conversations, and it can increase the potential for aggression.

Listen Carefully and Respond Properly

Communicate with an aggressor, listen to him/her, but make it clear that under no condition will physical aggression be tolerated. Communicate with the victim that there should not be any instigation on his/her part and that he/she should not take undue advantage of "being labelled as good".

Avoid Argument

Aggressive behaviours are mostly preceded by agitation. One should be aware of these early signs so that a right approach can be applied. Avoid arguments that can lead to aggression.

Do Not Remark

Shame results in aggression. People resort to violence when they think that they can wipe out shame by shaming others. It leads to aggression. Therefore, do not make such remarks or create situations that make someone feel ashamed and he/she decides to take revenge. A history of being victimised also leads to aggression later on. Therefore, victimised children/youth in a family or society should take professional help or join spiritual practices to resolve internal conflicts and to overcome the feelings of revenge.

Life Skill Training

Social competency skill curriculum such as life skills training (LST), which include stress management, problem solving, self-control and emotional intelligence reduce delinquency and substance abuse [18], and conduct related problems [19]. Young people who are able to manage their emotions and related behaviour are less likely to act aggressively [20] and more likely to act in socially competent ways [21].

Police Patrolling

Extra police patrolling in aggression-prone areas can also be helpful in controlling aggressive and violent acts [22].

Social Information Processing

Children with deficit social information processing react to social situations in maladaptive ways, such as representing or interpreting others' intentions as hostile even though the situation is ambiguous [23]. It is recognised as an integral component in the cause and maintenance of aggressive behaviour. Therefore, children should be guided to develop proper social information processing skills. Aggression is influenced by the ways in which children process information, interpret cues and utilise past experiences [24, 25]; all important parts of social reasoning. Therefore, social cognition intervention and early child rearing strategies like fostering socially competent behaviour can be very helpful in controlling aggression among children and the youth.

Intelligence

Low IQ is a known risk factor for crime and delinquency [26]. Goodman suggested some direct approach programmes to improve the self-esteem of children with low IQ. Various researchers, e.g. Giancola and Zeichner [27] have found that IQ and aggression are strongly linked even in non-criminal males.

Praise Children

Parents and teachers should praise children when the latter resolve their problems in constructive ways without resorting to violence. Children are more likely to repeat good behaviour when rewarded with attention and praise.

Avoid Punishment

Do not punish children. Hitting or slapping shows them the way to use similar behaviour with others to solve problems, and can encourage them to punish others in the same way as they were punished.

Keep Weapons Away from Children

Parents must make children aware of the dangers posed by firearms and other weapons if owned and/or used in the family. One should never store firearms where children can find them since it shows children the use of weapons in solving problems.

Do Not Blame Children

Do not blame and shame children as these actions may frighten and further isolate them, as well as make them more aggressive.

Regulate Emotions Properly

Both the aggressor and the victim need help. If the aggressor's emotions do not get addressed, it might further aggravate the situation and pent-up emotions can result in more aggressive and violent behaviour.

Sensation Seeking Personality

Sensation seeking is a prominent characteristic of adolescents that involves seeking novelty in behaviour. It is closely related to risky behaviour, such as drinking and smoking [28], drug use [29], and drunken driving [30]. Most of the college students are found to indulge in such risky behaviour. Therefore, we need programmes that can channelise their sensation seeking energy in constructive activities.

Impulse Control

Impulsiveness is a fundamental aspect of human personality. Impulsive people act on the spur of the moment and are unmindful of the consequences of their behaviour. People having difficulty in controlling their impulses may fall prey to many disruptive as well as risk taking behaviours like aggression, smoking, drinking, gambling etc. Behaviour modification, social skill training and psychologist's intervention can help in curbing such behaviour.

Avoid Noise

Crowds and loud noise also makes some people irritable, which turns into aggression. Therefore, travelling during rush-hour should be avoided. Noisy and quarrelsome neighbourhoods also force people to lose their peace. Therefore, such neighbours should be avoided.

Avoid Gang Membership

Gang membership also leads to aggression. Therefore, parents should keep a check on their children so that they do not fall prey to joining such gangs.

Right Displacement

Feelings of hostile aggression (act of harming others) should be displaced with instrumental aggression (act of obtaining or achieving something).

Parenting Style

Authoritarian parenting – high standards for proper behaviour, strict punishment in case of misconduct, low parent-child communication – should be replaced with authoritative parenting, i.e. parents set limits and provide guidance, but are willing to listen to the child's ideas and make compromises.

Beliefs

Studies have shown that children's exposure level to violence leads to changes in their belief about aggression, e.g. whether aggression is legitimate or not [31, 32]. It is also associated with increased aggression fantasy. Therefore, parents (at home) and teachers (at school) should resolve children's beliefs about violence so that such fantasies do not develop at a tender age.

Foster Positive Self-esteem

Low self-esteem also results in aggression. People strive to gain positive image of themselves. They do not have socially valued means to gain this image. So they organise their self-esteem around physical strength, power and superiority over others. Therefore, to avoid negative and low self-esteem, positive self-esteem should be fostered at school, college and family levels. Unrealistically high self-esteem paired with exposure to violence, a cognitive bias to attribute aggressive intent to others and an impulsive temperamental style may also lead to bullying behaviour [33]. Therefore, temperamental characteristics with a positive self-esteem in a realistic way should be developed in children by adopting proper intervention strategies.

Moral Development

Moral development plays an important role in behavioural regulation. Children begin to internalise moral values and standards early in life. If they imbibe bad experiences, chances are that they may develop some cues and schemas for such experiences. Therefore, moral values should be fostered in the children during early developmental stages.

Parental Monitoring

Poor parental monitoring is also linked with various behavioural problems including delinquency, risky sexual behaviour and lower academic achievement, in children [34]. Therefore, a great deal of work is required on the parts of parental monitoring.

Management of the AHA-Syndrome at Individual Level

1. Attack the *problem*, not the *person*.
2. Emphasise the *positive*, not the *negative*.
3. Do not let negative feelings accumulate over time.

4. Build bridges of positive communication so that negative emotions cannot have an effect. For instance, it is better to have husband and wife quarrelling, rather than a total unspoken relation where two partners 'exist' with a total breach of communication.
5. *Stop criticism* at any cost for a healthy and prosperous life. Criticism results in heated arguments, which then turn into aggression.
6. Express *positive feelings* just as one would express negative ones. It stops the development of negative emotions and hatred towards others.
7. Try to find solutions to problems in a cooperative and supportive manner, rather than engaging in fault-finding.
8. If there is a heated exchange between partners, peers or other relations with the intent to harm each other, one must stop immediately. This desire of harming another can result in serious relationship problems. Therefore, if one is hostile towards someone, the latter should calm down so that this phase passes out, and then discuss the problem.
9. Try to sort-out matters on a one-to-one basis.
10. Be assertive and tell others that what is bothering you about their behaviour.
11. Let an angry person 'cool down' and then discuss the situation rationally.
12. Understand the origin of anger and think what made you feel out of control and angry.
13. Develop empathy. The ability to empathise with others helps people in controlling anger, and is a hallmark of emotional maturity.
14. Think twice before saying something.
15. Think what will be achieved by saying or doing something inappropriate. (Does it resolve the problem?)
16. Recognise that all problems cannot be resolved immediately.
17. If you think you cannot control anger, try to change its frequency and intensity.
18. Sit back and analyse the situation neutrally without any emotional involvement. See others as playing their respective roles and analyse where things are going wrong.
19. Be simple, open and authentic.
20. Life is short; it is not to indulge in problems and solve mysteries. Live life in the true sense.
21. Recognise that *you* can be wrong.
22. Use a calm voice and gentle touch to calm down children.
23. Try the "Who Am I?" technique.
24. Admit mistakes and apologise when appropriate.
25. Use physical exercise like playing, running, or walking to divert attention and calming down.
26. Use muscular relaxation techniques to dissipate angry feelings.
27. Practice meditation in case one has an angry temperament.
28. Try to see a humorous serial/cartoon when angry. It puts our *red light* off.
29. Improve public awareness of effective intervention strategies.
30. Find sometime for yourself for being alone and do self-reflection.
31. Learn to trust others. By trusting others it is less likely that one would be angry with others.

Conclusion

It can be said that the problem of the AHA-Syndrome is evident in almost every aspect of life. It has a pervasive effect on one's life ranging from school to the workplace, family to peer relationships, and at all stages of life. It has cost a lot to human beings economically, biologically and psychologically, thereby reducing human potential in all fields. Since the costs of the AHA-Syndrome are clear, one must try to develop characteristics within oneself that can help in effectively dealing with such situations. At the same time, the aim should be to provide a healthy environment at home as well as the workplace, which fosters congenial attitudes and relations. Only then can one think of doing one's best, exploiting one's potential to the maximum possible so that one can be creative and productive in the true sense.

References

1. Spielberger, C.D., 1996, *Manual for the State-trait Anger Expression Inventory*, Psychological Assessment Resources, Odessa, Florida.
2. Berkowitz, L., 1962, *Aggression: A Social Psychological Analysis*, McGraw-Hill, New York.
3. Deffenbacher, J.L., Huff, M.E., Lynch, R.S., Oetting, E.R. and Salvatore, N.F., 2000, "Characteristics and Treatment of High Anger Drivers", *Journal of Counselling Psychology*, 47, pp. 5-17.
4. Spielberger, C.D., Jacobs, G., Russell, S. and Crane, R., 1983, "Assessment of Anger: The State-Trait Anger Scale (STAS)", In *Advances in Personality Assessment*, J.N. Butcher and C.D. Spielberger (Eds.), Lawrence Erlbaum Associates, Inc., New Jersey, pp. 2, 159-187.
5. Berkowitz, L., 1990, "On the Formation and Regulation of Anger and Aggression: A Cognitive Neo-associationistic Analysis", *American Psychologist*, 45, pp. 494-503.
6. Eaken, G.J., 2001, "State-trait Anger and Attributional Patterns Among Chronic and Violent Juvenile Offenders", *Dissertation Abstracts International*, 62, p. 2A.
7. Buss, A.H., 1961, *The Psychology of Aggression*, Wiley, New York.
8. Baron, R.A. and Richardson, D.R., 1994, *Human Aggression*, 2nd Ed., Plenum, New York.
9. Franz, C.E., McClelland, D.C. and Weinberger, J., 1991, "Childhood Antecedents of Conventional Social Accomplishment in Midlife Adults: A 36-year Prospective Study", *Journal of Personality and Social Psychology*, 60(4), pp. 586-595.
10. West, D. and Farrington, D.P., 1973, *Who Becomes Delinquent?* Heinemann, London.
11. Gottfredson, M.R. and Hirschi, T., 1990, *A General Theory of Crime*, Stanford University Press, California.
12. Keenan, K., Loeber, R. and Zhang, Q., 1995, "The Influence of Deviant Peers on the Development of Boys' Disruptive and Delinquent Behavior: A Temporal Analysis", *Development and Psychopathology*, 7, pp. 715-726.
13. Jambor, T., 1986, "Risk-taking Needs in Children: An Accommodating Play Environment", *Children's Environments Quarterly*, 3(4), pp. 22-25.
14. Catalano, R.F., Loeber, R. and McKinney, K.C., 1999, "School and Community Interventions to Prevent Serious and Violent Offending Juvenile", *Justice Bulletin*, pp. 1-12.
15. Kaufman, P., Chen, X., Choy, S.P., Peter, K., Ruddy, S.A., Miller, A.K., Fleury, J.K., Chandler, K.A., Planty, M.G. and Rand, M.R., 2001, "Indicators of School Crime and Safety", US Department of Education, Washington, D.C., NCES 2002-113/NCJ-190075.
16. Goldstein, A.D., 1999, *The PREPARE Curriculum (Revised Ed.)*, Research Press, Champaign, Illinois.
17. Andrews, D.A., Zinger, I., Hoge, R.D., Bonta, J., Gendreau, P. and Cullen, F.T., 1990, "Does Correctional Treatment Work? A Clinically Relevant and a Psychologically Informed Meta-analysis", *Criminology*, 28, pp. 369-404.
18. Botvin, G.J., Baker, E., Renick, N.L., Filazzola, A.D. and Botvin, E.M., 1984, "Cognitive Behavioral Substance Abuse Prevention", *Approach to Addictive Behaviors*, 9, pp. 137-147.

19. Greenberg, L. and Barling, J., 1999, "Predicting Employee Aggression Against Co-workers, Subordinates and Supervisors: The Roles of Person Behaviors and Perceived Workplace Factors", *Journal of Organisational Behavior*, 20, pp. 897-913.
20. Underwood, M.K., Coie, J.D. and Herbsman, C.R., 1992, "Display Roles for Anger and Aggression in School-age Children", *Child Development*, 63, pp. 366-380.
21. Eisenberg, N., Fabes, R., Shepard, S.A., Burphy, B.C., Guthrie, I.K., Jones, S., Friedman, J., Poulin, R. and Maszk, P., 1997, "Contemporaneous and Longitudinal Prediction of Children's Social Functioning from Regulation and Emotionality", *Child Development*, 68, pp. 642-664.
22. Koper, C., 1995, "Just Enough Police Presence: Reducing Crime and Disorderly Behavior by Optimizing Patrol Time in Crime Hot Spots", *Justice Quarterly*, 12, pp. 649-671.
23. Crick, N.R. and Dodge, K.A., 1994, "A Review and Reformulation of Social Information-processing Mechanisms in Children's Social Adjustment", *Psychological Bulletin*, 115, pp. 74-101.
24. Dodge, K.A. and Price, J.M., 1994, "On the Relation between Social Information Processing and Socially Competent Behavior in Early School-aged Children", *Child Development*, 65, pp. 1385-1397.
25. Huesmann, L.R. and Guerra, N.G., 1997, "Children's Normative Beliefs About Aggression and Aggressive Behavior", *Journal of Personality and Social Psychology*, 72, pp. 408-419.
26. Goodman, R., 1995, "The Relationship between Normal Variation in IQ and Common Childhood Psychopathology: A Clinical Study", *European Child and Adolescent Psychiatry*, 4, p. 3.
27. Giancola, P.R. and Zeichner, A., 1994, "Intellectual Ability and Aggressive Behavior in Non-clinical Non-forensic Males", *Journal of Psychopathology and Behavioral Assessment*, 16, p. 2.
28. Kraft, P. and Rise, J., 1994, "The Relationship between Sensation Seeking and Smoking, Alcohol Consumption and Sexual Behaviour Among Norwegian Adolescents", *Health Education Research*, 9, pp. 123-200.
29. Donohew, R.L., Hoyle, R.H., Clayton, R.R., Skinner, W.F., Colon, S.E. and Rice, R.E., 1999, "Sensation Seeking and Drug Use by Adolescents and their Friends: Models for Marijuana and Alcohol", *Journal of Studies on Alcohol*, 60(5), pp. 622-631.
30. Jonah, B., 1997, "Sensation Seeking and Risky Driving: A Review and Synthesis of the Literature", *Accident Analysis and Prevention*, 29, pp. 651-665.
31. Dodge, K.A. and Coie, J.D., 1987, "Social Information Processing Factors in Reactive and Proactive Aggression in Children's Peer Groups", *Journal of Personality and Social Psychology*, 53, pp. 1146-1158.
32. Slaby, R.G. and Guerra, N.G., 1988, "Cognitive Mediators of Aggression in Adolescent Offenders-I: Assessment", *Developmental Psychology*, 24, pp. 580-588.
33. Baumeister, R.F., Bushman, B.J. and Campbell, W.K., 2000, "Self-esteem", *Narcissism and Psychological Science*, 9, pp. 26-29.
34. Li, X., Feigelman, S. and Stanton, B., 2000, "Perceived Parental-child Relationships and Alcohol and Other Drug Use Among Teenagers in France and the United Kingdom", *Alcohol and Alcoholism*, 37(1), pp. 52-60.

The AHA-Syndrome and Cardiovascular Diseases
Editors: Swati Y. Bhave and Sunil Saini
Copyright © 2010 Anamaya Publishers, New Delhi, India

8. Anger, Hostility, Agonistic Behaviour and Coronary Heart Disease: A Biopsychosocial Synergistic Perspective

Randall S. Jorgensen and Kristin L. MacGregror
Department of Psychology and Center for Health and Behaviour, Syracuse University, Syracuse New York, USA

Abstract: Anger, hostility, and agonistic behaviour are implicated in stress related coronary heart disease (CHD). This chapter, firstly, gives an overview of the research concerning the association of CHD with anger and hostility, including reported inconsistencies. Then it discusses how a potential clustering of lifestyle as well as biological and interpersonal factors may underlie this association. The biological aspects relate to stress reactivity and immunity; the interpersonal aspects relate to conflict and loss of social support; and the lifestyle factors relate to diet, alcohol, obesity and smoking. Given the report of inconsistent findings and weak-to-modest associations, the traditional orientation of treating anger, hostility, or both as independent risk factors is problematic. In the end, the chapter argues for a biopsychosocial synergistic approach to studying anger, hostility and CHD.

Keywords: Anger, Hostility, Cardiovascular disease, Stress, Biopsychosocial.

Introduction

By causing one-third of the deaths globally, cardiovascular disease (CVD) ranks as the world's foremost cause of death [1]. Likewise, CVD is a major cause of a shorter lifespan, decreased quality of life, and economic burden [1, 2]. Given that at least one-third of all CVD is attributable to the five conventional risk factors of smoking, alcohol use, high blood pressure, high cholesterol and obesity [1], the psychosocial and stress related aspects of the CVD of coronary heart disease (CHD) has emerged as a significant area of inquiry, with a particular focus on anger and hostility [3]. Although trends exist, this area of research has yielded inconsistencies [4]. While discussing the covariation of CHD with anger and hostility, this chapter presents a biopsychosocial synergistic approach to the prediction of CHD.

William Harvey, in the 17th century, observed that cardiac activity is altered by either painful or pleasant emotions evoked by a "mental disturbance". Sir William Osler, in 1910, characterised cardiac patients as ambitious men who constantly overtaxed their body's machinery [5]. Due to the motivation of safeguarding social status and kinship, persons with high blood pressure of unknown origins (essential or primary hypertension), according to Alexander [6], are prone to a defensive inhibition of the cognitive and emotive aspects of anger while striving to avoid interpersonal conflict. With theoretical and methodological advances in medicine, physiology, psychology, and sociology, pre-scientific as well as 19th to 20th century speculations moved toward a rigorous examination of the scientific basis for the role of the experience, management and expression of anger and hostility in the development of CVD [7]. Recently, Korte et al. [8] discussed a Darwinian conceptualisation of behavioural strategies that are used widely in the animal kingdom to manage stressful social transactions. Briefly, 'hawks' show a preference for a fight-or-flight response when establishing a new territory or defending a current living domain, whereas 'doves' show a tendency to adapt to threat with caution, freezing and hiding. Based on their review of lab and ethological research of diverse animals (e.g. birds, rodents and primates), Korte et al. [8] conclude that hawks are more likely to be agonistic, aggressive, exhibit exaggerated sympathetic nervous system (SNS) hyperreactivity, CVD, and inflammatory disorders. While the hawk behavioural strategy is consistent with agonistic coronary prone behaviour (viz. high hostility and dispositional anger), the dove strategy is more in line with an avoidant management of social distress (e.g. denial, suppressed anger, defensive need for approval). In this chapter, we focus on the aspects of coronary prone behaviour characteristic of the hawk behavioural strategy.

As discussed by Smith et al. [9], anger relates to the tendency to experience this dysphoric emotion (ranging from annoyance and irritation to rage and fury), whereas hostility pertains to a cynical interpersonal outlook (distrust of others due to expectations of harmful social transactions) characterised by interpersonal conflict (e.g. argumentative, oppositional behaviour) as well as the desire to inflict harm or see others punished. Although inconsistent findings have been reported, a body of evidence supports the notion of relationships among anger, hostility and interpersonal conflict in the pathophysiology of stress related CVD [3, 9, 10]. We discuss the necessity of a biopsychosocial synergistic approach to the study of coronary prone agonistic reactions, i.e. the bi-directional links among biology, social and psychological factors, and lifestyle need to be addressed to increase the precision of prediction of CHD. We now overview fight-or-flight related stress reactivity.

Stress Reactivity

The involvement of the central nervous system (CNS) mediated SNS and neuroendococrine hyperreactivity in the pathophysiology of stress related CHD and, in general, CVD has been advanced for decades [11, 12]. This stress reactivity theory served as a heuristic for numerous inquiries into stress induced cardiovascular reactivity (CVR). As with the literature on hostility/ anger, attempts to longitudinally predict CVD from CVR has yielded mixed results. Nevertheless, in their review, Treiber et al. [13] concluded that "pre-clinical disease states" – defined as "pathogenic changes in CV structure or function that if continued, will often progress to overt manifestations of CVD, including MI and stroke" – were predicted from stress induced blood pressure (BP) reactivity. A report by Jennings et al. [14] replicated the prospective prediction of carotid atherosclerosis from BP reactivity. Likewise, Matthews et al. [15] showed systolic BP (SBP) reactivity to a videogame predicted coronary calcification after 13 years of follow-up. The link of CVR with neuroendocrine responses and possible vascular alterations has provided a theoretical base for the mechanisms associating CVR with CVD [12, 16, 17]. From a mechanical perspective, the increased blood flow turbulence and BP associated with frequent CVR bouts may contribute to arterial wall injury, thereby fostering such atherosclerotic processes as platelet adherence, smooth muscle wall proliferation, connective tissue formation, lipid accumulation, thrombosis, and calcification. Frequent bouts of associated stress evoked neuroendocrine activity (e.g. cortisol and catecholamine release) can augment lipoprotein metabolism and release of free fatty acids, elevate plasma glucose and circulating insulin levels, increase vascular constriction, and increase arteriolar as well as venous tone. Hyperlipidemia related to both diet and stress can impede arterial wall healing, thereby hastening development of atherosclerosis. Thus, a matrix of mechanical, CNS, SNS and neuroendocrine factors may link stress induced CVR to CVD and CHD, in particular [11, 16].

In their quantitative of review of trait hostility and CVR, Suls and Wan [18] concluded that the CVR hypothesis provides an incomplete explanation for the hostility and CVD correlation. Further, when stressors were categorised as "provocative vs. non-provocative", trait hostility correlated only with diastolic BP (DBP) reactivity induced by the provocative stressors. Subsequent research has shown results consistent with this person by situation interaction [19-21]. In addition to the high CVR of high trait hostility people being triggered only by the anagrams task with experimenter harassment, Suarez et al. [20] reported catecholamine, cortisol and testosterone reactivity for high trait hostility people in the harassment condition. However, other contextual factors (e.g. a public speaking task with evaluative threat having either a friendly or unfriendly experimenter manipulation) may obscure the emergence of this interaction [9].

Studies of ambulatory BP monitoring (ABPM) provide some evidence for the external validity of the above lab studies. A quantitative review by Schum et al. [22] showed trait anger measures to manifest a small but statistically significant effect for systolic BP. Thomas et al. [23] showed that hostility and anger correlate negatively with nocturnal BP dipping, a marker for CVD and end-organ damage. For a group of urban youth, Ewart and Jorgensen [24] showed an association of high DBP during social transactions with a profile of high agonistic striving (e.g. vigilance for potential harm from others, revenge for perceived harm, low affiliative striving, and pressured, emotional speech). Likewise, Brondolo et al. [25] reported that diastolic BP elevations evoked by negative social interactions were highest for high hostile participants.

Atherosclerosis is thought to reflect a chronic infectious disease [26, 27]. Kop [28] theorises that the chronic condition of dispositional hostility triggers acute stress reactions (e.g. angry reactions) and episodic stress reactions (e.g. depressed mood and exhaustion), linked to alterations of immune functioning (e.g. immune suppression, susceptibility to infection, phagocytosis, pro-inflammatory cytokines), which are conducive to atherogenesis. Low density lipoproteins (LDL) and hypertension can stimulate inflammatory responses [26, 27]. C-reactive protein, a marker of inflammation and risk for cardiovascular disease, has been correlated with an adverse lipid profile in children [29]. Further, cynical hostility has been correlated with elevated levels of LDL [20, 30]. For a marker of inflammatory status (the cytokine of interlukin-6), Suarez [31] showed high levels to be associated with high cynical hostility and high levels of depressed symptoms. Miller et al. [32] found that high interlukin-6 levels covary with high cynical hostility but low reports of depressed mood. In discussing the different pattern found by Miller et al. [32] and Suarez [31], the former suggested that the latter study's use of only male, non-smokers and the former study's use of a clinical sample could contribute to the observed discrepancy.

Interpersonal Relationships

Significant interpersonal relationships and social support have been shown to exert a stress buffering effect and relate to longevity [33]. However, hostility is thought to weaken this buffer [9]. The combined effects of hostility and strivings to dominate others are likely to be met with resistance by the other party. This resistance can trigger the interpersonal conflict commonly reported by hostile individuals. Accordingly, hostile people report lower levels of social support from friends, spouses and co-workers, i.e. high hostile people evoke conflict and, therefore, alienate those who would normally be providing social support [9].

Interpersonal conflict and low levels of social support also correlate with increased CVR, which could contribute to the development of CHD [34]. Studies have shown that the attempt to influence others has been associated with increased CVR [9]. Further, couples experiencing marital conflict involving hostile communications also show heightened CVR [35-37]. In short, stressful relationships can cause both stress reactivity and decreased social support – two factors that can lead to the development of CHD. Because of the complex nature of the interactions and the potential mediating effects of these psychological, interpersonal and biological factors, the investigation of bi-directional and interactive paths characteristic of biopsychosocial synergistic models is warranted.

Lifestyle

Hostility and related traits seem to be correlated with some of the major risk factors of CHD. As discussed now, these risk factors include high cholesterol, obesity, alcohol intake and smoking.

Diet

High cholesterol and obesity are two major CHD risk factors influenced by diet. According to the US Food and Drug Administration [38], in order to reduce the risk of developing CHD and related diseases, people should avoid foods high in fat (viz. saturated fat and trans fatty acids) and consume high amounts of fruits, vegetables and whole grains. Because diet contributes to CVD, diet could be a factor contributing to the apparent relationship between anger, hostility and aggression, and the development of CHD. Studies have shown a significant relationship between eating habits and hostility and related traits [39-41].

With a representative sample, relationships have been demonstrated between hostility and continued eating even when full [39]. This finding is of interest because, across the lifespan, continued eating following satiation can foster obesity later in life. However, this relationship was decreased following adjustment for other risks such as age, relationship status, exercise, smoking, and alcohol consumption. These results are consistent with biopsychosocial synergy; namely, hostility/anger and aggression likely relate to CVD through bi-directional linkages with a clustering of risk factors.

Hostility and the consumption of n-3 fatty acids have been examined. N-3 fatty acids are thought to serve a protective role in CVD [42]. Interestingly, the consumption of these fatty acids was associated with reduced levels of hostility in young adults [40]. Moreover, this relationship remained significant even after adjusting for traditional risk factors. The researchers concluded that n-3 fatty acid intake is associated with lower hostility, and that hostility could potentially mediate the relationship between these acids and cardiovascular disease. If others replicate these findings, incorporating n-3 fatty acids into the diet via more fish intake may contribute to lower hostility, which can lead to reduction in CHD risk. However, prevention may be more difficult if modification of eating habits is dependent on alteration of personality traits such as hostility. The complex interaction between these variables is not well understood and, therefore, warrants further investigation.

Multivitamin intake is another lifestyle habit of importance. In a sample of men, the relationship between plasma interleukin-6 and coronary risk factors was examined [43]. Higher levels of interleukin-6 are associated with increased risk of heart disease [44]. Results showed that taking a multi-vitamin daily significantly decreased this marker of immune functioning. Given associations suggesting links among CHD, hostility, anger and altered immune functioning, this finding is consistent with the notion of altering dietary habits to reduce the risk for CHD among angry, hostile people. Again, research is needed to investigate whether diet, including multi-vitamin intake, can buffer the CHD risk conferred by hostility/anger in both men and women.

Alcohol

It has also been determined that the relationship between alcohol consumption and CVD risk occurs in a U- or J-shaped relationship [45, 46]. The implications of this relationship are three-fold:

(i) Excessive drinkers are at a heightened risk for developing CHD.
(ii) Non-drinkers also appear to be at an increased risk for developing CVD.
(ii) Light-to-moderate drinking may lower risk of CHD development and, thus, serve as a protective factor.

While the definitions vary a bit, moderate drinking is generally defined in the research context as less than 1.05 ounces (30 g) of ethanol per day [46], whereas heavy drinking has been defined as anything above this amount. It is noteworthy that this definition of a heavy drinker places someone consuming three drinks per day in the same category as someone consuming 15 drinks per day. Also, note that the mechanisms underlying this association are unclear. Alcohol-related changes in serum lipids, lipoproteins, platelets, blood clotting proteins, insulin resistance and inflammatory cytokines have been discussed as possible underlying mechanisms [46].

Interestingly, heavy drinking, specifically intoxication, has also been demonstrated to be related to hostile and aggressive behaviour [47]. However, there seems to be some gender differences in these results; intoxicated men, in general, seem to show more aggressive behaviour than intoxicated women. Regarding interpersonal relationships and mood, young adults with less intimate and supportive friendships have been reported to drink more excessively after episodes of hostility and sadness [48]; such episodes of heavy drinking and negative mood were repeated a week later. These results are consistent with the notion of alcohol consumption being associated with hostility emanating from unsatisfying personal relationship, i.e. given the tendency to experience more hostility and interpersonal conflict, it seems reasonable to expect that high trait hostile/anger and aggressive people may drink as a means of dealing with the ill-will, anger, dissatisfaction and depressed mood related to poor social relationships. These possible connections, if verified and replicated across different populations, have important implications. Namely, given that drinking and hostility have been associated with heightened risk for CVD, cyclic connections of trait hostility/anger with unsatisfying personal relationships, agonistic reactions (anger, aggressive behaviour, resentment) and drinking could exacerbate CVD risk beyond the individual risk imposed by drinking or coronary prone traits alone. Again, more research on the linkages among anger, hostility, aggression and alcohol in the prevention and treatment of CHD is warranted.

Smoking

Smoking has been demonstrated to be a significant risk factor for many chronic diseases, including CHD and CVD in general. Therefore, it is important to understand the characteristics of smokers, both those who begin smoking and those who quit. Personality traits have often been investigated as they relate to the above smoking characteristics, including hostility. High levels of hostility have been associated with both current smoking behaviour and smoking initiation [49]. This evidence suggests that smoking could serve as a potential mediator between hostile characteristics and CHD development. Further, and perhaps more important to the prevention of CHD, smoking cessation has been related to lower hostility scores [50]. Perhaps, interventions taking into account both the smoking behaviour and the characteristics of the smoker could increase the likelihood of smoking cessation. Nevertheless, changing hedonistic habits – to the extent that such habits as smoking, drinking and eating reflect stable patterns of personality – could be quite resistant to alteration in high trait hostility/anger and aggressive people who are resistant to changing their hostile outlook.

Conclusions

Although anger and hostility are implicated in stress related CVD, this area of research is marked by inconsistency. A number of factors contribute to this state of affairs. Firstly, the simplistic approach of correlating a measure of hostility/anger with CVD assumes that the measure contains all the cognitive, affective and behavioural information necessary to predict stress related CVD. Likewise, the different measures of hostility and anger (e.g. interview vs. self-report) deployed across studies do not measure the same construct [3], thereby contributing a source of variation that may interact with variations in design (e.g. longitudinal study of persons without diagnosed CHD vs. the case-control study of persons with diagnosed CHD, samples varying in cultural and demographic characteristics etc.), i.e. the evanescent nature of this association likely varies with variations in assessment and design. Moreover, diatheses of lifestyle (diet, smoking and drinking), quality of social relations (an extended, supportive social network vs. social isolation) and biology (e.g. familial history of CVD linked to a tendency for stress induced psychoneuroimmunological and hemodynamic reactivity) are likely to buffer or augment the covariation of anger and hostility with CVD. Consequently, in line with Williams et al. [51], we conclude that as long as anger, hostility and agonistic behaviour utilise an independent risk factor approach in lieu of a biopsychosocial synergistic perspective, the linkages of hostility, anger, and aggression to CVD will be obscured, along with the development of strategies for prevention and treatment.

Key Points

- ❑ Consistent with the caveats of Williams et al. [51], attempts to examine hostility, anger and agonistic behaviour as independent risk factors are likely to perpetuate imprecise prediction and inconsistent findings.

- Consistent with the available literature [11, 51, 52], we propose that biopsychosocial synergistic models of hostility, anger and agonistic behaviour be examined for the profiling of CVD risk and developing strategies for prevention and treatment.
- In both cross-sectional and prospective studies, investigation of bi-directional causal linkages among genetic diatheses (e.g. CVD family history), biological factors (e.g. impaired LDL clearance, CNS mediated CVR, neuroendocrine reactivity and immune function), environmental stressors (e.g. interpersonal conflict at work, home, or both), and lifestyle (e.g. excessive drinking and smoking, little exercise, and high fat diet low in vegetables, fruits and vitamins) is necessary to accurately identify the means by which markers of agonistic, coronary-prone personal characteristics augment the risk for CVD and CHD, in particular.

References

1. Mackay, J. and Mensah, G. (Eds.), 2004, *The Atlas of Heart Disease and Stroke*, World Health Organisation, Geneva, Switzerland.
2. AHA, 2003, *Heart Disease and Stroke Statistics: 2004 Update*, American Heart Association, USA.
3. Dembroski, T.M. and Costa, P.T., Jr., 1987, "Coronary Prone Behavior: Components of the Type A Pattern and Hostility", *Journal of Personality*, 55(2), pp. 211-235.
4. Miller, T.Q., Smith, T.W., Turner, C.W., Guijarro, M.L. and Hallet, A.J., 1996, "A Meta-analytic Review of Research on Hostility and Physical Health", *Psychol Bull.*, 119(2), pp. 322-348.
5. Williams, R.B. and Barefoot, J.C., 1988, "Coronary-prone Behavior: The Emerging Role of the Hostility Complex", In *Type A Behavior Pattern: Research, Theory and Intervention*, B.K. Houston and C.R. Snyder (Eds.), Wiley, New York, pp. 189-211.
6. Alexander, F., 1939, "Emotional Factors in Essential Hypertension", *Psychosomatic Medicine*, 1, pp. 175-179.
7. Jorgensen, R.S. and Thibodeau, R., 2006, "Defensive Hostility and Cardiovascular Disease: Theoretical and Empirical Basis for an Interpersonal Approach-avoidance Conflict Perspective", In *Clinical Psychology and Heart Disease*, E. Molinari, A. Compare and G. Parati (Eds.), Springer, Milan, Italy, pp. 217-232.
8. Korte, S.M., Koolhaas, J.M., Wingfield, J.C. and McEwen, B.S., 2005, "The Darwinian Concept of Stress: Benefits of Allostasis and Costs of Allostatic Load and the Trade-offs in Health and Disease", *Neuroscience and Biobehavioral Review*, 29(1), pp. 3-38.
9. Smith, T.W., Glazer, K., Ruiz, J.M. and Gallo, L.C., 2004, "Hostility, Anger, Aggressiveness and Coronary Heart Disease: An Interpersonal Perspective on Personality, Emotion and Health", *Journal of Personality*, 72(6), pp. 1217-1270.
10. Jorgensen, R.S., Johnson, B.T., Kolodziej, M.E. and Schreer, G.E., 1996, "Elevated Blood Pressure and Personality: A Meta-analytic Review", *Psychological Bulletin*, 120, pp. 293-320.
11. Lovallo, W.R., 2005, "Cardiovascular Reactivity: Mechanisms and Pathways to Cardiovascular Disease", *Int. J. Psychophysiol.*, 58(2-3), pp. 119-132.
12. Rozanski, A., Blumenthal, J.A. and Kaplan, J., 1999, "Impact of Psychological Factors on the Pathogenesis of Cardiovascular Disease and Implications for Therapy", *Circulation*, 99(16), pp. 2192- 2217.
13. Treiber, F.A., Kamarck, T., Schneiderman, N., Sheffield, D., Kapuku, G. and Taylor, T., 2003, "Cardiovascular Reactivity and Development of Preclinical and Clinical Disease", *Psychosomatic Medicine*, 65, pp. 46-62.
14. Jennings, J.R., Kamarck, T.W., Everson-Rose, S.A., Kaplan, G.A., Manuck, S.B. and Salonen, J.T., 2004, "Exaggerated Blood Pressure Responses During Mental Stress are Prospectively Related

to Enhanced Carotid Atherosclerosis in Middle-aged Finnish Men", *Circulation*, 110(15), pp. 2198-2203.

15. Matthews, K.A., Zhu, S., Tucker, D.C. and Whooley, M.A., 2006, "Blood Pressure Reactivity to Psychological Stress and Coronary Calcification in the Coronary Artery Risk Development in Young Adults Study", *Hypertension*, 47(3), pp. 391-395.
16. Herd, J.A., 1984, "Cardiovascular Disease and Hypertension", In *Handbook of Behavioral Medicine*, W.D. Gentry (Ed.), Guilford, New York, pp. 222-281.
17. Herd, J.A., 1991, "Cardiovascular Response to Stress", *Physiological Review*, 71(1), pp. 305-330.
18. Suls, J. and Wan, C.K., 1993, "The Relationship between Trait Hostility and Cardiovascular Reactivity: A Quantitative Review and Analysis", *Psychophysiology*, 30(6), pp. 615-626.
19. Miller, S.B., Friese, M., Dolgoy, L., Sita, A., Lavoie, K. and Campbell, T., 1998, "Hostility, Sodium Consumption and Cardiovascular Response to Interpersonal Stress", *Psychosomatic Medicine*, 60(1), pp. 71-77.
20. Suarez, E.C., Kuhn, C.M., Schanberg, S.M., Williams, R.B., Jr. and Zimmermann, E.A., 1998, "Neuroendocrine, Cardiovascular and Emotional Responses of Hostile Men: The Role of Interpersonal Challenge", *Psychosomatic Medicine*, 60(1), pp. 78-88.
21. Smith, B.D., Cranford, D. and Green, L., 2001, "Hostility and Caffeine: Cardiovascular Effects During Stress and Recovery", *Personality and Individual Differences*, 30(7), pp. 1125-1137.
22. Schum, J.L., Jorgensen, R.S., Verhaeghen, P., Sauro, M. and Thibodeau, R., 2003, "Trait Anger, Anger Expression and Ambulatory Blood Pressure: A Meta-analytic Review", *J. Behav. Med.*, 26(5), pp. 395-415.
23. Thomas, K.S., Nelesen, R.A. and Dimsdale, J.E., 2004, "Relationships between Hostility, Anger Expression and Blood Pressure Dipping in an Ethnically Diverse Sample", *Psychosomatic Medicine*, 66(3), pp. 298-304.
24. Ewart, C.K. and Jorgensen, R.S., 2004, "Agonistic Interpersonal Striving: Social Cognitive Mechanism of Cardiovascular Risk in Youth", *Health Psychology*, 23, pp. 75-85.
25. Brondolo, E., Rieppi, R., Erickson, S.A., Bagiella, E., Shapiro, P.A., McKinley, P. et al., 2003, "Hostility, Interpersonal Interactions and Ambulatory Blood Pressure", *Psychosomatic Medicine*, 65(6), pp. 1003-1011.
26. Fahdi, I.E., Gaddam, V., Garza, L., Romeo, F. and Mehta, J.L., 2003, "Inflammation, Infection and Atherosclerosis", *Brain Behaviour and Immunity*, 17(4), pp. 238-244.
27. Ross, R., 1999, "Atherosclerosis: An Inflammatory Disease", *New England Journal of Medicine*, 340(2), pp. 115-126.
28. Kop, W.J., 2003, "The Integration of Cardiovascular Behavioral Medicine and Psychoneuroimmunology: New Developments based on Converging Research Fields", *Brain Behav. Immun.*, 17(4), pp. 233-237.
29. Wu, D.M., Chu, N.F., Shen, M.H. and Chang, J.B., 2003, "Plasma c-reactive Protein Levels and their Relationship to Anthropometric and Lipid Characteristics Among Children", *Journal of Clinical Epidemiology*, 56(1), pp. 94-100.
30. Brindley, D.N., McCann, B.S., Niaura, R., Stoney, C.M. and Suarez, E.C., 1993, "Stress and Lipoprotein Metabolism: Modulators and Mechanisms", *Metabolism*, 42(9 Suppl. 1), pp. 3-15.
31. Suarez, E.C., 2003, "Joint Effect of Hostility and Severity of Depressive Symptoms on Plasma Interleukin-6 Concentration", *Psychosomatic Medicine*, 65(4), pp. 523-527.
32. Miller, G.E., Freedland, K.E., Carney, R.M., Stetler, C.A. and Banks, W.A., 2003, "Cynical Hostility, Depressive Symptoms and the Expression of Inflammatory Risk Markers for Coronary Heart Disease", *Journal of Behavioral Medicine*, 26(6), pp. 501-515.
33. Berkman, L.F., Glass, T., Brissette, I. and Seeman, T.E., 2000, "From Social Integration to Health: Durkheim in the New Millennium", *Social Science Medicine*, 51(6), pp. 843-857.

34. Kamarck, T.W., Peterman, A.H. and Raynor, D.A., 1998, "The Effects of the Social Environment on Stress-related Cardiovascular Activation: Current Findings, Prospects and Implications", *Annals of Behavioral Medicine*, 20(4), pp. 247-256.
35. Ewart, C.K., Taylor, C.B., Kraemer, H.C. and Agras, W.S., 1991, "High Blood Pressure and Marital Discord: Not Being Nasty Matters More than Being Nice", *Health Psychology*, 10(3), pp. 155-163.
36. Smith, T.W. and Brown, P.C., 1991, "Cynical Hostility, Attempts to Exert Social Control and Cardiovascular Reactivity in Married Couples", *Journal of Behavioral Medicine*, 14(6), pp. 581-592.
37. Smith, T.W. and Gallo, L.C., 1999, "Hostility and Cardiovascular Reactivity During Marital Interaction", *Psychosomatic Medicine*, 61(4), pp. 436-445.
38. USFDA, 2006, US Food and Drug Administration, Cited 20 July 2006, available at *www.fda.gov*
39. van den Bree, M.B.M., Przybeck, T.R. and Cloninger, C.R., 2006, "Diet and Personality: Associations in a Population-based Sample", *Appetite*, 46, pp. 177-188.
40. Iribarren, C., Markovitz, J.H., Jacobs, D.R., Jr., Schreiner, P.J., Daviglus, M. and Hibbeln, J.R., 2004, Dietary Intake of n-3, n-6 Fatty Acids and Fish: Relationship with Hostility in Young Adults – The CARDIA Study", *European Journal of Clinical Nutrition*, 58, pp. 24-31.
41. Milligan, R.A., Burke, V., Beilin, L.J., Richards, J., Dunbar, D., Spencer, M. et al., 1997, "Health-related Behaviours and Psycho-social Characteristics of 18 year-old Australians", *Social Science and Medicine*, 45(10), pp. 1549-1562.
42. Hallgren, C.G., Hallmans, G., Jansson, J.H., Marklund, S.L., Huhtasaari, F., Schutz, A. et al., 2000, "Markers of High Fish Intake are Associated with Decreased Risk of a First Myocardial Infarction", *British Journal of Nutrition*, 86, pp. 397-404.
43. Suarez, E.C., 2003, "Plasma Interleukin-6 is Associated with Psychological Coronary Risk Factors: Moderation by Use of Multivitamin Supplements", *Brain, Behavior and Immunity*, 17, pp. 296-303.
44. Ridker, P.M., Rifai, N., Stampfer, M.J. and Hennekens, C.H., 2000, "Plasma Concentration of Interleukin-6 and the Risk of Future Myocardial Infarction Among Apparently Healthy Men", *Circulation*, 101, pp. 1767-1772.
45. Beilin, L., 2005, "Alcohol and Hypertension: Balancing the Risks and Benefits", *Journal of Hypertension*, 23, pp. 1953-1955.
46. Lucas, D.L., Brown, R.A., Wassef, M. and Giles, T.D., 2005, "Alcohol and the Cardiovascular System: Research Challenges and Opportunities", *Journal of the American College of Cardiology*, 45(12), pp. 1916-1924.
47. Ogle, R.L., Miller, W.R., 2004, "The Effects of Alcohol Intoxication and Gender on the Social Information Processing of Hostile Provocations Involving Male and Female Provocateurs", *Journal of Studies on Alcohol*, 65, pp. 54-62.
48. Hussong, A.M., Hicks, R.E., Levy, S.A. and Curran, P.J., 2001, "Specifying the Relations between Affect and Heavy Alcohol Use Among Young Adults", *Journal of Abnormal Psychology*, 110(3), pp. 449-461.
49. Jeanne, A., van Loone, M., Tijhuis, M., Surtees, P.G. and Ormel, J., 2005, "Determinants of Smoking Status: Cross-sectional Data on Smoking Initiation and Cessation", *European Journal of Public Health*, 15(3), pp. 256-261.
50. Lipkus, I.M., Barefoot, J.C., Williams, R.B. and Siegler, I.C., 1994, "Personality Measures as Predictors of Smoking Initiation and Cessation in the UNC Alumni Heart Study", *Health Psychology*, 13, pp. 149-155.
51. Williams, R.B., Barefoot, J.C. and Schneiderman, N., 2003, "Psychosocial Risk Factors for Cardiovascular Disease: More than One Culprit at Work", *Journal of the American Medical Association*, 290(16), pp. 2190-2202.
52. Belardinelli, R., 2005, "The Whole is Greater than its Parts", *European Heart Journal*, 26(18), pp. 1820-1821.

The AHA-Syndrome and Cardiovascular Diseases
Editors: Swati Y. Bhave and Sunil Saini
Copyright © 2010 Anamaya Publishers, New Delhi, India

9. Hostility and Aggression in the Marital Relationship: Links to Children's Cardiovascular Reactivity and Sensitisation

Peggy S. Keller,[1] E. Mark Cummings[2] and Mona El-Sheikh[3]
[1]University of Kentucky, Lexington, KY 40506, USA
[2]University of Notre Dame, Notre Dame, Indiana 46556, USA
[3]Auburn University, Auburn, Alabama 36849, USA

Abstract: This chapter provides a brief overview of the emotional security theory and how this theory explains the effects of marital conflict on children. It discusses the current understanding of physiological response to stress and considers the ways in which children's emotional insecurity is tied to cardiovascular reactivity. Studies regarding children's cardiovascular functioning in the context of hostile and aggressive marital conflict, and the relations with emotional security are reviewed, including the implications for children's adjustment.

Keywords: Marital conflict, Emotional security, Vegal regulation, Child health.

Introduction

Hostility and aggression in the marital relationship is often manifested in high rates of intense and unresolved marital conflict. Marital conflict, in turn, has important implications for the whole family and child functioning. Over the past few decades, researchers have repeatedly demonstrated that exposure to hostile marital conflict can lead to physical and psychological problems among children. The next frontier in research in this field is to consider possible theoretical explanations for this relationship. Recently, investigators have begun to explore how children's cardiovascular reactivity serves as a mechanism of risk in the context of aggressive marital relations. The present chapter reviews this research, particularly from a significant emerging theoretical perspective, i.e. *emotional security theory*.

Emotional Security Theory

Emotional security theory (EST) [1-3] proposes that children have a sense of security about the family that reflects their confidence in family stability and the ability of parents to provide a warm and safe environment. EST grew out of *attachment theory* [4], which proposes that children's sense of security about the parent-child relationship influences their social and emotional development and adjustment. EST extended attachment theory to reflect the evidence that multiple dimensions of family functioning affect children's assessments of their security. In particular, disruptions to the marital relationship and marital discord signal to children that family stability is in jeopardy, i.e. problems in marital functioning lead to less than adequate parenting, marital hostility places children directly into harm's way by exposing them to aggressive and intense social contexts, and the dissolution of the marital relationship is associated with multiple stressful life changes [5]. EST contends that children exposed to hostile and aggressive marital conflict develop emotional insecurity about the marital relationship, viewing parents as unable to solve problems and control their tempers. Children exposed to constructive and resolved conflict, on the other hand, develop a strong sense of security because they are confident about parents' abilities to handle disagreements and maintain a healthy relationship.

Emotional security is reflected in multiple and inter-related regulatory processes such as children's emotional reactions to conflict, their behavioural regulation in response to conflict, and their cognitive representations of family relationships. Children who are emotionally insecure have more intense negative emotional reactions to conflict, including anger, fear and sadness. As a result, they are more likely to try to behaviourally regulate their exposure to conflict, or become behaviourally dysregulated in the context of marital conflict. For example, emotionally insecure children may interrupt parents or endeavour to help them with the disagreement in an effort to end the conflict and reduce the threat to their emotional security, or they may become more aggressive in response to the emotional dysregulation induced by exposure to conflict. Insecure children also represent the marriage as threatening and unstable, expecting minor disagreements to blow up into major ones, or even blaming themselves for the conflict. In contrast, secure children are emotionally regulated in response to marital conflict. They may even evidence positive emotions, and are less likely to intervene or mediate conflict or become aggressive, because they are emotionally well-regulated and have representations of the marriage as stable.

Children repeatedly exposed to hostile and aggressive marital conflict become sensitised to marital discord over time [6, 7]. In other words, children do not "get used" to conflict between the parents. On the contrary, because their emotional security is threatened, they are vigilant regarding interparental interactions and are quick to exhibit exaggerated responses to marital disagreements. Over time, these children's elevated vigilance may contribute to chronic anxiety and depression, as well as somatic complaints. Children who act out or become aggressive in response to their parents' fights may generalise such disruptive behaviour to peer and school settings. In this way, children's emotional insecurity may contribute to the development of long-term physical and psychological problems both at home and at school.

Emotional Security and Cardiovascular Reactivity

A new frontier in research on children's emotional security about the marital relationship concerns the role of children's cardiovascular functioning. Cardiovascular functioning has been hypothesised as a regulatory system(s) affected by marital conflict, and related to children's emotional security [2], but empirical research has only recently begun to explore these issues, including relations between cardiovascular reactivity and regulatory processes of emotional security. Towards advancing a psychophysiological perspective on relations between marital conflict and children's cardiovascular reactivity, Whitson and El-Sheikh [8] extended the Polyvagal Theory developed by Porges [9] to the study of relations between marital conflict and children's cardiovascular reactivity. Polyvagal Theory proposes three response systems:

(i) The reptilian vagus reduces the use of oxygen and energy in response to threat by reducing the heart rate and redirecting energy resources, often resulting in the reorientation of attention or freezing.
(ii) The sympathetic nervous system (SNS) prepares the body for action in response to threat by increasing cardiac output and slowing digestion.
(iii) The parasympathetic nervous system (PNS) controls facial expression, vocalisation, and slows heart rate to promote calm and pro-social behaviour. The PNS is hypothesised to be the most advanced system from an evolutionary perspective, and is likened to a 'brake', so that activation of the PNS slows down heart rate while deactivation speeds up the heart rate.

The PNS and SNS both affect heart rate and blood pressure, but they do so via different processes. PNS arousal is often assessed via the activity of the vagus nerve, the cranial nerve connecting the brain with the heart and other organs. Vagal tone is often measured via respiratory sinus arrhythmia (RSA), the difference between heart rate during inhalation and heart rate during exhalation. Higher RSA is related to lower vagal tone and higher heart rate. Therefore, higher baseline vagal tone indicates that the vagus nerve is promoting a lower heart rate and reduced physiological arousal. Conversely, a lower baseline vagal tone suggests that individuals are more likely to suffer from emotional and behavioural problems, including aggression, depression and anxiety [10]. The Polyvagal Theory proposes that when confronted with danger, mammals immediately orient themselves toward the threat and then deactivate the PNS (vagal suppression), which raises the heart rate and physiological arousal, allowing them to focus their attention and meet more complex environmental demands. However, when an already low baseline vagal tone is suppressed even further in response to stress, the individual can become dysregulated and experience a panic attack [10].

An especially dangerous or sustained threat will activate the SNS, which permits "fight or flight" responses but is more physically taxing. Results of SNS arousal include higher heart rate and greater blood pressure. In terms of cardiovascular reactivity, activation of the SNS can be assessed via pre-ejection period, the time interval between the beginning of the heart beat to the ejection of blood into the aorta, and total peripheral resistance, the mean arterial pressure relative to cardiac output. Shorter pre-ejection period and greater total peripheral resistance are associated with SNS arousal. Although SNS arousal may be considered adaptive in response to danger, chronic activation of the SNS has important negative implications for physical and psychological health [11, 12].

Viewed from this perspective, one can conclude there is emerging evidence that both the PNS and SNS may play a role in the adverse effects of children's exposure to marital conflict.

Hostile and aggressive marital conflict strategies are stressors for children; exposure to stress affects cardiovascular reactivity and regulation in children. In response to acute stress, their blood pressure, heart rate and cardiac output increase while pre-ejection period and stroke volume decrease [13]. In comparison to girls, boys experience greater blood pressure and longer pre-ejection period, engaging in greater vasoconstriction, i.e. constriction of the blood vessels, reducing blood flow and increasing blood pressure. Girls experience greater stroke volume and cardiac output reactivity, engaging in greater myocardial reaction, i.e. changes in the activity of the heart muscle, than boys in response to stress [13, 14].

Persons exposed to persistent background stress have heightened cardiovascular reactivity to acute stress [15, 16]. Cardiovascular reactions may thus be heightened in the context of background stress. For example, a study of children's acute stress response following the terrorist attacks of September 11, 2001 found that controlling for child gender, stroke volume and cardiac output in response to a reaction time task and a star tracing task were increased following the attacks [17]. After one year, children's cardiovascular reactivity returned to normal levels. However, normalisation of reactivity may not take place when the stressor is persistent. Marital conflict, particularly hostile and aggressive conflict, may represent a persistent background stressor that is associated with heightened cardiovascular responses to stress in children. This is consistent with the sensitisation hypothesis within EST, which proposes that children who are exposed to higher rates of hostile and aggressive marital conflict become increasingly reactive to conflict over time in an effort to remain vigilant to potential threats to emotional security.

EST, therefore, provides a conceptual basis for understanding how marital conflict may have detrimental effects on cardiovascular functioning in children. EST posits that emotional insecurity among children is related to negative emotional reactivity, behavioural regulation, and cognitive appraisals in response to marital conflict. Notably, each has been associated with cardiovascular reactivity. For example, with regard to emotional reactivity, Buss, Goldsmith and Davidson [18] found that two-year-old children's greater negative emotional reactivity to stressful laboratory tasks (e.g., stranger approach; toy removal tasks etc.) was associated with higher heart rate and also that the relationship between heart rate and negative affect was stronger for girls. Other research suggests that dysregulated fear responding to stranger approach tasks is associated with shorter baseline pre-ejection period [19]. Given that many children have intense emotional reactions to hostile and aggressive marital conflict [5], it follows that children's cardiovascular reactivity may play a role in their response in the context of exposure to marital conflict.

With regard to cognitive representations, Chen and Matthews [15] explored how children's and adolescents' appraisals of ambiguous and non-ambiguous negative social situations might explain why the stress associated with lower SES is related to greater cardiovascular response to challenging tasks. Results indicated that appraisals of hostility helped account for the cross-sectional relationship between lower SES and total peripheral resistance, and the longitudinal relationship between SES and blood pressure. Thus, one reason why some children may experience greater cardiovascular reactivity in response to stress is their tendency for perceived hostile intentions in others. Additional research has explored children's cardiovascular reactivity to story stem completion tasks, an innovative method for assessing children's cognitive representations. In this methodology, children are presented with the beginning of a story, acted out with dolls or action figures and then asked to finish the story however they like. Stories likely to elicit threats to children's sense of emotional security (such as separation and reunion from caregivers) elicited faster heart rates and decreased vagal tone in children. In contrast, vagal suppression was associated with more coherent and positive narratives during the story stem battery [20].

Finally, research has also examined relations between behavioural regulation and cardiovascular functioning in children. A study of two- and three-year-olds found that greater vagal suppression was associated with children's behavioural orientation (looking at and talking to) toward experimenters during tasks in which an attractive toy was taken away and in which they were required to wait before beginning a fun activity [21]. Less vagal suppression was related to children orienting more toward the attractive object. Thus, children who choose to focus their attention on frustrated goals or ruminate on negative events (i.e. look at the toy) experience a pattern of cardiovascular regulation different from children who are able to distract themselves (i.e. look at the experimenters).

These studies, in demonstrating that children's emotion reactivity, behavioural regulation, and cognitive representations are associated with patterns of cardiovascular functioning, support cardiovascular functioning as a feature of children's emotional insecurity about marital relations. A small but growing literature has specifically addressed this topic. One of the first studies examining this issue was conducted by El-Sheikh [22], in which preschoolers were assessed during exposure to an audiotaped disagreement between adults. Results indicated that girls in homes with lower marital satisfaction and higher levels of marital aggression experienced greater heart rate reactivity than those from homes with higher marital satisfaction and lower levels of aggression. This pattern of cardiovascular reactivity was associated with increased distress among girls in response to the argument.

Subsequent studies shed more light on these findings. Using a similar methodology, El-Sheikh and Harger [23] found that children who perceived marital conflict as threatening and tended to blame themselves for their parents' arguments showed greater cardiovascular reactivity to an audiotaped disagreement between two adults. Children with lower baseline vagal tone and lower vagal suppression in response to inter-adult arguments were at greater risk of internalising problems, externalising problems, and health problems such as chronic and acute illness, respiratory problems, digestive problems and fatigue [8, 24]. Most convincing, these relations were found when these processes were assessed longitudinally [25]. Leary and Katz [26] found that for children with low vagal suppression, hostile and withdrawn marital conflict was associated with greater peer conflict over time.

Conclusion

The chronic physiological arousal that is associated with children's exposure to hostile and aggressive marital conflict can have serious implications for children's long-term physical and psychological well-being. EST offers a useful theoretical framework for understanding why marital conflict affects cardiovascular reactivity, particularly PNS and SNS arousal, and how this may be related to children's functioning and adjustment.

Key Points

- Children do not become desensitised to marital conflict. Rather, exposure to hostile and aggressive marital conflict erodes their sense of security about the family, resulting in heightened sensitivity to family disagreements.
- Children have a sense of security about the marital relationship that is reflected in their emotional reactions to conflict, their behavioural regulation in response to conflict, and their cognitive representations of the marital relationship.
- Children's greater sensitisation to conflict and emotional insecurity are reflected in their cardiovascular reactivity to conflict, including PNS and SNS arousal.
- Research has directly implicated cardiovascular regulation in the relationship between hostile and aggressive marital conflict and children's physical and psychological health.

References

1. Davies, P.T. and Cummings, E.M., 1994, "Marital Conflict and Child Adjustment: An Emotional Security Hypothesis", *Psychological Bulletin*, 116(3), pp. 387-411.
2. Cummings, E.M. and Davies, P.T., 1996, "Emotional Security as a Regulatory Process in Normal Development and the Development of Psychopathology", *Development and Psychopathology*, 8(1), pp. 123-139.
3. Cummings, E.M. and Keller, P.S., 2006, "Marital Discord and Children's Emotional Self-regulation", In *Emotion Regulation in Couples and Families: Pathways to Dysfunction and Health*, D.K. Snyder, J.A. Simpson and J.N. Hughes (Eds.), American Psychological Association, Washington, D.C., pp. 163-182.
4. Bowlby, J., 1969, *Attachment and Loss, Vol. 1: Attachment*, Basic Books, New York.
5. Cummings, E.M. and Davies, P.T., 2002, "Effects of Marital Conflict on Children: Recent Advances and Emerging Themes in Process-oriented Research", *Journal of Child Psychology and Psychiatry*, 43(1), pp. 31-63.
6. Davies, P.T., Myers, R.L., Cummings, E.M. and Heindel, S., 1999, "Adult Conflict History and Children's Subsequent Responses to Conflict: An Experimental Test", *Journal of Family Psychology*, 13, pp. 610-628.
7. Cummings, E.M., Kouros, C.D. and Papp, L.M., 2007, "Marital Aggression and Children's Responses to Everyday Inter-Parental Conflict", *European Psychologist*, 12, pp. 17-28.
8. Whitson, S. and El-Sheikh, M., 2003, "Marital Conflict and Health: Processes and Protective Factors", *Aggression and Violent Behavior*, 8, pp. 283-312.
9. Porges, S.W., 1995, "Orienting in a Defensive World: Mammalian Modifications of Our Evolutionary Heritage – A Polyvagal Theory", *Psychophysiology*, 32, pp. 301-318.
10. Beauchaine, T., 2001, "Vagal Tone, Development and Gray's Motivational Theory: Toward an Integrated Model of Autonomic Nervous System Functioning in Psychopathology", *Development and Psychopathology*, 13, pp. 183-214.
11. Baker, D.G., Geracioti, T.G., Kaschow, J.W., Zoumakis, E. and Chrousos, G.P., 2003, "Cytokines and Post-traumatic Stress Disorders", In *Cytokines and Mental Health*, Z. Kronfol (Ed.), Kluwer Academic Publishers, Dordrecht, Netherlands, pp. 301-338.
12. Goldman, N., Weinstein, M., Cornman, J., Singer, B., Seeman, T. and Chang, M.C., 2004, "Sex Differentials in Biological Risk Factors for Chronic Disease: Estimates from Population Based Surveys", *Journal of Women's Health*, 13(4), pp. 393-403.
13. Matthews, K.A., Salomon, K., Kenyon, K. and Allen, M.T., 2002, "Stability of Children's and Adolescents' Hemodynamic Responses to Psychological Challenge: A Three-year Longitudinal Study of a Multiethnic Cohort of Boys and Girls", *Psychophysiology*, 39, pp. 826-834.
14. Kudielka, B.M., Buske-Kirschbaum, A., Hellhammer, D.H. and Kirschbaum, C., 2004, "Differential Heart Rate Reactivity and Recovery After Psychosocial Stress (TSST) in Healthy Children, Younger Adults and Elderly Adults: The Impact of Age and Gender", *International Journal of Behavioral Medicine*, 11(2), pp. 116-131.
15. Chen, E. and Matthews, K.A., 2001, "Cognitive Appraisal Biases: An Approach to Understand the Relation Between Socioeconomic Status and Cardiovascular Reactivity in Children", *Annals of Behavioral Medicine*, 23(2), pp. 101-111.
16. Matthews, K.A., Gump, B.B., Block, D.R. and Allen, M.T., 1997, "Does Background Stress Heighten or Dampen Children's Cardiovascular Responses to Acute Stress?" *Psychosomatic Medicine*, 59, pp. 488-496.
17. Gump, B.B., Reihman, J., Stewart, P., Lonky, E. and Darvill, T., 2005, "Terrorism and Cardiovascular Responses to Acute Stress in Children", *Health Psychology*, 24(6), pp. 594-600.

18. Buss, K.A., Goldsmith, H.H. and Davidson, R.J., 2005, "Cardiac Reactivity is Associated with Changes in Negative Emotion in 24-month-olds", *Developmental Psychobiology*, 46(2), pp. 118-132.
19. Buss, K.A., Davidson, R.J., Kalin, N.H. and Goldsmith, H.H., 2004, "Context-specific Freezing and Associated Physiological Reactivity as a Dyregulated Fear Response", *Developmental Psychology*, 40(4), pp. 583-594.
20. Bar-Haim, Y., Fox, N.A., VanMeenen, K.M. and Marshall, P.J., 2004, "Children's Narratives and Patterns of Cardiac Reactivity", *Developmental Psychobiology*, 44(4), pp. 238-249.
21. Calkins, S.D., 1997, "Cardiac Vagal Tone Indices of Temperamental Reactivity and Behavioral Regulation in Young Children", *Developmental Psychobiology*, 31(2), pp. 125-135.
22. El-Sheikh, M., 1994, "Children's Emotional and Physiological Responses to Interadult Angry Behavior: The Role of History of Interparental Hostility", *Journal of Abnormal Child Psychology*, 22(6), pp. 661-678.
23. El-Sheikh, M. and Harger, J., 2001, "Appraisals of Marital Conflict and Children's Adjustment, Health, and Physiological Reactivity", *Developmental Psychology*, 37(6), pp. 875-885.
24. El-Sheikh, M., Harger, J. and Whitson, S.M., 2001, "Exposure to Interparental Conflict and Children's Adjustment and Physical Health: The Moderating Role of Vagal Tone", *Child Development*, 72(6), pp. 1617-1636.
25. El-Sheikh, M. and Whitson, S.A., 2006, "Longitudinal Relations Between Marital Conflict and Child Adjustment: Vagal Regulation as a Protective Factor", *Journal of Family Psychology*, 20(1), pp. 30-39.
26. Leary, A. and Katz, L.F., 2004, "Coparenting, Family-level Processes and Peer Outcomes: The Moderating Role of Vagal Tone", *Development and Psychopathology*, 16, pp. 593-608.

The AHA-Syndrome and Cardiovascular Diseases
Editors: Swati Y. Bhave and Sunil Saini
Copyright © 2010 Anamaya Publishers, New Delhi, India

10. Anger, Hostility and Heart Disease

K.K. Aggarwal
President, Heart Care Foundation of India, New Delhi - 110 065; Department of Cardiology
Moolchand Medcity, New Delhi - 110 024, India

Abstract: Stress management courses are mushrooming all over India. It is high time that doctors also learn this aspect of mental health. There is no way a psychiatrist or counsellor can handle all the children, adolescents and young adults going through various behavioural problems and/or mental stress. The present chapter outlines a new risk factor for heart disease – anger, hostility and aggression (AHA). All of them are invariably related to unfulfilled desires either acutely or over a period of time. The chapter is based on a single saying from the Vedic *Upanishads*, "You are what your deep-rooted desires are". Evidence-based examples are given about the relationship of AHA with heart disease, and on its pathogenesis. At the end, brief principles of management are outlined, which allopathic doctors should learn from the yogic sciences in the management of stress.

Keywords: Anger, Hostility, Cynicism and recall of anger, AHA, Stress, Heart disease.

Introduction

Darkness is absence of light. While darkness cannot be removed physically, it can be removed by bringing the light back. Similarly, negative thoughts are absence of positive thoughts. The former can only be removed by bringing back the latter. A newborn baby is free of all negative emotions. Actions over time lead to experiences at the level of senses. An action leads to memory and memory leads to desires. Action, memory and desires are the basic triad of life's experiences. Desires are the root cause for every medical illness. If everytime a desire is produced, it is fulfilled, the person will become proud, egoistic and will end up into the *chakravyuh* (encirclement) of *lobh* (greed) and *moha* (attachments). All addictions and lust start at this level. However, if desire is not fulfilled, the first reaction is anger. If not managed well, an episode of anger would lead to an impulsive reaction or an aggressive behaviour. Non-fulfillment of desires over time will manifest itself as persistent negative behaviour, defined as *hostility*, which again, if not managed well, will end up with all the grades of aggressive behaviours.

Chronic suppression of anger, hostility and aggression (AHA) can lead to frustration, despondency, depression and suicide. The scientific answer for these is to learn yoga, meditation, *pranayama* and undergo regular counselling. The seeds of atherosclerosis are sowed in adolescence. If one has to prevent coronary artery disease in middle age, one has to modify the diet, exercise regularly and teach the right attitude and behaviours to fellow humans in this group of population.

AHA and Heart Disease

Type (D) distressed personality comprises people with negative emotions and social inhibitions. It correlates with the triad of AHA [1].

In women, higher plasma levels of tryptopham, the precursor to 5-HT are associated with AHA [2]. Anger, hostility and verbal (not physical) aggression are associated with high total serum cholesterol levels [3]. Anger and severity of depressive symptoms, either alone or in combination, are associated with high C-reactive protein (CRP) levels [4].

The triad of AHA is now accepted as new risk factors for coronary artery disease (CAD) [5]. Hostility scores are associated with increased risk of cardiovascular events in women undergoing coronary angiography [6]. Type A behaviour and hostility are also linked to CAD [7]. A meta-analytical review of some 45 studies has concluded that hostility is an independent risk factor for all-cause mortality and also for CAD mortality and morbidity [8].

Not only in younger men, a high level of expressed anger is also shown to be a risk factor for CAD among older men [9]. Even recall of anger has been shown to produce significant decreases in left ventricular ejection fraction as measured by radionuclide ventriculography [10], as well as coronary artery vasoconstriction in already narrowed segments [11].

Anger and hostility have been linked with CAD, which is shown by the following:

(i) In a three-year follow-up study of 3,750 Finnish men aged 40 to 59 years, high ratings of hostility (assessed from self-ratings of irritability and ease of anger arousal) were associated with increased CAD mortality, although the excess risk was confined to men with pre-existing heart disease [12].
(ii) In the Multiple Risk Factor Intervention Trial, men with high "potential for hostility", a behavioural rating correlated with high verbal and physical expression of anger, had an adjusted relative risk of incident CAD of 1.5 ($p = 0.03$) [13].
(iii) In the Determinants of Myocardial Infarction (MI) Onset Study, a case-crossover study involving 1,623 patients, episodes of anger were found to be potent triggers of acute MI. The relative risk of MI in 2 h after an episode of anger was 2.3 [14].

Post-menopausal women with high Cook-Medley hostility scores are at a two-fold increased risk for recurrent CAD events. Among HERS women, the risk associated with high levels of hostility was greater than that associated with elevated serum low-density lipoprotein cholesterol levels, tobacco use, hypertension, and diabetes [15].

Hostility, a construct that includes cynicism, anger, mistrust and aggression, has been correlated with carotid atherosclerosis, angiographic CAD, exercise-induced ischemia, and restenosis after mechanical revascularisation in women. High hostility scores have also been associated with an increased risk of non-fatal MI among older women, but not with fatal events in patients with documented CAD [16].

Pathogenesis

Exaggerated adrenergic responses to stress can increase heart rate and blood pressure, induce coronary vasoconstriction in atherosclerotic arteries, and activate platelets. Anger outburst may trigger acute rupture of vulnerable plaques, increasing the risk of non-fatal MI or CAD death [17].

Feelings of chronic cynicism and mistrust may result in continual sympathetic nervous system arousal. In the Canadian Amlodipine/Atenolol in Silent Ischemia Study (CASIS), high levels of hostility diminished the benefits of anti-ischemic medications, i.e. amlodipine, atenolol etc. [18].

Both low social support and high hostility increase a person's risk of developing CAD and to die from it. Psychological factors hyperactivate neuroendocrine systems, especially the sympathetic nervous system, and activate platelets.

Hostility predicts restenosis and anger recurrent events, after PTCA [19]. Anger is frequent in acute stroke patients. In such patients, anger can disturb management and rehabilitation and create a stressful situation for family, health-care providers and other patients [20].

The Time Tested Principles for Managing the AHA Parameters Are Based on Ancient Indian Texts

- You are incomplete in your dress unless you are wearing a smile on your face. Both smile and laughter are associated with reduced hostility scores.
- Law of giving and sharing: never go empty handed to meet someone. Even a smile or compliment can make all the difference.
- Everyone has a weakness for being appreciated: appreciate people.
- Communication is the key to de-stressing.
- Practice the detachment exercise: give someone a thing you love the most.
- When angry, count one to ten or do deep left nostril breathing. Simple deep breathing, laughing, crying and walking also helps.
- Learn to change the perceptions in life. Every situation has two ends, search for the other message and path.
- *Pranayama* and meditation are the journeys which shift one from sympathetic to para sympathetic modes; learn them. *Pranayama* is slower and deeper breathing. Meditation is the process of concentrating over the object of concentration and while doing so giving preference to that object over the thoughts.
- Reward and punish yourself; do this exercise every night before retiring while reviewing the day long actions.
- Write your emotions freely and destroy the evidence.

Conclusion

Stress, for years, has been described as a risk factor for atherosclerosis and CAD. However, it is only negative stress alone or its recall, which has been linked to this illness and not positive stress, which is required for a successful life. Stress is nothing but the reaction of the body and/ or the mind to the interpretation of a known situation. Stress management, therefore, involves either changing the situation, changing its interpretation or preparing the body the yogic way so that the stress does not create any imbalance.

Until now, Type A or Type D personalities were linked to heart diseases. Now evidence-based medicine has shown that it is the triad of AHA, which relates to coronary atherosclerosis. They all occur due to acute expression or suppression of negative emotions, which invariably arise when acutely or, over a period of time the desires are not met. Unfulfilled desires, therefore, are the root cause of coronary atherosclerosis and should be tackled while they are at their infancy.

Key Points

- "You are what your deep-rooted desires": An old *Upanishad* saying.
- Unmanaged stress can precipitate acute heart attack and, over a period of time, can cause coronary thrombosis.
- You get what you deserve and not what you desire.
- Learn to manage stress as both suppression and acute expression of anger can cause heart disease.
- *Pranayama* – deeper and slower breathing – is the best remedy for stress management.
- Meditation – giving preference to the object of concentration over thoughts – if done 20 min in the morning and evening, can even reverse existing coronary atherosclerosis.
- Attachment leads to anger, greed leads to attachment and egocentric desires lead to over sympathetic reactions in the body.

References

1. Perbandt, K., Hodapp, V., Wendt, T. and Jordan, J., 2006, *Psychother. Psychosom. Med. Psychol.*, August, 56(8), pp. 310-317; E-published on 22 May 2006.
2. Suarez, E.C. and Krishnan, K.R., 2006, *Ann. Behav. Med.*, June, 31(3), pp. 254-260.
3. Hillbrand, M., Waite, B.M., Rosenstein, M., Harackiewicz, D., Lingswiler, V.M. and Stehney, M., 2005, "Serum Cholesterol Concentrations and Non-physical Aggression in Healthy Adults", *J. Behav. Med.*, June, 28(3), pp. 295-299.
4. Suarez, E.C., 2004, "C-reactive Protein is Associated with Psychological Risk Factors of Cardiovascular Disease in Apparently Healthy Adults", *Psychosom. Med.*, September-October, 66(5), pp. 684-691.
5. Glazer, K., Ruiz, J.M., Gallo, L.C. and Smith, T.W., 2004, "Hostility, Anger, Aggressiveness and Coronary Heart Disease: An Interpersonal Perspective on Personality, Emotion and Health", *J. Pers.*, December, 72(6), pp. 1217-1270.
6. Marian, B., Olson, M.S., Krantz, D.S., Kelsey, S.F., Pepine, C.J., Sopko, G., Handberg, E., Rogers, W.J., Gierach, G.L., McClure, C.K. and Merz, C.N.B., 2002, "Hostility Scores are Associated with Increased Risk of Cardiovascular Events in Women Undergoing Coronary Angiography: A Report from the NHLBI-Sponsored WISE Study", *International Journal of Epidemiology*, WISE Study Group, 31, pp. 1227-1234.
7. Sykes, D.H., Arveiler, D., Salters, C.P., Ferrieres, J., McCrum, E., Amouyel, P., Bingham, A., Montaye, M., Ruidavets, J.-B., Haas, B., Ducimetiere, P. and Evans, A.E., "Psychosocial Risk Factors for Heart Disease in France and Northern Ireland: The Prospective Epidemiological Study of Myocardial Infarction (PRIME)".
8. Miller, T.Q., Smith, T.W., Turner, C.W., Guijarro, M.L. and Hallet, A.J., 1996, "A Meta-analytic Review of Research on Hostility and Physical Health", *Psychol. Bull.*, 119, pp. 322-348.
9. Kawachi, I., Sparrow, D., Spiro III, A., Vokonas, P. and Weiss, S.T., 1996, "A Prospective Study of Anger and Coronary Heart Disease: The Normative Aging Study", *Circulation*, 94, p. 2090.
10. Ironson, G., Taylor, C.B., Boltwood, M., Bartzokis, T., Dennis, C., Chesney, M., Spitzer, S. and Segall, G.M., 1992, "Effects of Anger on Left Ventricular Ejection Fraction in Coronary Artery Disease", *Am. J. Cardiol.*, 70, pp. 281-285.
11. Boltwood, M.D., Taylor, C.B., Burke, M.B., Grogin, H. and Giacomini, J., 1993, "Anger Report Predicts Coronary Artery Vasomotor Response to Mental Stress in Atherosclerotic Segments", *Am. J. Cardiol.*, 72, pp. 1361-1365.

12. Kawachi, I., Sparrow, D., Kubzansky, L.D., Spiro III, A., Vokonas, P.S. and Weiss, S.T., 1998, "Prospective Study of a Self-Report Type A Scale and Risk of Coronary Heart Disease Test of the MMPI-2 Type A Scale", *Circulation*, 98, p. 405.
13. Chaput, L.A., Adams, S.H., Simon, J.A., Blumenthal, R.S., Vittinghoff, E., Lin, F., Loh, E. and Matthews, K.A., 2002, "Hostility Predicts Recurrent Events Among Postmenopausal Women with Coronary Heart Disease", *Am. J. Epidemiol.*, 156, pp. 1092-1099.
14. Barefoot, J.C., Dodge, K.A., Peterson, B.L. et al., 1989, "The Cook-Medley Hostility Scale: Item Content and Ability to Predict Survival", *Psychosom. Med.*, 51, pp. 46-57.
15. Matthews, K.A., Owens, J.F., Kuller, L.H. et al., 1998, "Are Hostility and Anxiety Associated with Carotid Atherosclerosis in Healthy Postmenopausal Women?" *Psychom. Med.*, 60, pp. 633-638.
16. Barefoot, J.C., Peterson, B.L., Harrell, F.E. et al., 1989, "Type A Behavior and Survival: A Follow-up Study of 1,467 Patients with Coronary Artery Disease", *Am. J. Cardiol.*, 64, pp. 427-432.
17. Mittleman, M.A., Maclure, M., Sherwood, J.B. et al., 1995, "Triggering of Acute Myocardial Infarction Onset by Episodes of Anger: Determinants of Myocardial Infarction Onset Investigators", *Circulation*, 92, pp. 1720-1725.
18. Rozanski, A., Blumenthal, J.A. and Kaplan, J., 1999, "Impact of Psychological Factors on the Pathogenesis of Cardiovascular Disease and Implications for Therapy", *Circulation*, 99, pp. 2192-2217.
19. Knox, S.S., Siegmund, K.D., Weidner, G., Ellison, R.C., Adelman, A. and Paton, C., 1998, "Hostility, Social Support and Coronary Heart Disease in the National Heart, Lung, and Blood Institute Family Heart Study", *Am. J. Cardiol.*, 82, pp. 1192-1196.
20. Santos, C.O., Caeiro, L., Ferro, J.M., Albuquerque, R. and Figueira, M.L., 2006, "Anger, Hostility and Aggression in the First Days of Acute Stroke", *Eur. J. Neurol.*, April, 13(4), pp. 351-358.

The AHA-Syndrome and Cardiovascular Diseases
Editors: Swati Y. Bhave and Sunil Saini
Copyright © 2010 Anamaya Publishers, New Delhi, India

11. Individual Differences in Displaced Aggression as a Risk Factor for Poor Cardiovascular Health

Thomas F. Denson
School of Psychology, University of New South Wales, Sydney, NSW 2052, Australia

Abstract: Much evidence now supports the notion that high levels of anger-hostility-aggression (AHA) are a risk factor for cardiovascular disease. The present chapter discusses a related yet distinct personality dimension *trait displaced aggression* and its potential associations with poor cardiovascular health. Trait displaced aggression is characterised by the general tendency to ruminate and harm innocent others following interpersonal provocation. Because the distinction between general trait aggression and trait displaced aggression has emerged only recently, researchers have not yet investigated the role that individual differences in displaced aggression might play in cardiovascular diseases. In this chapter, it is argued that those high in trait displaced aggression may be at risk for experiencing poor cardiovascular health, perhaps even to a greater extent than those high in general AHA. Three pathways to poor cardiovascular outcomes are discussed. Specifically, individuals high in trait displaced aggression tend to (i) ruminate about provocations, (ii) alienate importance sources of social support such as romantic partners, and (iii) are likely to engage in maladaptive, health-compromising self-regulatory behaviours. It also discusses possible harm reduction mechanisms including distraction, the mental activation of social support, and increasing forgiveness.

Keywords: Displaced aggression, Aggression, Cardiovascular health, Cardiovascular disease, Aggressive personality, Trait displaced aggression, Social support, Rumination.

Introduction

One of the most well-documented findings in health psychology is the relationship between individual differences in anger-hostility-aggressiveness (AHA) and negative cardiovascular outcomes. A large body of meta-analytic evidence supports a small-to-moderate positive relationship between AHA and poor cardiovascular health. For instance, a meta-analysis of Type A and B personalities indicated that the AHA component of the personality type was responsible for an increased occurrence of coronary heart disease [1]. Other meta-analytic reviews have also revealed positive relationships between trait anger and elevated blood pressure [2, 3] and between trait hostility and blood pressure reactivity to provocations [4].

The present chapter explores the potential effects of an additional personality dimension, namely trait displaced aggression (DA), on cardiovascular outcomes. Trait DA is a recently developed personality construct that is related to, yet distinct from AHA. I shall first discuss the conceptualisation of trait DA, followed by a discussion of the possible pathways associated with high levels of trait DA that may place these individuals at risk for poor cardiovascular outcomes. In conclusion we will discuss implications for research on AHA and cardiovascular health, as well as several suggestions for future research.

Trait DA

Trait DA refers to stable individual differences in the tendency to aggress against undeserving targets in response to prior provocation [5]. Evidence suggests that when provoked, individuals high in trait DA tend not to deal immediately and directly with the provocateur. Instead, when confronted with an interpersonal provocation (e.g. an insult), they are behaviourally inhibited, yet continue to experience extended anger and hostility. Specifically, those high in trait DA ruminate and dedicate extensive mental effort to planning revenge in the aftermath of the provocation [5]. Moreover, those high in trait DA often harm those closest to them, including their romantic partners [5].

Trait DA consists of three highly correlated, yet distinct affective, cognitive and behavioural components:

- Angry rumination (affect; e.g. "I keep thinking about events that angered me for a long time")
- Revenge planning (cognition; e.g. "When someone makes me angry, I cannot stop thinking about how to get back at this person")
- Behavioural DA (behaviour; e.g. "I take my anger out on innocent others")

These three components comprise the DA questionnaire (DAQ), a reliable and valid 31-item self-report measure used to assess individual differences in trait DA [5]. Thus, those high in trait DA experience anger over an extended period of time (angry rumination), experience hostile cognition over an extended period of time (revenge planning), and harm those close to them (behavioural DA), thereby eliminating important sources of social support. Any one of these factors is likely to impair cardiovascular health. Individuals high in trait DA possess all three of these risk factors. As discussed below, it appears likely then, that those high in trait DA are at especially high risk for suffering from poor cardiovascular outcomes, perhaps even to a greater degree than those high in general AHA.

Pathways to Poor Cardiovascular Health

Because trait DA is a recently developed construct, prior research on aggressive personality and health outcomes has not differentiated among individuals high in general AHA from those who tend to aggress against innocent others (i.e. trait DA). Although general AHA and trait DA are moderately correlated [5], there is good reason to suspect that those high in trait DA may be especially prone to negative cardiovascular health. Based on some of the author's research and related empirical work by others, three possible pathways associated with trait DA that might contribute to poor cardiovascular health are discussed. Specifically, those high in trait DA are likely to (i) engage in angry and hostile rumination, (ii) alienate important sources of social support, and (iii) engage in poor self-regulatory strategies.

Rumination

Because trait DA consists of angry and hostile rumination, this implies that anger and hostility are experienced for extended periods of time (e.g. potentially even days or weeks). Thus, whereas individuals high in general AHA may experience frequent anger and hostility that dissipates relatively quickly, those high in trait DA also experience these frequent emotional states but for longer periods of time, thereby increasing the harmful effects associated with AHA. For instance, when confronted with an inter-personal provocation, those high in general AHA might experience a brief activation of the physiological stress response, whereas when those high in trait DA are confronted with the same provocation, they likely experience an extended hyperactivation of the stress response. According to the reactivity hypothesis of disease, individuals who tend to demonstrate high levels of cardiovascular reactivity to stressful experiences may be at increased risk for negative cardiovascular outcomes [6]. Therefore, this extended activation of the stress response is likely to lead to poor cardiovascular health [7].

Empirical evidence is emerging suggesting that it is not the immediate reaction to a stressful experience that is the most important determinant of chronic, poor cardiovascular health, but rather the cognitive-affective experience following a stressor that may be an important risk factor. One such experience is rumination. Indeed, reviews of the empirical literature suggest that rumination may play a role in cardiovascular disease [8, 9]. Thus, examining cardiovascular recovery in the aftermath of a stressful experience may provide insight into long-term cardiovascular outcomes. For instance, in one experiment, Brosschot and Thayer [10] found that heart rate responses were longer after negative emotions than positive emotions and speculated that rumination may be responsible for this effect. Of more relevance to trait DA are the findings that individual differences in angry rumination predicted delayed cardiovascular recovery following a provocation [11] and after recalling angry life episodes [12]. Glynn, Christenfeld and Gerin [13] (experiment 1) exposed participants to somewhat hostile emotional stressors or non-emotional stressors, and then instructed participants to ruminate about their experiences. They found that only rumination following the hostile emotional stressors produced elevated systolic and diastolic blood pressure. In another study, Bermúdez and Pérez-García [14] administered Caprara's [15] Dissipation-Rumination scale – a measure of vengeance and very similar to the Revenge Planning sub-scale of the DAQ – and exposed them to a hostile emotional stressor. Those high in trait rumination demonstrated increased systolic and diastolic blood pressure reactivity.

How might rumination lead to a hyperactivation of cardiovascular activity? According to one account, it is perseverative cognition, a feature characteristic of rumination that may exacerbate cardiovascular, endocrine and immune responses to stress [16]. Specifically, repeatedly thinking about a stressor may lead to an extended stress response entailing hyperstimulation of the cardiovascular and hypothalamic-pituitary-adrenal (HPA) axis. In more cognitive terms, rumination maintains the likelihood of angry affect, physiological arousal and aggressive cognition [17] via an associative network of aggression-related concepts [18]. Such a network is characterised by activation of aggression-related concepts and inhibition of incompatible responses such as positive affect or empathy. Brosschot, Gerin and Thayer [16] conducted a review of literature on perseverative cognition and concluded that individual differences in rumination are associated with exacerbated cardiovascular, cortisol and immune reactivity. It is also important to note that dysregulation of the HPA axis is associated with cardiovascular disease [19].

In summary, emerging literature indicates that rumination, and especially the hostile-angry rumination that characterises those high in trait DA, may represent a risk factor for poor cardiovascular outcomes.

Loss of Social Support

In addition to the exacerbated stress response linked to angry and hostile rumination, a second factor associated with trait DA is the tendency to aggress against close others – a phenomenon which is intricately connected with rumination. By maintaining the accessibility of aggressive constructs and angry affect, rumination makes subsequent aggression more likely to 'transfer' to undeserving others – a finding that has been experimentally demonstrated [20]. Over time, such aggressive behaviour is likely to push away close others, thereby reducing the availability of important sources of social support. Sources of social support such as romantic partners are capable of providing a buffer to life's provocations [21]. Indeed, a survey of American adults that simultaneously examined the relative effects of trait DA and general AHA revealed that trait DA accounted for a substantial proportion of the explained variance in self-reported acts of romantic partner abuse whereas the effect of general AHA did not reach statistical significance [5].

The consequences of loss of social support for cardiovascular health can be quite serious. Those who lack social support demonstrate increased mortality, largely from cardiovascular disease [22-24]. In contrast, high levels of social support are associated with lower ambulatory blood pressure [25] and less underlying atherosclerosis [26].

In light of the reactivity hypothesis [6], researchers have proposed that social support should buffer the effects of life stressors (including inter-personal provocations), thereby attenuating cardiovascular reactivity [21]. Several experiments support the notion that when individuals provide supporting comments during laboratory stress manipulations cardiovascular reactivity is indeed reduced [27, 28], but not always among those high in AHA [29]. Thus, although in general, social support is associated with better cardiovascular outcomes, no study to date has investigated the buffering role of social support on cardiovascular reactivity in individuals high in trait DA specifically. Therefore, it remains to be seen whether social support buffers the effects of acute stress on these outcomes among those high in trait DA. Nonetheless, those high in trait DA harm those close to them, which presumably leads to alienation of social support over time. Initial self-report data indicate that high levels of trait DA are related to lower social support, which in turn is related to more stress and subsequent increased negative health problems [30].

In addition to buffering emotional and cardiovascular reactivity to acute stress, there is a second mechanism through which social support may affect cardiovascular health [24]. Specifically, social support may also promote healthy behaviours and medication adherence [31]. Thus, those high in trait DA are unlikely to enjoy these additional benefits of social support.

Maladaptive Self-regulation

A third pathway through which individual differences in trait DA may affect cardiovascular health is through maladaptive self-regulation. When individuals high in trait DA are provoked, they are likely to experience a complex negative emotional response including anxiety, anger and hostility. In addition, rumination is associated with increased self-awareness [32]. Indeed, a large body of research demonstrates that a heightened state of self-awareness often intensifies negative feelings

[33], including anger [34]. Presumably, individuals are motivated to reduce this self-awareness and negative affect. One way to accomplish this is to stop the ruminative process. However, because rumination is characterised by uncontrollable, repetitive thoughts, this may prove difficult. The uncomfortable state that individuals high in trait DA find themselves in may lead them to engage in unhealthy behaviours intended to provide relief from the cognitive and affective sequelae of a provocation.

Individuals might engage in several types of self-regulatory behaviours in order to reduce self-awareness and improve mood. Unfortunately, these behaviours might also harm one's cardiovascular health. For instance, abusing alcohol or binging on unhealthy foods are both common mechanisms of reducing self-awareness [35, 36]. Because of their awareness-altering effects, using hard drugs that affect the cardiovascular system such as cocaine or methamphetamine may be another common coping mechanism among those high in trait DA. Also, given that trait DA is related to behavioural inhibition [5], which has been linked with avoidant coping strategies [37], those high in trait DA may be more likely to engage in avoidant coping strategies (such as binge drinking) rather than problem-solving coping.

There is indeed some preliminary support that high levels of trait DA are associated with unhealthy self-regulatory behaviours. In a survey of 827 adult American Internet respondents, it was found that trait DA predicted symptoms of alcohol dependence, eating an unhealthy diet, and use of hard drugs (but not marijuana or tobacco), when controlling for age, gender and income [38]. In this same study, participants were asked to answer questions about how they coped with a recent anger-inducing provocation. Those high in trait DA reported using more avoidant behaviours and fewer problem-solving behaviours in response to the provocation [38].

Implications and Suggestions for Future Research

In light of the current review, it is likely that individuals high in trait DA are at risk for poor cardiovascular health, perhaps even to a greater extent than those high in general AHA. However, further research is necessary to empirically validate whether those high in trait DA relative to those high in general AHA differ in terms of cardiovascular health, and if so, to what extent. If trait DA is demonstrated to be a potent predictor of cardiovascular health, models of AHA should incorporate trait DA. Another implication drawn for the present review is that it is not only the immediate reaction to a provocation that impacts cardiovascular outcomes, but also that rumination delays recovery from interpersonal stress.

Future work could focus on cardiovascular reactivity to acute provocation in the laboratory as well as examining real world longitudinal disease outcomes and mortality. Longitudinal data are especially relevant to trait DA because it is expected that there may be a cumulative negative effect of the personality dimension on cardiovascular health as one ages. Specifically, when one is young and healthy, trait DA may exert little influence on one's cardiovascular state (including laboratory reactivity to stressful situations). However, as one becomes older, a lifetime of experiencing extended angry and hostile rumination coupled with harming key sources of social support, may take its toll on the cardiovascular system. Indirect support for this was found in the cross-sectional survey reported previously [38]. An interaction was observed between trait DA and age such that whereas trait DA remained a significant predictor across all three age groups (i.e. 21, 34 and 47 years), the effect of trait DA on self-reported physical health symptoms (including cardiovascular symptoms) increased with age. Additional work should also focus on the relationships between cardiovascular disease, immune dysregulation, and endocrine dysregulation among those high in trait DA.

Reducing the Harm

There is some evidence in the literature to support the notion that targeted interventions may eventually aid in decreasing the proposed harmful cardiovascular consequences associated with trait DA. Specifically, these interventions may include distraction techniques, the mental activation of social support and forgiveness. The General Aggression Model [39] describes aggressive cognition, angry affect and physiological arousal as three possible mediators of personality on aggression. Presumably, all three interventions discussed below operate by inhibiting aggressive cognition as well as affecting and promoting cardiovascular recovery to inter-personal stressors.

Distracting oneself following an inter-personal provocation may be an especially promising research avenue to explore. Distraction should be especially helpful because it is affectively neutral, non-arousing and cognitively demanding, thereby permitting little room for aggressive thoughts or angry affect. Experimental evidence supports this notion. For instance, in the laboratory, when participants were provoked and subsequently asked to write about a neutral topic for 20 min, trait DA no longer predicted physical harm against an innocent participant [5]. Directly relevant to cardiovascular disease, in one experiment, participants were exposed to a hostile emotional stressor and then either completed a cognitively engaging, yet non-stressful moral dilemma task for 10 min or just sat quietly for 10 min [13] (Experiment 2). Those exposed to the distracting task evidenced faster cardiovascular recovery following the stressor than those who were simply asked to sit quietly. It is speculated that the distracting task prevented participants from ruminating. Similarly, in another experiment, participants who read a neutral, distracting article following an anger recall task displayed faster heart rate recovery than those instructed to do nothing for 10 min [40]. Distraction was associated with lower anger and rumination during the experiment. Thus, even brief (e.g. 10 min) distraction tasks may be effective.

Another strategy that may prove useful is the mental activation of social support [41]. In one laboratory study, participants who wrote about supportive people in their lives prior to being exposed to a public speech stressor had lower heart rate and blood pressure compared to those participants who wrote about casual acquaintances [41]. This held true for all participants except women high in trait hostility (although men high in trait hostility still benefitted from the mental activation of social support). There is one important caveat, however. Because those high in trait DA tend to harm close others, it may be more difficult for them to spontaneously activate an important source of social support.

A third strategy would be to increase forgiveness among those high in trait DA. Forgiveness is negatively associated with rumination [42] and positively associated with marital quality [43]. In one study, participants underwent a stressful interview about a time when someone had betrayed them [44]. Those high in trait forgiveness had faster blood pressure recovery following the stressful interview. These findings suggest that training those high in trait DA to be more forgiving when confronted with inter-personal provocation may protect their cardiovascular health and increase satisfaction with their romantic partners.

Conclusion

Much evidence now supports the notion that high levels of AHA are a risk factor for cardiovascular disease. Although recent empirical work has differentiated between general trait AHA and trait DA [5], no work to date has directly investigated the role that individual differences in displaced aggression might play in cardiovascular health. Based on a review of the empirical literature, it appears that those high in trait DA are likely at risk for poor cardiovascular outcomes, perhaps even to a greater extent than those high in general AHA. Specifically, individuals high in trait DA tend to ruminate about provocations, alienate important sources of social support, and engage in maladaptive self-regulatory behaviours. All three pathways are likely to negatively impact cardiovascular outcomes. Those high in trait DA likely engage in all three behaviours, thus, further compounding their risk for poor cardiovascular health.

Key Points

- Although recent empirical work has differentiated between general trait AHA and trait DA [5, 45], no work to date has directly investigated the role that individual differences in displaced aggression might play in cardiovascular health.
- Based on a review of the empirical literature, it appears that those high in trait DA are likely at risk for poor cardiovascular outcomes, perhaps even to a greater extent than those high in general AHA.
- Specifically, individuals high in trait DA tend to ruminate about provocations, alienate important sources of social support, and engage in maladaptive self-regulatory behaviours.
- All three pathways are likely to negatively impact cardiovascular outcomes.
- Those high in trait DA likely engage in all three behaviours, thus, further compounding their risk for poor cardiovascular health.

Acknowledgements

The author thanks Nida Denson, William C. Pedersen and Eduardo A. Vasquez for providing comments on an earlier draft of this chapter.

References

1. Booth-Kewley, S. and Friedman, H.S., 1987, "Psychological Predictors of Heart Disease: A Quantitative Review", *Psychological Bulletin*, 101, pp. 343-362.
2. Jorgensen, R.S., Johnson, B.T., Kolodziej, M.E. and Schreer, G.E., 1996, "Elevated Blood Pressure and Personality: A Meta-analytic Review", *Psychological Bulletin*, 120, pp. 293-320.
3. Schum, J.L., Jorgensen, R.S., Verhaeghen, P., Sauro, M. and Thibodeau, R., 2003, "Trait Anger, Anger Expression and Ambulatory Blood Pressure: A Meta-analytic Review", *Journal of Behavioral Medicine*, 26, pp. 395-415.
4. Suls, J. and Wan, C.K., 1993, "The Relationship Between Trait Hostility and Cardiovascular Reactivity: A Quantitative Review and Analysis", *Psychophysiology*, 30, pp. 615-626.
5. Denson, T.F., Pedersen, W.C. and Miller, N., 2006, "The Displaced Aggression Questionnaire", *Journal of Personality and Social Psychology*, 90, pp. 1032-1051.
6. Lepore, S.J., 1998, "Problems and Prospects for the Social Support-reactivity Hypothesis", *Annals of Behavioral Medicine*, 20, pp. 257-269.

7. Sapolsky, R.M., 1998, *Why Zebras Don't Get Ulcers: An Updated Guide to Stress, Stress-related Diseases and Coping*, Freeman and Company, New York, USA.
8. Kubazansky, L.D., Davidson, K.W. and Rozanski, A., 2005, "The Clinical Impact of Negative Psychological States: Expanding the Spectrum of Risk for Coronary Artery Disease", *Psychosomatic Medicine*, 67, pp. S10-S14.
9. Pieper, S. and Brosschot, J., 2005, "Prolonged Stress-related Cardiovascular Activation: Is There Any?", *Annals of Behavioral Medicine*, 30, pp. 91-103.
10. Brosschot, J.F. and Thayer, J.F., 2003, "Heart Rate Response is Longer After Negative Emotions Than After Positive Emotions", *International Journal of Psychophysiology*, 50, pp. 181-187.
11. Suchday, S., Carter, M.M., Ewart, C.K., Larkin, K.T. and Desiderato, O., 2004, "Anger Cognitions and Cardiovascular Recovery Following Provocation", *Journal of Behavioral Medicine*, 27, pp. 319-341.
12. Gerin, W., Davidson, K.W., Christenfeld, N.J., Goyal, T. and Schwartz, J., 2006, "The Role of Angry Rumination and Distraction in Blood Pressure Recovery from Emotional Arousal", *Psychosomatic Medicine*, 68, pp. 64-72.
13. Glynn, L.M., Christenfeld, N. and Gerin, W., 2002, "The Role of Rumination in Recovery from Reactivity: Cardiovascular Consequences of Emotional States", *Psychosomatic Medicine*, 64, pp. 714-726.
14. Bermúdez, J. and Pérez-García, A.M., 1996, "Cardiovascular Reactivity, Affective Responses and Performance Related to the Risk Dimensions of Coronary-prone Behaviour", *Personality and Individual Differences*, 21, pp. 919-927.
15. Caprara, G.V., 1986, "Indicators of Aggression: The Dissipation-rumination Scale", *Personality and Individual Differences*, 7, pp. 763-769.
16. Brosschot, J.F., Gerin, W. and Thayer, J.F., 2006, "The Perseverative Cognition Hypothesis: A Review of Worry, Prolonged Stress-related Physiological Activation and Health", *Journal of Psychosomatic Research*, 60, pp. 113-124.
17. Pedersen, W.C., Denson, T.F., Goss, R.J., Vasquez, E.A. and Miller, N., 2006, "The Impact of Rumination on Aggressive Thoughts, Feelings, Behavior and Arousal", *Unpublished Manuscript*.
18. Berkowitz, L., 1993, *Aggression: Its Causes, Consequences and Control*, McGraw-Hill, New York.
19. Lundberg, U., 2005, "Stress Hormones in Health and Illness: The Roles of Work and Gender", *Psychoneuroendocrinology*, 30, pp. 1017-1021.
20. Bushman, B.J., Bonacci, A.M., Pedersen, W.C., Vasquez, E.A. and Miller, N., 2005, "Chewing on It Can Chew You Up: Effects of Rumination on Triggered Displaced Aggression", *Journal of Personality and Social Psychology*, 88, pp. 969-983.
21. Cohen, S. and Willis, T.A., 1985, "Stress, Social Support and the Buffering Hypothesis", *Psychological Bulletin*, 98, pp. 310-357.
22. Brummett, B.H., Barefoot, J.C., Siegler, I.C., Clapp-Channing, N.E., Lytle, B.L., Bosworth, H.B., Williams, R.B. and Mark, D.B., 2001, "Characteristics of Socially Isolated Patients with Coronary Artery Disease Who Are at Elevated Risk for Mortality", *Psychosomatic Medicine*, 63, pp. 267-272.
23. Kaplan, G.A., Salonen, J.T., Cohen, R.D., Brand, R.J., Syme, S.L. and Puska, P., 1988, "Social Connections and Mortality from all Causes and from Cardiovascular Disease: Prospective Evidence from Eastern Finland", *American Journal of Epidemiology*, 128, pp. 370-380.
24. Uchino, B.N., 2006, "Social Support and Health: A Review of Physiological Processes Potentially Underlying Links to Disease Outcomes", *Journal of Behavioral Medicine*, 29, pp. 377-387.
25. Linden, W., Chambers, L., Maurice, J. and Lenz, J.W., 1993, "Sex Differences in Social Support, Self-deception, Hostility and Ambulatory Cardiovascular Activity", *Health Psychology*, 12, pp. 376-380.
26. Seeman, T.E. and Syme, L., 1987, "Social Networks and Coronary Artery Disease: A Comparison of the Structure and Function of Social Relations as Predictors of Disease", *Psychosomatic Medicine*, 49, pp. 341-354.

27. Christenfeld, N., Gerin, W., Linden, W., Sanders, M., Mathur, J., Deich, J.D. and Pickering, T.G., 1997, "Social Support Effects on Cardiovascular Reactivity: Is a Stranger as Affective as a Friend?", *Psychosomatic Medicine*, 59, pp. 388-398.
28. Lepore, S.J., Allen, K.A.M. and Evans, G.W., 1993, "Social Support Lowers Cardiovascular Reactivity to an Acute Stressor", *Psychosomatic Medicine*, 55, pp. 518-524.
29. Lepore, S.J., 1995, "Cynicism, Social Support and Cardiovascular Reactivity", *Health Psychology*, 14, pp. 210-216.
30. Pedersen, W.C., Zapata, C. and Denson, T.F., "Trait Displaced Aggression and Perceived Social Support", Manuscript under Preparation.
31. DiMatteo, M.R., 2004, "Social Support and Patient Adherence to Medical Treatment: A Meta-analysis", *Health Psychology*, 23, pp. 207-218.
32. Trapnell, P.D. and Campbell, J.D., 1999, "Private Self-consciousness and the Five-factor Model of Personality: Distinguishing Rumination from Reflection", *Journal of Personality and Social Psychology*, 76, pp. 284-304.
33. Duval, S. and Wicklund, R.A., 1972, "A Theory of Objective Self-awareness", Academic Press, Oxford, UK.
34. Rusting, C.L. and Nolen-Hoeksema, S., 1998, "Regulating Responses to Anger: Effects of Rumination and Distraction on Angry Mood", *Journal of Personality and Social Psychology*, 74, pp. 790-803.
35. Baumeister, R.F., 1991, *Escaping the Self: Alcoholism, Spirituality, Masochism and Other Flights from the Burden of Selfhood*, Basic Books, New York, USA.
36. Heatherton, T.F. and Baumeister, R.F., 1991, "Binge Eating as Escape from Self-awareness", *Psychological Bulletin*, 110, pp. 86-108.
37. Litman, J.A., 2006, "The COPE Inventory: Dimensionality and Relationships with Approach and Avoidance-motives and Positive and Negative Traits", *Personality and Individual Differences*, 41, pp. 273-284.
38. Denson, T.F., Pedersen, W.C., Ronquillo, J., Curtis, M., Borders, A. and Miller, N., In Press, "Trait Displaced Aggression, Physical Health and Life Satisfaction: A Process Model", In *Personality Down Under: Perspectives from Australasia*, S. Boag (Ed.), Nova Science Publishers, New York.
39. Anderson, C.A. and Bushman, B.J., 2002, "Human Aggression", *Annual Review of Psychology*, 53, pp. 27-51.
40. Neumann, S.A., Waldstein, S.R., Sollers, J.J., Thayer, J.F. and Sorkin, J.D., 2004, "Hostility and Distraction Have Differential Influences on Cardiovascular Recovery from Anger Recall in Women", *Health Psychology*, 23, pp. 631-640.
41. Smith, T.W., Ruiz, J.M. and Uchino, B.N., 2004, "Mental Activation of Supportive Ties, Hostility and Cardiovascular Reactivity to Laboratory Stress in Young Men and Women", *Health Psychology*, 23, pp. 476-485.
42. Berry, J.W., Worthington, E.L., Parrott, L., O'Connor, L.E. and Wade, N.G., 2005, "Forgivingness, Vengeful Rumination and Affective Traits", *Journal of Personality*, 73, pp. 183-225.
43. Paleari, F.G., Regalia, C. and Fincham, F., 2005, "Marital Quality, Forgiveness, Empathy and Rumination: A Longitudinal Analysis", *Personality and Social Psychology Bulletin*, 31, pp. 368-378.
44. Lawler, K.A., Younger, J.W., Piferi, R.L., Billington, E., Jobe, R., Edmondson, K. and Jones, W.H., 2003, "A Change of Heart: Cardiovascular Correlates of Forgiveness in Response to Interpersonal Conflict", *Journal of Behavioral Medicine*, 26, pp. 373-393.
45. Denson, T.F., Pedersen, W.C., Ronquillo, J. and Nandy, A.S., In Press, "The Angry Brain: Neural Correlates of Anger, Angry Rumination and Aggressive Personality", *Journal of Cognitive Neuroscience*.

The AHA-Syndrome and Cardiovascular Diseases
Editors: Swati Y. Bhave and Sunil Saini
Copyright © 2010 Anamaya Publishers, New Delhi, India

12. Aggression, Cardiovascular Disease and Genetics

Ana Butkovic and Denis Bratko
Department of Psychology, Faculty of Humanities and Social Sciences, University of Zagreb, Croatia

Abstract: The present chapter begins with a brief overview of the foundations and the methods used in behaviour and molecular genetics. That is followed by an overview of results from behaviour genetic studies of aggression, including information about heritability of aggression, genetic overlap between different types of aggression, sex differences in heritability, stability and change in aggression, contextual factors associated with individual differences in aggression, and an overview of results from molecular genetic studies of aggression. Then it gives an overview of results from behaviour and molecular genetic studies of risk factors for developing cardiovascular disease, including blood pressure, obesity, cholesterol, smoking, and physical activity, as well as their covariation. Finally, the association between aggression and cardiovascular disease is addressed and recommendations for future research are given.

Keywords: Aggression, Cardiovascular disease, Genetics, Twin study, Personality.

Introduction

When it comes to any behavioural characteristic, one of the questions that has been of interest to mankind for a long time is why people are different or, in a more scientific manner, why are there individual differences for that characteristic? For a long time people were trying to answer this question by simply attributing individual differences to one factor. Some thought individual differences exist because people are born a certain way (nature) and some thought they exist because people are brought up in a certain way (nurture). However, it became apparent that both factors play a role in the existence of individual differences and that what needs to be determined is a relative contribution of each factor for every characteristic.

Behaviour and Molecular Genetics

Behaviour genetics is a fast growing and relatively new field of research investigating the relative contribution of genetic and environmental factors to individual differences. The theoretical basis of behaviour genetics is a quantitative genetic theory which provides an expectation that individuals will differ in complex behavioural traits [1]. The quantitative genetic theory begins with a model in which observed (phenotypic) differences in a population are a function of genetic and environmental differences ($V_P = V_G + V_E$). The genetic variance is then decomposed into additive genetic variance due to variation in number of particular allele present in a genotype, and non-additive genetic variance not predicted by the number of particular allele present in a genotype

($V_G = V_A + V_{NA}$). Non-additive genetic variance can be decomposed into dominance variance due to the interaction of alleles at the same locus and variance resulting from epistatic interactions due to the interaction of alleles at different loci ($V_{NA} = V_D + V_I$). The environmental variance can also be decomposed into shared and non-shared environmental variance ($V_E = V_{SH} + V_{NSH}$). Shared environmental influences are those environmental influences that make family members similar, while non-shared ones are those making family members different from one another.

The proportion of phenotypic variance attributable to genotypic variance is called *heritability* ($h^2 = V_G/V_P$). There are two types of heritability, a *broad-sense heritability* representing the proportion of phenotypic variance due to all genetic influences ($h^2 = V_A + V_{NA}/V_P$) and a *narrow-sense heritability* representing the proportion of phenotypic variance due only to additive genetic influences ($h^2 = V_A/V_P$). A few important things that need to be kept in mind when interpreting heritability estimates are:

(i) There is an error of estimation linked with every heritability estimate. This error of estimation is dependent on the size of a measured effect and the sample size [2].
(ii) Heritability estimate refers to genetic contribution to individual differences and does not say anything about a single individual. In sum, heritability refers to the contribution of genetic differences to observed differences among individuals for a particular trait in a particular population at a particular time.
(iii) Heritability does not imply genetic determinism, which means that even highly heritable traits can be changed, or be under environmental influence.

There are a variety of methods used in behaviour genetics to estimate the relative contribution of genetic and environmental influences to individual differences. The most widely used is a *twin study*, which takes advantage of the natural occurrence of two types of twins who differ in their degree of genetic similarity to estimate heritability of a measured characteristic. *Monozygotic* (MZ) twins develop from one fertilised egg and, therefore, share all their genetic material. *Dizygotic* (DZ) twins develop from two fertilised eggs and, therefore, on an average share 50% of their genetic material, same as other siblings. If MZ twins correlate more for a measured characteristic than DZ twins, this is an indication that genetic effects influence the measured characteristic. A rough estimate of heritability can be obtained from Falconer's formula by doubling the difference between MZ and DZ twins correlation ($h^2 = 2\ (r_{MZ} - r_{DZ})$) [3]. For a more precise estimate model-fitting procedures are used. Another method used in behaviour genetics is an *adoption study*, in which adopted children can be compared in a measured characteristic with their biological parents with whom they share genes but not the environment, or with their adopting parents with whom they share environment but not genes. Similarity between adopted children and their biological parents in a measured characteristic suggests the importance of genetic influences, while similarity between adopted children and their adopting parents in a measured characteristic suggests the importance of shared environmental influences. The third behavioural genetic method, *family study*, is the least powerful of behavioural genetic methods because parents and their biological children who share both genes and environment are compared on a measured characteristic. Their similarity can be used to get an estimate of upper-limit heritability, but influences of genes and shared environment cannot be disentangled. Each of these methods has specific limitations and, therefore, behaviour geneticists use combination of methods to arrive at more precise estimates of heritability, like twins raised apart, families with both biological and adopted children, parents of twins and twins, twins and their children.

Following the finding that a measured characteristic is heritable and under genetic influence, the next step includes trying to identify specific genes responsible for that genetic influence. Molecular genetic approach is used with two different strategies, linkage analysis and association analysis. Because we cannot manipulate human genotypes to see the effects that would have on their phenotypes, we have to search for genes indirectly. *Association analysis* is used to link an allele with a trait for individuals in population, while *linkage analysis* is used to link an allele with a trait for individuals in families, tracing co-inheritance of genes and disorders within families [2]. In other words, the data about the measured characteristic (phenotype) are correlated with a specific combination of genes (genotype). However, these efforts to identify specific genes responsible for different complex traits have not been as successful as everyone expected. Although there have been many positive findings of genetic association, less than 1% of them have been replicated because of a number of reasons, including small sample sizes, use of complex, not well-measured phenotypes, and population stratification. Population stratification refers to analysis of mixed samples having different allele frequencies due to systematic differences in ancestry rather than association of genes with a measured trait. It leads to false evidence for allelic association. However, efforts are being made to solve all the potential problems, like using large samples and better designs, which will hopefully enable us to find true genetic associations and determine which genes are responsible for different complex traits.

Aggression

Aggression can be defined as any behaviour directed towards another individual and is carried out with the immediate intent to cause harm [4]. However, the term 'aggression' covers a whole range of different manifestations including verbal aggression, physical aggression and different forms of violence [5]. Also, the distinction is made between two types of aggression depending on their underlying function or motivation:

(i) Proactive: Instrumental and requires neither provocation nor anger.
(ii) Reactive: Affective and includes angry outbursts in response to actual or perceived provocations or threats [6, 7].

Aggression can also come in more subtle forms of social exclusion or gossip for which different labels have been used including indirect, relational or social aggression [8].

Aggression is one of the traits whose development can be traced from the infancy to adulthood. In their review of development of aggression, Loeber and Hay [5] say that the earliest manifestations of aggression occur during infancy with most infants showing signs of frustration and rage. During the second and third year behavioural signs of temper tantrums and aggression toward adults can be observed, while from early to middle childhood aggression decreases as children develop interpersonal skills. However, in this period, sex differences become apparent with males showing higher rates of physical aggression, while females tend to use more verbal and indirect aggression. During adolescence and early adulthood several changes occur in level and pattern of aggression including increase in impact of aggressive acts, engagement of peer groups in collective forms of violence, increase in parent-child conflict, increase in cross-gender aggression and onset of abuse toward partner or children. Use of physical aggression is highest early in life and then, subsequently, decreases during adolescence, but more serious violence increases with age especially during adolescence. Many longitudinal studies have shown that early aggression in childhood or adolescence and later aggression are highly correlated and stable in time and that early aggression is predictive of different manifestations of later violence.

Because of its early manifestation, stability and individual differences, aggression has been of interest to behavioural genetic research. Miles and Carey [9] performed a meta-analysis on data from 24 twin and adoption studies on aggression, in which they concluded that:

- Heritability and common environment were responsible for individual differences in aggression, with heritability accounting for as much as 50% of the variance.
- Different estimates are obtained depending on the method (self-report, parental report or observational methods).
- Genetic and family environmental architecture of aggression may change over time.
- In adulthood common environmental influences are not important.

Another review of behaviour genetic research of aggression in children by DiLalla [10] reached a similar conclusion. It concluded that one of the biggest problems in aggression research is the lack of consistent definition of aggression across studies. Also, different conclusions about the heritability of aggression are obtained with different methods of data collection. When distinction is made between aggression and delinquency, it becomes apparent that their etiology is different, with more genetic and less shared environmental influences for aggression and less genetic and more shared environmental influences for delinquency. It seems that behaviour genetic analysis should be performed separately for different manifestations of aggression.

Several studies have shown the importance of measuring different types of aggression separately. Brendgen et al. [11] examined genetic and environmental influences to proactive and reactive aggression. They found that both are influenced by genes (41% vs. 39%) and non-shared environmental influences to a similar extent. They also found that proactive and reactive aggression share 76% of their genetic influences and 12% of environmental influences. However, they showed that much of the overlap could be explained by a shared underlying form such as physical aggression. In another study, Brendgen et al. [8] examined genetic and environmental influences to social and physical aggression. The results for physical aggression were similar to previous studies with 50-60% of the variance explained by genetic factors and the rest by unique environmental factors, but for social aggression genetic factors only accounted for 20% of the variance, shared environmental influences for another 20% and unique environmental factors for 60% of the variance. The overlap between physical and social aggression was explained mostly by overlapping genetic influences and small amount of overlapping environmental influences. Ligthart et al. [12] examined genetic and environmental influences to relational and direct aggression. For relational aggression, 66% of the variance was due to additive genetic influences, 16% to shared environment and 18% to non-shared environment. For direct aggression, additive genetic effects accounted for 53% of the variance in males and 60% in females, shared environment explained 23% of the variance in males and 13% in females, and non-shared environmental effects explained 24% of the variance in males and 27% in females. Covariance between the aggression subtypes was mostly accounted for by additive genetic and shared environmental influences. Both relational and direct aggression were influenced by one underlying set of shared environmental factors, but only partly by the same genes.

Sex differences in aggression were also explored using behaviour genetic research. However, results differed from study to study. Silberg et al. [13] found significant sex differences in the magnitude of genetic and environmental effects using maternal ratings of externalising behaviour of twins aged 8-16 years. Eley, Lichtenstein and Stevenson [14] found no sex differences using maternal ratings of aggressive anti-social behaviour in Swedish (7- to 9-year-olds) and British (8- to 16-year-olds) samples of twins. Hudziak et al. [15] assessed aggression in a cross-sectional sample of Dutch twins aged 3, 7 and 10 years using mother, father and teacher ratings. They found evidence for moderate to high genetic influence (51-72%) by all three informants at all ages with only small sex differences in heritability estimates. The largest sex differences in heritabilities were seen at age 10. Vierikko et al. [16] used teacher and parent ratings of aggression in the Finnish population based twin sample aged 12 years and found sex differences in the magnitude of genetic and environmental effects for parental ratings, and sex differences in the magnitude of genetic and environmental effects as well as sex-specific common environmental or additive genetic effects for teacher ratings. Sex differences in environmental contributions to aggression, as well as either sex-specific common environmental or additive genetic effects were evident in the same sample using teacher ratings 2 years later [17]. In contrast to the previous studies that measured aggression in childhood or adolescence using informants, Jacobson, Prescott and Kendler [18] collected retrospective reports of anti-social behaviour from adult twins over three periods: prior to 15 years (childhood), 15-17 years (adolescence), and 18 years and older (adulthood). They found sex differences in the magnitude of genetic and environmental influences to childhood aggression, but those sex differences diminished with age and were not found in adolescence and adulthood. Taken together these findings suggest that sex differences in genetic and environmental influences to aggression might arise at a specific period of development, somewhere between ages of 10 and 15 years and might be linked with sex differences in the timing of puberty.

Genetic and environmental contributions to stability of aggression were explored using longitudinal behavioural genetic studies. O'Connor et al. [19] examined the genetic as well as environmental origins of the stability and change of anti-social and depressive symptoms in adolescence using twins and full, half and unrelated siblings from non-divorced and stepfamilies. They found that stability of anti-social behaviour could be accounted for by genetic, shared and non-shared environmental factors. Genetic factors also contributed to change in anti-social behaviour. Eley, Lichtenstein and Moffitt [20] explored the genetic and environmental influences on aggressive and non-aggressive anti-social behaviour in twins when they were 8-9 years and 13-14 years old. In childhood, aggressive anti-social behaviour was highly heritable and showed little influence of shared environment, while in adolescence it was influenced by both genes and shared environment. The continuity in aggressive anti-social behaviour symptoms from childhood to adolescence was largely mediated by genetic influences. Bratko [21] has presented the results of a longitudinal twin study of verbal and physical aggressiveness. The twin sample was followed from adolescence (17 years) to early adulthood (21 years) and the data were analysed to assess:

(i) Phenotypic stability and change of verbal and physical aggressiveness.
(ii) Relative contribution of the genetic and environmental influences to the individual differences in aggressiveness.

(iii) Genetic and environmental contribution to the phenotypic stability.

The results indicate increase of means in verbal aggressiveness and decrease in physical aggressiveness at the phenotypic level. Phenotypic stability was moderate with test retest correlations of 0.49 for verbal and 0.57 for physical aggressiveness. The heritability was 58 and 48% for verbal aggressiveness in adolescence and early adulthood, respectively, while for physical aggressiveness it was 49 and 48%. Longitudinal behavioural genetic analyses indicate that both genes and shared environmental influences contribute to the phenotypic stability of verbal and physical aggressiveness. van Beijsterveldt et al. [22] examined the causes of stability of aggression from early childhood to adolescence on Dutch twins aged 3, 7, 10 and 12 years. They found that genetic factors accounted for approximately 65% of stability and that there was a transmission of existing genetic effects which interact with new genetic influences. Shared environmental factors accounted for approximately 25% of phenotypic stability and it seemed that these shared environmental factors were the same during development. Non-shared environmental factors were age specific. Vierikko et al. [17] examined stability of teacher-rated aggression in 12- to 14-years-old Finnish twins. Sources of stability of aggression differed by sex including genes and common environmental factors for boys and shared environmental and, to lesser degree, non-shared environmental factors for girls. For both sexes, change in aggression was due to genes and non-shared environmental factors. These studies suggest that marked stability of aggression is largely attributed to genetic factors and, to a lesser degree, to shared environmental factors.

Behaviour genetic research has also been useful in exploring different contextual or specific factors associated with individual differences in aggression. Bratko and Zuzul [23] tried to identify some specific non-shared environmental influences which are related to individual differences in aggression. They explored the relation between differential experience of MZ twins and their aggression scores. It was found that two differential experiences, *maternal affection* and *peer delinquency*, were significant predictors of difference in aggression scores of MZ twins. Rowe, Almeida and Jacobson [24] tried to evaluate the effect of two moderator variables, racial-ethnic heterogeneity in schools and family warmth on a school-level, on genetic and environmental influences on aggression. They found that environmental context measured at school-level moderated mean level of aggression because they found higher levels of aggression in schools with greater racial and ethnic heterogeneity and in schools with lower average levels of family warmth. Genetic and environmental influences on variation in aggression were also moderated because heritability was higher in schools with higher average levels of family warmth, while shared and non-shared environmental influences were higher in schools with lower average levels of family warmth. The same sample of adolescents was used in another study that explored differences in genetic and environmental influences on adolescent aggression across adequate and disadvantaged neighbourhoods [25]. Results showed that although genetic influences on aggression were important in both adequate and disadvantaged neighbourhoods, shared environmental influences were important only in disadvantaged neighbourhoods. This suggests that differences in family environment are more important for expression of adolescent aggression in disadvantaged than in adequate neighbourhood contexts.

Following findings of heritability of aggression, molecular genetic studies tried to discover specific genes responsible for aggression. Although research findings are mixed, it seems that several genes and systems are involved in shaping individual differences in aggression. Several serotonergic genes have been implicated in impulsivity and aggression-related behaviours in pharmacologic studies on rats or mice, knockout studies on mice and in studies of gene variation or deletion in humans [26]. In a review of the role serotonergic system plays in aggression Olivier and van Oorschot [27] concluded that this system seemed to be involved in either performance or the termination of aggressive behaviours. The enzyme monoamine oxidase A (MAOA), which has a direct regulatory impact on the serotonin, norepinephrine and dopamine systems, was also implicated in aggression-related behaviours. Functional polymorphisms and mouse knockout models suggest that MAOA activity affects the expression of aggressive behaviour, while in human studies the link was also found but in different directions [28]. Chen et al. [29] hypothesised that polymorphisms of the dopaminergic system are involved in a predisposition to pathological aggression. Several important studies have shown the importance of gene-environment interactions for aggressive behaviours. Caspi et al. [30] studied the association between childhood maltreatment and development of anti-social behaviour in a large sample of male children. They found that functional polymorphism in the gene encoding MAOA moderated the effect of maltreatment and that maltreated children with a genotype conferring high levels of MAOA expression were less likely to develop anti-social problems. Verona et al. [31] examined gene-environment interactive effects on aggressive behaviour among men and women genotyped for the serotonin transporter gene using experimental laboratory paradigm. They found that serotonin transporter gene is linked to risk for externalising reactivity (aggression) in men under acute stress conditions. Further studies are of course needed in this area of research but results so far encourage hopes of discovering mechanisms associated with aggressive behaviours.

Cardiovascular Disease

Cardiovascular disease (CVD) is one of the leading causes of death throughout the world. It is known that there are a number of risk factors for developing CVD, like high blood pressure, obesity, smoking, family history of heart disease, inactive lifestyle and high cholesterol [32].

Behaviour genetic research of blood pressure (BP) has shown that both systolic and diastolic blood pressures are heritable. Hottenga et al. [33] examined genetic and environmental influences on BP in participants from four twin studies carried out between 1986 and 2003. Heritabilities ranged from 48 to 60% for systolic BP (SBP) and from 34 to 67% for diastolic BP (DBP). Also, there was little evidence for sex differences in BP heritability. They also found that across an average period of 7 years BP tracking was entirely explained by the same genetic factors. Similar heritabilities of BP were obtained on Australian twins participating in three different studies with heritabilities of SBP ranging from 19 to 56% and of DBP from 37 to 52% [34]. Also, in this sample, the BP tracking was explained by the same set of genetic factors over an average period of 12 years. In an extended twin design that used twins and their singleton siblings it was found that there were no differences between singletons and twins and that estimates of heritability of ambulatory BP from twin studies can be generalised to the singleton population [35]. Heritability of hypertension was 61%, while heritabilities of BP became lower when medicated hypertensive subjects were excluded. It was concluded that exclusion of medicated hypertensive subjects removes part of the true genetic variance in ambulatory BP. Since hypertension prevalence is much higher in African-Americans than in European-Americans several studies tested if there were ethnic differences in the relative contribution of genes and environment to population variation in BP. Brandon et al. [36] studied heritability of BP in a sample of adult African-American twins and found heritabilities similar to those obtained in other samples, between 44 and 52% for SBP and between 27 and 36% for DBP. Snieder, Harshfield and Treiber [37] studied African- and European-American youth and found difference in heritability only for DBP with African-Americans having higher heritability than European-Americans. Also, they found no sex differences in heritabilities of BP. Kupper et al. [38] studied heritability of BP in a sample of European-American and African-American twins, with an intervening period of 4.1 years. Heritabilities were moderate to high (25-64%) and relatively stable over time, genetic influences accounted for 60 to 100% of the phenotypic tracking correlations and novel genetic influences accounted for a significant part of the variance (17-33%) at the second measurement occasion. They also found significant ethnic differences for both SBP and DBP, with non-shared environmental influences becoming larger over time for African-Americans than European-Americans.

Obesity is a condition characterised by increased body weight caused by excessive accumulation of fat. There are a number of indicators used for obesity and they include body mass index (BMI), waist circumference, waist-hip ratio, skinfold thicknesses and body fat measurement. Schousboe et al. [39] investigated the genetic and environmental influences on adult body size, shape and composition in a sample of Danish twins. They found that genetic contributions were significant in both women and men for all phenotypes – BMI, body fat percentage, total skinfolds, extremity skinfolds, truncal skinfolds, suprailiac skinfolds, waist and hip circumference, lean body mass/height^2 and height – and they were all in 50-70% range. Since the prevalence of obesity among African-Americans is higher than among whites, Nelson et al. [40] investigated genetic and environmental influences among African-American twins. Heritability estimates for waist circumference, waist-to-hip ratio and BMI were for both men and women in the 50-70% range, similar to findings among white twin samples. So, heritability estimates for obesity are high, typically around 70% [41]. Obesity genetic researchers were, at first, mainly interested in monogenic or syndromic obesity and that led to the identification of many genes involved in the regulation of appetite via the leptin-melanocortin pathway. As for common polygenic obesity, there are currently 22 gene associations supported by at least five positive studies which include members of the leptin-melanocortin pathway, proinflammatory cytokines and uncoupling proteins [41].

Several studies tried to establish if covariation between obesity indicators and BP could be explained by genetic factors. McCaffery et al. [42] analysed the correlation among SBP, DBP, BMI, fasting total cholesterol and triglycerides in a sample of twins. Their results indicated that all measures were individually influenced by genetic and non-shared environmental effects and that common genetic and, to a lesser extent, common non-shared environmental effects contributed to the covariation of these measures. However, these common influences accounted for a relatively small percentage of the variance in each risk factor compared to the genetic and environmental factors that were specific for each risk factor. Nelson et al. [43] examined the covariation between body fat and BP measures in a sample of African-American twins. Again, both common genetic and environmental variance between these measures were very small and majority of the variance was accounted for by genetic and environmental influences unique to each measure. Livshits, Pantsulaia and Gerber [44] used a pedigree-based cross-sectional study to ascertain the extent to which relationships between obesity and BP could be explained by an individual's leptin plasma levels. They found that this covariation was substantially mediated by circulating leptin levels. Only genetic variation of DBP in their sample shared very little with that of leptin. A number of twin studies found that leptin levels were also heritable [45-49].

Cholesterol is a soft, waxy substance found among the lipids (fats) in the bloodstream and in all body cells. Cholesterol, like fats, cannot dissolve in the blood and has to be transported to and from the cells by special carriers called *lipoproteins*. There are several kinds, but the most well known and often mentioned are *low-density lipoprotein* (LDL) and *high-density lipoprotein* (HDL). The apolipoproteins forming the surface of the given lipoprotein particle determine from what cells cholesterol will be removed and to where it will be supplied. Behaviour genetic research has examined genetic and environmental influences to variation in cholesterol, lipid, lipoprotein and apolipoprotein levels. Boomsma et al. [50] examined plasma lipid, lipoprotein and apolipoprotein levels in adolescent twins and their parents. They found large inter-generational differences in heritabilities with no sex differences. Heritabilities for children were between 65 and 87%, while heritabilities for their parents were between 10 and 50%. This pattern of results was best explained by the increase in non-shared environmental variance with increasing age. Iliadou et al. [51] examined variation of lipids and apolipoproteins in a sample from Swedish Twin Registry aged 17-85 years. Heritabilities for lipids and apolipoproteins ranged from 35 to 74% and consistent sex differences were found only in triglycerides with higher heritabilities for females across the age groups. They also found differences in phenotypic variation for cholesterol and apolipoprotein B across the age groups due to an increase in non-shared environmental influences. Beekman et al. [52] investigated the influence of genes and environment on the variation of apolipoprotein and lipid levels in three twin samples from the Netherlands, Australia and Sweden. The variation of apolipoprotein and lipid levels depended largely on the influences of additive genetic factors in each twin sample, with heritabilities in the 48-87% range. They found no significant evidence for the influence of common environment and no sex differences in heritability estimates. Similar heritability estimates for total, LDL and HDL cholesterol, ranging from 36 to 64%, were found in a sample of Polish twins [53]. Iliadou et al. [54] examined ethnic differences in genetic and environmental influences on lipids and found high heritabilities with no sex differences for all measures and no ethnic differences for total cholesterol, triglycerides and HDL, with LDL showing higher heritability in African-Americans (92%) than in European-Americans (69%). Researchers have stressed on the importance of measuring cholesterol levels more than once per participant because of the confounding effects of biological variation measurement error and ageing. Results from longitudinal studies indicate that an individual's long-term cholesterol values are strongly genetically determined, but that some of these genes are age-specific in their effects [55] and also that more than one genetic factor influence HDL and LDL components of cholesterol and triglycerides over time [56]. Because of its important role in atherogenesis, special attention has been given to apolipoprotein E (apoE), which comes in three slightly different versions encoded by three different alleles – epsilon 2, epsilon 3 and epsilon 4. Different studies of the impact of apoE polymorphism on risk for CVD reached different conclusions, but in their meta-analysis of 48 studies Song, Stampfer and Liu [57] and Kharrazi et al. [58] found that epsilon 4 allele is a significant risk factor for CVD. The apoE plays a central role in plasma lipoprotein metabolism and in lipid transport. Because apoE gene affects a lipid level, it seems that apoE 4 allele can be considered as a 'thrifty allele' to the coronary artery disease [59].

Smoking is also one of the risk factors for developing CVD. Behaviour genetic research on smoking has explored different smoking related phenotypes. In their meta-analysis of genetic and environmental effects in male and female adult twins, Li et al. [60] used two different phenotypes, smoking initiation (SI) and smoking persistence (SP). For SI they found that genetic factors were more important (55% vs. 37%) and shared environmental influences less important (30% vs. 49%) for females than for males, while for SP the situation was reversed with genetic factors being more important (57% vs. 46%) and shared environmental influences less important (8% vs. 27%) for males than for females. These findings suggest that genetic and environmental factors may contribute differently to smoking initiation and persistence in male and female smokers. Czerwinski et al. [61] tested for gene *x* smoking interaction effects on plasma triglyceride levels, HDL cholesterol level and median LDL particle diameter in Mexican-American families enrolled in the San Antonio Family Heart Study. They found a significant gene *x* smoking interaction effect on triglyceride level and median LDL particle diameter as well as possible evidence for an effect on HDL cholesterol level, which indicates that the gene or suite of genes regulating each of these phenotypes is likely to be the same in smokers and non-smokers but that smoking may alter the expression of those genes. Hozawa et al. [62] tested the hypothesis that smoking is a stronger risk factor for CVD when LDL cholesterol is high. They found that both smoking and increased LDL cholesterol were risk factors for CVD and that the relative hazard of CVD in relation to smoking tended to be larger among higher LDL categories compared with lower LDL categories.

Regular physical activity can help prevent heart and blood vessel disease by controlling blood cholesterol, diabetes and obesity and by lowering BP in some people. The study of familial aggregation of physical activity phenotypes showed that physical activity level is characterised by a significant degree of familial resemblance and that inactivity has a slightly higher heritability level than moderate to strenuous physical activity or total physical activity phenotypes [63]. Spinath et al. [64] objectively assessed motor activity level in a sample of twins and found moderate genetic influence of 40%. Joosen et al. [65] investigated the relative contribution of genetic and environmental factors to activity-induced energy expenditure and physical activity in a small sample of twins and found that 78% of the variance in physical activity can be explained by genetic factors. Eriksson, Rasmussen and Tynelius [66] examined the genetic contribution to physical activity on a nationwide male twin sample and found heritability of 49% for total physical activity and genetic contributions between 40 and 65% for all physical activity dimensions. Muldoon et al. [67] tested the hypothesis that individual differences in serotonergic function are associated with the metabolic syndrome and physical inactivity. Across the sample, low serotonergic function was associated with greater BMI, higher concentrations of triglycerides, glucose and insulin, higher SBP and DBP, greater insulin resistance and less physical activity.

Behaviour genetic research done so far on risk factors for developing CVD consistently shows that all these risk factors – high BP, obesity, cholesterol, smoking and inactive lifestyle – are influenced by genetic factors. Another conclusion is that there is a complex and interactive relationship between these factors that can alter their influence and impact on CVD.

Aggression and CVD

In the 1960s cardiologists Meyer Friedman and Ray Rosenman noticed that many of their patients exhibited similar pattern of behaviour that included competitiveness, aggression, hostility and achievement strivings, and named that pattern *Type A personality* [32]. Later on, it was noticed that not all components of Type A personality are related to development of CVD and hostility component was identified as a pathogenic agent. Why is that so? Strong feelings of hostility and aggression produce the "fight-or-flight" response which leads to increase in BP, constriction of the arteries and increase in the heart rate and amount of blood pumped out with each heartbeat. Because more blood is pumped through small arteries during the fight-or-flight response, this can, with time, cause microscopic tears and abrasions on the inside lining of the arteries at which cholesterol and fat can become attached. Stress hormones released into the blood during the fight-or-flight response may also lead to artery damage. Build-up of fatty deposits on artery walls leads to narrowing, hardening or blocking of the arteries and when arteries that feed the heart muscle become blocked, heart attack occurs.

In their review of the studies that examined the associations between measures of anger, hostility and aggressiveness with increased risk of CVD and reduced longevity, Smith et al. [68] concluded that although findings are mixed, there is enough evidence that anger, hostility and aggressiveness contribute to the development of CVD. There are a number of mechanisms linking anger, hostility and aggression with CVD. People with higher levels of anger, hostility and aggression are more psychophysiologically reactive, as described earlier. They are psychosocially vulnerable because they experience greater levels of interpersonal conflict and stress and lower levels of social support. They also lead a less healthy life-style which includes known risk factors for CVD like smoking and physical inactivity.

It is possible that similar systems that are associated with aggression-related behaviours play an important role in CVD. Even more so, polymorphisms involved in serotonergic systems have been related to individual differences in hostility and aggressiveness as well as to cardiovascular responses to psychological stress [68]. Serotonin has been implicated in cardiovascular function as blood, blood vessels and the heart are targets for circulating serotonin signalling. Cardiovascular dysfunction is observed when serotonin signalling is altered or when variation in serotonin concentration occurs. Components of the serotonergic system that have been implicated in both aggression and cardiovascular system are $5\text{-}HT_{1B}$ receptor and MAOA [69]. Lung, Fan and Chen [70] investigated the possible association between MAOA gene promoter polymorphisms and telomere length as influenced by age and gender in a sample from Taiwan because both telomere shortening and increased MAOA gene activity occur with aging. It has been shown that telomere length is associated with CVD, although it remains to be seen whether telomere shortening is a cause or a consequence of CVD [71, 72]. The results suggest that high-activity MAOA promoter gene polymorphisms, as in aging, are a risk factor for telomeric shortening. Since serotonergic activity correlates with human aggressive behaviour and depression in many studies, it was concluded that the MAOA promoter gene may also serve as a clinical marker in the treatment of CVD.

Conclusion

There is an increased recognition among experts in the field about the importance of psychosocial factors for CVD. Personality traits like aggression, mistrust or proneness to anger have an important role in predisposing people to CVD. However, the biological process that underlies disease and also the connection between personality and disease, is less often recognised. This process is usually long and related to the aging. For example, Iribarren et al. [73] assessed the hostility in a sample of 374 young adults. After 10 years they checked the participant's coronary arteries for calcification – an early sign of atherosclerosis. Results indicated that hostile participants were more likely to have coronary calcification. How can personality traits like aggressiveness or hostility affect the development of coronary heart disease? Aggression and hostility can produce flight-or-fight response, including increase in BP and constriction of arteries. Blood flow through the constricted arteries can produce microscopic tears and abrasions, which then become sites at which cholesterol and fat can become attached. Hormonal changes during the flight-or-fight reaction may also lead to artery damage. There is compelling evidence suggesting that both aggression and hostility, on the one side, and CVD, on the other, are heritable. Also, there is compelling evidence about the phenotypic association of aggressiveness and hostility with CVD. However, we are not aware of any multivariate behavioural genetic study which includes both, cardiovascular and personality phenotypes. Do genetic and environmental influences on aggression, hostility and CVD overlap? Also, it is possible to hypothesise the gene-gene interaction in the probability for developing CVD. For example, a group of people with epsilon 4 allele, which have genes that contribute to aggressiveness, would be at a higher risk for early development of CVD. Genotype-environment interaction is also possible. For example, we may hypothesise that stress would have a more negative effect on people with epsilon 4 in genotype, because hormonal changes may affect more the group with higher cholesterol level. That may be one of the possible topics in a future research. A recommendation for future research of aggression and CVD would be to include information about known genetic markers or to use genetically informative populations like twins.

Key Points

- ❑ Observed (phenotypic) differences in a population are a function of genetic and environmental differences ($V_P = V_G + V_E$).
- ❑ The proportion of phenotypic variance attributable to genotypic variance is called heritability ($h^2 = V_G/V_P$).
- ❑ Methods used in behaviour genetics to estimate the relative contribution of genetic and environmental influences to individual differences are twin study adoption and family studies.
- ❑ Molecular genetic approach is used with two different strategies, viz. linkage analysis and association analysis.
- ❑ Behaviour genetic studies of aggression examined heritability, sex differences in heritability, stability and change and contextual factors associated with individual differences in aggression.
- ❑ Molecular genetic studies of aggression indicate that serotonergic genes and monoamine oxidase A (MAOA) could be associated with aggressive behaviours.
- ❑ Risk factors for developing cardiovascular disease, i.e. BP, obesity, cholesterol, smoking, and physical activity, have been examined using behaviour genetic studies and results consistently show that they are all influenced by genetic factors.
- ❑ Personality traits like aggression, mistrust, or proneness to anger have an important role in predisposing people to CVD because they can produce flight-or-fight response and lead to artery damage.
- ❑ Multivariate behavioural genetic studies, which include both cardiovascular and personality phenotypes, are needed.

References

1. Plomin, R., DeFries, J.C., McClearn, G.E. and Rutter, M., 1997, *Behavioral Genetics*, W.H. Freeman and Co., New York.
2. Plomin, R., DeFries, J.C., McClearn, G.E. and McGuffin, P., 2000, *Behavioral Genetics*, Worth Publishers, New York.
3. Plomin, R., DeFries, J.C. and McClearn, G.E., 1990, *Behavioral Genetics: A Primer*, W.H. Freeman and Co., New York.
4. Anderson, C.A. and Bushman, B.J., 2002, "Human Aggression", *Annual Review of Psychology*, 53, pp. 27-51.
5. Loeber, R. and Hay, D., 1997, "Key Issues in the Development of Aggression and Violence from Childhood to Early Adulthood", *Annual Review of Psychology*, 48, pp. 371-410.
6. Crick, N.R. and Dodge, K.A., 1996, "Social Information-processing Mechanisms on Reactive and Proactive Aggression", *Child Development*, 67, pp. 993-1002.
7. Dodge, K.A. and Coie, J.D., 1987, "Social-information-processing Factors in Reactive and Proactive Aggression in Children's Peer Groups", *Journal of Personality and Social Psychology*, 53, pp. 1146-1158.
8. Brendgen, M., Dionne, G., Girard, A., Boivin, M., Vitaro, F. and Pérusse, D., 2005, "Examining Genetic and Environmental Effects on Social Aggression: A Study of 6-year-old Twins", *Child Development*, 76, pp. 930-946.
9. Miles, D.R. and Carey, G., 1997, "Genetic and Environmental Architecture of Human Aggression", *Journal of Personality and Social Psychology*, 72, pp. 207-217.
10. DiLalla, L.F., 2002, "Behavior Genetics of Aggression in Children: Review and Future Directions", *Developmental Review*, 22, pp. 593-622.
11. Brendgen, M., Vitaro, F., Boivin, M., Dionne, G. and Pérusse, D., 2006, "Examining Genetic and Environmental Effects on Reactive Versus Proactive Aggression", *Developmental Psychology*, 42, pp. 1299-1312.
12. Ligthart, L., Bartels, M., Hoekstra, R.A., Hudziak, J.J. and Boomsma, D.I., 2005, "Genetic Contributions to Subtypes of Aggression", *Twin Research and Human Genetics*, 8, pp. 483-491.
13. Silberg, J.L., Erickson, M.T., Meyer, J.M., Eaves, L.J., Rutter, M.L. and Hewitt, J.K., 1994, "The Application of Structural Equation Modeling to Maternal Ratings of Twins' Behavioral and Emotional Problems", *Journal of Consulting and Clinical Psychology*, 62, pp. 510-521.
14. Eley, T.C., Lichtenstein, P. and Stevenson, J., 1999, "Sex Differences in the Etiology of Aggressive and Nonaggressive Antisocial Behavior: Results from Two Twin Studies", *Child Development*, 70, pp. 155-168.
15. Hudziak, J.J., van Beijsterveldt, C.E.M., Bartels, M., Rietveld, M.J.H., Rettew, D.C., Derks, E.M., and Boomsma, D.I., 2003, "Individual Differences in Aggression: Genetic Analyses by Age, Gender and Informant in 3-, 7-, and 10-year-old Dutch Twins", *Behavior Genetics*, 33, pp. 575-589.
16. Vierikko, E., Pulkkinene, L., Kaprio, J., Viken, R. and Rose, R.J., 2003, "Sex Differences in Genetic and Environmental Effects on Aggression", *Aggressive Behavior*, 29, pp. 55-68.
17. Vierikko, E., Pulkkinene, L., Kaprio, J. and Rose, R.J., 2006, "Genetic and Environmental Sources of Continuity and Change in Teacher-rated Aggression During Early Adolescence", *Aggressive Behavior*, 32, pp. 308-320.
18. Jacobson, K.C., Prescott, C.A. and Kendler, K.S., 2002, "Sex Differences in the Genetic and Environmental Influences on the Development of Antisocial Behavior", *Development and Psychopathology*, 14, pp. 395-416.
19. O'Connor, T.G., Neiderhiser, J.M., Reiss, D., Hetherington, E.M. and Plomin, R., 1998, "Genetic Contributions to Continuity, Change and Co-occurrence of Antisocial and Depressive Symptoms

in Adolescence", *Journal of Child Psychology and Psychiatry and Allied Disciplines*, 39, pp. 323-336.

20. Eley, T.C., Lichtenstein, P. and Moffitt, T.E., 2003, "A Longitudinal Behavioral Genetic Analysis of the Etiology of Aggressive and Nonaggressive Antisocial Behavior", *Development and Psychopathology*, 15, pp. 383-402.
21. Bratko, D., 2000, "Genetic and Environmental Contribution to the Individual Differences in Aggressiveness", *Conference Abstracts*, 10th European Conference on Personality, Krakow.
22. van Beijsterveldt, C.E.M., Bartels, M., Hudziak, J.J. and Boomsma, D.I., 2003, "Causes of Stability of Aggression from Early Childhood to Adolescence: A Longitudinal Genetic Analysis in Dutch Twins", *Behavior Genetics*, 33, pp. 591-605.
23. Bratko, D. and Zuzul, M., 1994, "Genetic and Environmental Contribution to Individual Differences in Aggressiveness: Exploring Some Non-shared Environmental Factors", In *Personality Psychology in Europe*, B. De Raad, W.K.B. Hofstee and G.L. van Heck (Eds.), Tilburg University Press, pp. 133-137.
24. Rowe, D.C., Almeida, D.M. and Jacobson, K.C., 1999, "School Context and Genetic Influences on Aggression in Adolescence", *Psychological Science*, 10, pp. 277-280.
25. Clevelend, H.H., 2003, "Disadvantaged Neighborhoods and Adolescent Aggression: Behavioral Genetic Evidence of Contextual Effects", *Journal of Research on Adolescence*, 13, pp. 211-238.
26. Lesch, K.P. and Merschdorf, U., 2000, "Impulsivity, Aggression and Serotonin: A Molecular Psychobiological Perspective", *Behavioral Sciences and the Law*, 18, pp. 581-604.
27. Olivier, B. and van Oorschot, R., 2005, "5-HT_{1B} Receptors and Aggression: A Review", *European Journal of Pharmacology*, 526, pp. 207-217.
28. Beithcman, J.H., Mik, H.M., Ehtesham, S., Douglas, L. and Kennedy, J.L., 2004, "MAOA and Persistent, Pervasive Childhood Aggression", *Molecular Psychiatry*, 9, pp. 546-547.
29. Chen, T.J.H., Blum, K., Mathews, D., Fisher, L., Schnautz, N., Braverman, E.R., Schoolfield, J., Downs, B.W. and Comings, D.E., 2005, "Are Dopaminergic Genes Involved in a Predisposition to Pathological Aggression? Hypothesizing the Importance of "Super Normal Controls" in Psychiatricgenetic Research of Complex Behavioral Disorders", *Medical Hypotheses*, 65, pp. 703-707.
30. Caspi, A., McClay, J., Moffitt, T.E., Mill, J., Martin, J., Craig, I.W., Taylor, A. and Poulton, R., 2002, "Role of Genotype in the Cycle of Violence in Maltreated Children", *Science*, 297, pp. 851-854.
31. Verona, E., Joiner, T.E., Johnson, F. and Bender, T.W., 2006, "Gender Specific Gene-environment Interactions on Laboratory-assessed Aggression", *Biological Psychology*, 71, pp. 33-41.
32. Larsen, R.J. and Buss, D.M., 2005, *Personality Psychology: Domains of Knowledge About Human Nature*", McGraw Hill, New York.
33. Hottenga, J.J., Boomsma, D.I., Kupper, N., Posthuma, D., Snieder, H., Willemsen, G. and de Geus, E.J.C., 2005, "Heritability and Stability of Resting Blood Pressure", *Twin Research and Human Genetics*, 8, pp. 499-508.
34. Hottenga, J.J., Whitfield, J.B., de Geus, E.J.C., Boomsma, D.I. and Martin, N.G., 2006, "Heritability and Stability of Resting Blood Pressure in Australian Twins", *Twin Research and Human Genetics*, 9, pp. 205-209.
35. Kupper, N., Willemsen, G., Riese, H., Posthuma, D., Boomsma, D.I. and de Geus, E.J.C., 2005, "Heritability of Daytime Ambulatory Blood Pressure in an Extended Twin Design", *Hypertension*, 45(1), pp. 80-85.
36. Brandon, D.T., Whitfield, K.E., Sollers, J.J., Wiggins, S.A., West, S.G., Vogler, G.P., McClearn, G.E. and Thayer, J.F., 2003, "Genetic and Environmental Influences on Blood Pressure and Pulse Pressure Among Adult African Americans", *Ethnicity and Disease*, 13(2), pp. 193-199.
37. Snieder, H., Harshfield, G.A. and Treiber, F.A., 2003, "Heritability of Blood Pressure and Hemodynamics in African- and European-American Youth", *Hypertension*, 41(6), pp. 1196-1201.

38. Kupper, N., Ge, D.L., Treiber, F.A. and Snieder, H., 2006, "Emergence of Novel Genetic Effects on Blood Pressure and Hemodynamics in Adolescence: The Georgia Cardiovascular Twin Study", *Hypertension*, 47(5), pp. 948-954.
39. Schousboe, K., Visscher, P.M., Erbas, B., Kyvik, K.O., Hopper, J.L., Henriksen, J.E., Heitmann, B.L. and Sørensen, T.I.A., 2004, "Twin Study of Genetic and Environmental Influences on Adult Body Size, Shape and Composition", *International Journal of Obesity*, 28, pp. 39-48.
40. Nelson, T.L., Brandon, D.T., Wiggins, S.A. and Whitfield, K.E., 2002, "Genetic and Environmental Influences on Body-fat Measures Among African-American Twins", *Obesity Research*, 10, pp. 733-739.
41. Walley, A.J., Blakemore, A.I.F. and Froguel, P., 2006, "Genetics of Obesity and the Prediction of Risk for Health", *Human Molecular Genetics*, 15, pp. R124-R130.
42. McCaffery, J.M., Pogue-Geile, M.F., Debski, T.T. and Manuck, S.B., 1999, "Genetic and Environmental Causes of Covariation Among Blood Pressure, Body Mass and Serum Lipids During Young Adulthood: A Twin Study", *Journal of Hypertension*, 17, pp. 1677-1685.
43. Nelson, T.L., Brandon, D.T., Wiggins, S.A. and Whitfield, K.E., 2006, "Genetic and Environmental Influences on Body-fat and Blood Pressure in African-American Adult Twins", *International Journal of Obesity*, 30, pp. 243-250.
44. Livshits, G., Pantsulaia, I. and Gerber, L.M., 2005, "Association of Leptin Levels with Obesity and Blood Pressure: Possible Common Genetic Variation", *International Journal of Obesity*, 29, pp. 85-92.
45. Narkiewicz, K., Szczech, R., Winnicki, M., Chrostowska, M., Pawlowski, R., Lysiak-Szydlowska, W., Choe, I., Kato, M., Sivitz, W.I., Krupa-Wojciechowska, A. and Somers, V.K., 1999, "Heritability of Plasma Leptin Levels: A Twin Study", *Journal of Hypertension*, 17, pp. 27-31.
46. Kaprio, J., Eriksson, J., Lehtovirta, M., Koskenvuo, M. and Tuomilehto, J., 2001, "Heritability of Leptin Levels and the Shared Genetic Effects on Body Mass Index and Leptin in Adult Finnish Twins", *International Journal of Obesity*, 25, pp. 132-137.
47. Wallace, A.M., Banfield, E., Ingram, M., Fraser, R., Swan, L., Hillis, W.S. and Connell, J.M.C., 2004, "Glucocorticoids Contribute to the Heritability of Leptin in Scottish Adult Female Twins", *Clinical Endocrinology*, 61, pp. 149-154.
48. Jordan, J., Brabant, G., Brinsuk, M., Tank, J., Horn, R., Luft, F.C. and Busjahn, A., 2005, "Heritability of Free and Receptor-bound Leptin in Normal Twins", *American Journal of Physiology*, 288, pp. 1411-1416.
49. Li, H.J., Ji, C.Y., Wang, W. and Hu, Y.H., 2005, "A Twin Study for Serum Leptin, Soluble Leptin Receptor and Free Insulin-like Growth Factor-I in Pubertal Females", *Journal of Clinical Endocrinology and Metabolism*, 90, pp. 3659-3664.
50. Boomsma, D.I., Kempen, H.J.M., Leuven, J.A.G., Havekes, L., de Knijff, P. and Frants, R.R., 1996, "Genetic Analysis of Sex and Generation Differences in Plasma Lipid, Lipoprotein and Apolipoprotein Levels in Adolescent Twins and Their Parents", *Genetic Epidemiology*, 13, pp. 49-60.
51. Iliadou, A., Lichtenstein, P., de Faire, U. and Pedersen, N.L., 2001, "Variation in Genetic and Environmental Influences in Serum Lipid and Apolipoprotein Levels Across the Lifespan in Swedish Male and Female Twins", *American Journal of Medical Genetics*, 102, pp. 48-58.
52. Beekman, M., Heijmans, B.T., Martin, N.G., Pedersen, N.L., Whitfield, J.B., DeFaire, U., van Baal, G.C.M., Snieder, H., Vogler, G.P., Slagboom, P.E. and Boomsma, D.I., 2002, "Heritabilities of Apolipoprotein and Lipid Levels in Three Countries", *Twin Research*, 5, pp. 87-97.
53. Jedrusik, P., Januszewicz, A., Busjahn, A., Zawadzki, B., Wocial, B., Ignatowska-Switalska, H., Berent, H., Kuczynska, K., Oniszczenko, W., Strelau, J., Luft, F.C. and Januszewicz, W., 2003, "Genetic Influence on Blood Pressure and Lipid Parameters in a Sample of Polish Twins", *Blood Pressure*, 12, pp. 7-11.

54. Iliadou, A., Snieder, H., Wang, X.L., Treiber, F.A. and Davis, C.L., 2005, "Heritabilities of Lipids in Young European American and African American Twins", *Twin Research and Human Genetics*, 8, pp. 492-498.
55. Middelberg, R., Heath, A.C., Martin, N.G. and Whitfield, J.B., 2005, "Evidence of Age-dependent Genetic Influences on Plasma Total Cholesterol", *European Journal of Cardiovascular Prevention and Rehabilitation*, 12, pp. 380-386.
56. Middelberg, R., Martin, N.G. and Whitfield, J.B., 2006, "Longitudinal Genetic Analysis of Plasma Lipids", *Twin Research and Human Genetics*, 9, pp. 550-557.
57. Song, Y.Q., Stampfer, M.J. and Liu, S.M., 2004, "Meta-analysis: Apolipoprotein E Genotypes and Risk for Coronary Heart Disease", *Annals of Internal Medicine*, 141, pp. 137-147.
58. Kharrazi, H., Raygani, A.V., Sabokroh, A.R. and Pourmotabbed, T., 2006, "Association Between Apolipoprotein E Polymorphism and Coronary Artery Disease in the Kermanshah Population in Iran", *Clinical Biochemistry*, 39, pp. 613-616.
59. Corbo, R.M. and Scacchi, R., 1999, "Apolipoprotein E (APOE) Allele Distribution in the World: Is APOE*4 a 'Thrifty' Allele?" *Annals of Human Genetics*, 63, pp. 301-310.
60. Li, M.D., Cheng, R., Ma, J.Z. and Swan, G.E., 2003, "A Meta-analysis of Estimated Genetic and Environmental Effects on Smoking Behavior in Male and Female Adult Twins", *Addiction*, 98, pp. 23-31.
61. Czerwinski, S.A., Mahaney, M.C., Rainwater, D.L., Vandeberg, J.L., Maccluer, J.W., Stern, M.P. and Blangero, J., 2004, "Gene by Smoking Interaction: Evidence for Effects on Low-density Lipoprotein Size and Plasma Levels of Triglyceride and High-density Lipoprotein Cholesterol", *Human Biology*, 76, pp. 863-876.
62. Hozawa, A., Folsom, A.R., Sharrett, A.R., Payne, T.J. and Chambless, L.E., 2006, "Does the Impact of Smoking on Coronary Heart Disease Differ by Low-density Lipoprotein Cholesterol Level? The Atherosclerosis Risk in Communities (ARIC) Study", *Circulation Journal*, 70, pp. 1105-1110.
63. Simonen, R.L., Perusse, L., Rankinen, T., Rice, T., Rao, D.C. and Bouchard, C., 2002, "Familial Aggregation of Physical Activity Levels in the Quebec Family Study", *Medicine and Science in Sports and Exercise*, 34, pp. 1137-1142.
64. Spinath, F.M., Wolf, H., Angleitner, A., Borkenau, P. and Riemann, R., 2002, "Genetic and Environmental Influences on Objectively Assessed Activity in Adults", *Personality and Individual Differences*, 33, pp. 633-645.
65. Joosen, A.M.C.P., Gielen, M., Vlietinck, R. and Westerterp, K.R., 2005, Genetic Analysis of Physical Activity in Twins", *American Journal of Clinical Nutrition*, 82, pp. 1253-1259.
66. Eriksson, M., Rasmussen, F. and Tynelius, P., 2006, "Genetic Factors in Physical Activity and the Equal Environment Assumption: The Swedish Young Male Twins Study", *Behavior Genetics*, 36, pp. 238-247.
67. Muldoon, M.F., Mackey, R.H., Williams, K.V., Korytkowski, M.T., Flory, J.D. and Manuck, S.B., 2004, "Low Central Nervous System Serotonergic Responsivity is Associated with the Metabolic Syndrome and Physical Inactivity", *Journal of Clinical Endocrinology and Metabolism*, 89, pp. 266-271.
68. Smith, T.W., Glazer, K., Ruiz, J.M. and Gallo, L.C., 2004, "Hostility, Anger, Aggressiveness and Coronary Heart Disease: An Interpersonal Perspective on Personality, Emotion and Health", *Journal of Personality*, 72, pp. 1217-1270.
69. Côté, F., Fligny, C., Fromes, Y., Mallet, J. and Vodjdani, G., 2004, "Recent Advances in Understanding Serotonin Regulation of Cardiovascular Function", *Trends in Molecular Medicine*, 10, pp. 232-238.
70. Lung, F., Fan, P. and Chen, N.C., 2005, "Telomeric Length Varies with Age and Polymorphisms of the MAOA Gene Promoter in Peripheral Blood Cells Obtained from a Community in Taiwan", *Psychiatric Genetics*, 15, pp. 31-35.

71. Serrano, A.L. and Andres, V., 2004, "Telomeres and Cardiovascular Disease: Does Size Matter?" *Circulation Research*, 94, pp. 575-584.
72. Fuster, J.J. and Andres, V., 2006, "Telomere Biology and Cardiovascular Disease", *Circulation Research*, 99, pp. 1167-1180.
73. Iribarren. C., Sidney, S., Bild, D.E., Liu, K., Markovitz, M.H., Roseman, R.M. and Matthew, K., 2000, "Association of Hostility with Coronary Artery Calcification in Young Adults: The CARDIA Study", *The Journal of the American Medical Association*, 283, pp. 2546-2551.

The AHA-Syndrome and Cardiovascular Diseases
Editors: Swati Y. Bhave and Sunil Saini
Copyright © 2010 Anamaya Publishers, New Delhi, India

13. Sex Differences in Biological and Psychological Risk Factors for Coronary Artery Disease

Kim L. Lavoie,[1,2,3] Roxanne Pelletier[1,3] and Simon L. Bacon[2,3,4]

[1]Department of Psychology, University of Quebec at Montreal, P.O. Box 8888, Succursale Centre-Ville, Montreal, Quebec, H3C 3P8, Canada

[2]Research Centre, Division of Chest Medicine, Hôpital du Sacré-Cœur de Montréal – A University of Montreal Affiliated Hospital, 5400 Gouin West, Montreal, Quebec, H4J 1C5, Canada

[3]Research Centre, Montreal Heart Institute – A University of Montreal Affiliated Hospital, 5000 Belanger, Montreal, Quebec, H1T 1C8, Canada

[4]Department of Exercise Science, Concordia University, 7141 Sherbrooke, St. West SP16535, Montreal, Quebec, H4B 1R6, Canada

Abstract: The present chapter reviews the unique presentation of coronary artery disease (CAD) and the challenges associated with diagnosing CAD in women. It also discusses in detail the major sex differences in both biological and psychological risk factors for CAD.

Keywords: Sex differences, Coronary artery disease, Risk factors, Depression, Anxiety, Anger.

Introduction

Coronary artery disease (CAD) is the leading cause of mortality in the western world, accounting for over one-third of all deaths [1, 2]. In 2006, this disease cost the United States (US) alone an estimated US$ 142.5 billion [2]. Despite major advances in our understanding of the pathophysiology, diagnosis and management of CAD, there remain important sex differences in mortality rates of women and men with CAD. Although CAD has been traditionally considered a "man's disease", it remains the number one cause of death among women [1, 2] with mortality rates due to CAD (38%) [2] far exceeding those due to breast cancer (22-25%) [2, 3]. In Canada, not only did the 2002 mortality rate due to CAD in women (37,848) exceed that of men (36,778), but CAD accounted for a greater proportion of the death toll in women (34.3%) compared to men (32.5%) [1, 4]. Though overall mortality rates due to CAD have declined substantially over the past two decades, this decline has been less dramatic in women than in men [5]. Women have also been shown to have worse CAD outcomes relative to their male counterparts: more women (38%) than men (25%) die within one year of having their first myocardial infarction (MI) [6]. Hospital mortality rates following an acute MI have been shown to be higher in women (16%) than in men (11%) [7]. The following three main reasons for this sex disparity in CAD mortality and outcome have been suggested:

(1) Unique presentation of CAD in women [8, 9].
(2) Sex differences in the prevalence and impact of both biological and psychological risk factors for CAD [10, 11].
(3) A general under-representation and lack of sex-specific data from clinical trials and research [9, 12].

For example, it was not until 1999 that the first female-specific recommendations for preventative cardiology were published [13]. Put together these factors have left major gaps in our ability to identify and properly treat women with CAD.

Sex Differences in CAD Presentation and Diagnosis

One of the greatest challenges to the proper diagnosis and treatment of CAD in women is that the disease itself, and its risk factors have been defined based on men's experience with the disease [14]. The clearest sex difference associated with CAD is highlighted by the initial presentation of the disease. In general, classic symptoms of CAD are uncommon in pre-menopausal women (< 55 years of age), with symptom onset typically occurring about 10 years later than in men [15]. However, once CAD has been diagnosed in women, their rate of disease progression is much quicker than in their male counterparts [1, 15-17]. Moreover, women with acute coronary syndromes (ACS) – defined as having a history of MI, non-Q-wave MI, or unstable angina – present with very different symptoms compared to men. Women are less likely to have a chief complaint of chest pain, which is the 'classic' sign of CAD among men, and are more likely to report non-classic symptoms such as shortness of breath, weakness and unusual fatigue [14, 18, 19]. Unfortunately, these 'atypical' symptoms often go unrecognised by physicians [19-22], thus, resulting in women being referred for comparably fewer diagnostic tests (e.g. exercise stress tests, coronary angiography) and revascularisation procedures (e.g. percutaneous coronary interventions, PCI's) [18, 19, 23]. The fact that fewer women are being referred for diagnostic tests and procedures may, in part, explain why they have worse CAD outcomes than men, including increased in-hospital complications following acute MI, increased 30-day mortality following MI and increased rates of refractory (treatment-resistant) ischemia [23, 24]. However, the healthcare system may not be the only one to blame for women's poorer outcomes; women themselves may also fail to recognise the significance of their symptoms [25] and, as a result, may delay seeking medical treatment [26, 27].

Biological Explanations for Sex Differences in CAD Symptom Onset and Presentation

There are a number of hypotheses regarding the delayed onset and unique presentation of CAD in women. The most widely accepted biological explanation for the delayed onset of CAD in women relative to men is related to elevated levels of pre-menopausal endogenous estrogen, which has been shown to have important anti-atherosclerotic effects [28]. For example, a review [10] identified numerous animal studies finding evidence of estrogen's anti-oxidative and anti-inflammatory properties and its ability to increase the elasticity of the vessel wall, which may be beneficial during times of high physical and/or mental stress when oxygen demands are high. During menopause, levels of endogenous estrogen drop drastically to approximately one-tenth of their pre-menopausal levels, likely accounting for the sharp increase in CAD incidence in women aged 50-55 years or older [10]. A study by the Women's Ischemia Syndrome Evaluation (WISE) investigators linked estrogen deficiencies in younger, pre-menopausal women to increased risk for ischemic heart disease. Specifically, they reported that stress-induced disruptions in ovulation leading to decreased estrogen levels were associated with a 7.4-fold increased risk of CAD in women under investigation for myocardial ischemia [29]. In fact, estrogen deficiencies were the most powerful predictors of CAD in this study, and highlighted the cardio-protective (and, potentially, cardio-toxic) effects of alterations in estrogen levels in women. The strength of the estrogen-CAD association has led to hormone replacement therapy (HRT) interventions designed to increase estrogen levels in menopausal and post-menopausal women. Though numerous benefits have been associated with HRT, including regulation of vasomotor tone and response to injury (which may protect against the development of atherosclerosis and ischemic heart diseases), reductions in low density lipoprotein (LDL) and increases in high density lipoprotein (HDL) and antioxidant effects, HRT is not without important risks. These risks include venous embolisms, gallbladder disease and possibly breast cancer [28], all of which need to be weighed against the potential benefits of hormone replacement before initiating therapy.

With respect to sex differences in the presentation of CAD, there are a number of anatomical differences between men and women, including smaller left ventricular mass and cavity size [30] and smaller left main (LM) and proximal left anterior descending (LAD) coronary artery diameters [31], that have been proposed to explain the unique challenges of detecting and diagnosing CAD in women. It has been hypothesised that smaller vessel diameters in women may increase their risk of acute cardiac events associated with coronary occlusion (e.g. ischemia or MI) [11]. Interestingly, women appear to be at lower risk for events related to complete occlusion of the coronary arteries (e.g. MI) [14, 24], but there is evidence linking smaller vessel diameter to increased risk of operative mortality. For example, the Collaborative Study in Coronary Artery Surgery (CASS) reported that higher rates of coronary artery bypass graft (CABG) operative mortality in women (4.5%) compared to men (1.9%) were, in part, attributable to the smaller diameter of the coronary arteries in women [32].

The unique presentation of CAD in women may also be explained by sex differences in the prevalence and impact of both biological and psychological risk factors. Like the definition of CAD itself, the classic CAD risk factor profile has been determined primarily from observations in men [10]. A review of the literature reveals that there is substantial sex-related variability in the prevalence and impact of both biological and psychological risk factors that have often been overlooked in previous research. The following sections will review these differences in greater detail and discuss the potential implications on CAD outcomes.

Biological Risk Factors for CAD

Biological risk factors for CAD may be divided into two classes: *non-modifiable* and *modifiable*. Non-modifiable biological risk factors include sex, age and family history of CAD. Although being male has been traditionally considered a risk factor for CAD, CAD risk projection algorithms (e.g. Framingham Score) now estimate risk separately for men and women [33]. As mentioned earlier, CAD typically emerges an average of 10 years later in women, relative to men, around the age of menopause [34]. With respect to family history of CAD, there is little evidence of any sex differences in prevalence or impact of this risk factor. However, there are several sex differences in the prevalence and impact of *modifiable* biological risk factors for CAD, which include hypertension (high blood pressure), smoking, hyperlipidemia, poor diet and physical inactivity (obesity) and diabetes.

Sex Differences in Biological Risk Factors for CAD

Hypertension

Hypertension – having a resting systolic and/or diastolic blood pressure ≥ 140/90 – affects nearly 28% of Americans and 27% of Canadians [35]. However, these rates are substantially higher in Western Europe, ranging from 37.7% (Italy) to 55.3% (Germany) [35]. In individuals between the ages of 35 to 64 years, rates of hypertension are generally higher in men (30-60%) than in women (25-50%) [35], though rates among women tend to be higher than in men from age 45 years onward [2]. Oral contraceptive use appears to be an important risk factor for the development of hypertension in women, which can be two-three fold higher in users vs. non-users, particularly if taken over extended periods [36]. Hypertension rates may also vary considerably depending on one's race. According to statistics from the US, hypertension is particularly prevalent among blacks, with black females having the highest rates (45.4%), followed by black males (41.8%), white females (31%) and white males (30.6%) [2]. These figures highlight the importance of considering race and ethnicity when assessing CAD risk.

Smoking

Smoking has been recognised as an important risk factor for CAD since the first Surgeon General's Report on Tobacco was issued in 1964 [37]. Though rates of smoking have declined significantly since then, it is estimated that over 23 and 18% of adult men and women, respectively, are current smokers [38]. Contrary to rates among adults, smoking rates among teenagers are similar in both male and female adolescents. Results from the Global Youth Tobacco Survey (GYTS), initiated in 1999 by the World Health Organisation (WHO), the Centre for Disease Control (CDC) and the Canadian Public Health Association revealed that nearly 20% of teens reported currently using a tobacco product [39]. Nonetheless, there may still be additional cardiac risks conferred to women who smoke, particularly in those using oral contraceptives. One review reported that oral contraceptive use in pre-menopausal women who smoked was associated with an increased risk of non-fatal MI and that this risk increased 128-fold if these women had at least three other CAD risk factors [40]. It has also been reported that those at highest risk for MI are female smokers under the age of 55 years [2]. Finally, smoking has been shown to reduce life expectancies more in women than in men. Another report by the US Surgeon General reported that while male smokers die an average 13.2 years earlier than male non-smokers, female smokers die an average 14.5 years earlier than female non-smokers [41]. This data suggests that despite the fact that smoking rates are moderately higher among men than among women, smoking may confer greater CAD risk in women.

Hyperlipidemia

Dysregulated cholesterol levels affect approximately 100 million Americans [2]. The negative effects of cholesterol are associated with having high total cholesterol, high low-density lipoprotein

(LDL, "bad cholesterol") levels, or low high-density lipoprotein (HDL, "good cholesterol") levels. Although total cholesterol levels are generally higher in men until the age of 50 years, after which these levels are higher among women [10], the prevalence of hypercholesterolemia (total cholesterol ≥ 200 mg/dL) appears to be similar in men (48.9%) and women (50.2%) [2]. Likewise, high LDL cholesterol (LDL ≥ 130 mg ml/dL) affects a comparable number of men (39.1%) and women (37.0%). The most notable sex differences in lipids are observed in HDL cholesterol levels, which are generally lower in men than in women throughout the lifespan [10]. For example, recent US statistics reveal a far greater prevalence of low HDL (< 40 mg/dL) in men (33.2%) relative to women (12.8%) [2], suggesting that women may be somewhat protected from the negative effects of cholesterol through their disproportionately elevated HDL levels. This has been supported by at least one study showing that higher levels of HDL appear to be more strongly associated with CAD risk reduction in older women relative to older men [42]. Cholesterol levels have also been shown to differentially predict CAD risk according to sex, with elevated LDL levels being less predictive of CAD risk in women compared to men [42, 43]. Given the resources currently allocated to improving cholesterol screening and treatment, it seems crucial to consider the differential impact of this risk factor in men vs. women.

Diabetes Mellitus

This is a condition related to abnormal carbohydrate metabolism, affects over 21 million Americans [44] and has increased in prevalence by over 54% between 1994 and 2002 from 4.8 to 7.3% in the US alone [2]. Though the prevalence of diabetes (90-95% of which is accounted for by Type 2 diabetes), is comparable between men (7%) and women (7.1%) [2], the cardiovascular risks and complications associated with diabetes appear to be more severe in women than in men. According to a publication from the CDC [45], diabetic women are at greater risk for developing CAD and blindness (a common complication of diabetes), compared to diabetic men. Moreover, women with diabetes who have suffered a heart attack have lower survival rates and worse quality of life relative to their male counterparts [45]. A review by the WISE investigators also reported marked elevations in CAD mortality rates in diabetic women relative to diabetic men [10]. Death rates in pre-menopausal women with diabetes are also more than three-fold greater than for women without diabetes [45]. Taken together, this data suggest that diabetes is a particularly powerful CAD risk factor in women and may even eliminate women's pre-menopausal protective advantage relative to men.

Poor Diet and Physical Inactivity

These are two intricately linked risk factors for CAD as they contribute to one of the world's most important and rising health crises: obesity. Over the past 30 years, the prevalence of obesity has risen drastically in North America and costs the US healthcare system about US$ 70 billion per year [46]. Obesity, defined as having a body mass index (BMI) ≥ 30 kg/m^2, affects nearly 30% [2] of the US and 15% [47] of the Canadian population. When one also considers those who are overweight (BMI ≥ 25 kg/m^2), these rates as much as triple, reaching 65% of Americans [2] and nearly 50% of Canadians [47]. According to US statistics, rates of obesity are comparable between men (27.6%) and women (28.2%) [2]. However, women appear to be at greater risk for weight gain throughout the lifespan compared to men, whose BMI increases until the age of 50 years and then reaches a plateau [48]. This may be partially explained by the fact that as women age, they lose more physical functioning and become less physically active than men [49]. Less women (20.0%) than men (31.4%) of all ages appear to participate in regular leisure-time physical activity [2], and up to 25% of adult women admit to participating in no regular physical activity [50]. Another factor contributing to increased weight gain in women is related to a loss in ovarian estrogen at the onset of menopause, which is associated with the development of an 'apple'-shaped body profile and an increase in the deposition of abdominal or visceral fat. An increase in abdominal fat has been linked to greater risk for CAD in women [48] and there is evidence that waist circumference (WC), which is a measure of abdominal or visceral fat, is associated with numerous health risks in women. For example, a study found that women with a high (> 88 cm) vs. low (≤ 88 cm) WC were at greater risk of developing hypertension, Type 2 diabetes, hypercholesterolemia, hypertriglyceridemia and the metabolic syndrome [51][#]. Moreover, this study found that the health risks associated with having a high WC were greater in women compared to men. For example, the risk of Type 2 diabetes was over twice as high among women with a high WC compared to men with a high (> 102 cm) WC. Finally, high abdominal or central fat has also been associated with premature mortality in women [52], making obesity, and central obesity, in particular, a highly potent CAD risk factor in women.

Psychological Risk Factors for CAD

Though biological risk factors explain a significant proportion of the variance in CAD, they do not explain it fully. This has led researchers to consider the potential impact of alternative risk factors, particularly psychological factors, on CAD development and progression. One of the most important and influential studies to date to document a link between psychological factors and CAD is the INTERHEART Study [53], which is one of the largest, international, standardised, case-control studies designed to assess the relative importance of various risk factors for CAD (and MI in particular). It included 15,152 cases and 14,820 controls from 52 countries worldwide and found that psychological factors (including depression, perceived life stress, low locus of control and major life events) were the third most important risk factors for incident MI (odds ratio, OR = 2.67, PAR[*] = 32.5%), after elevated apolipoproteins (lipids) (OR = 3.25, PAR = 49.2%) and current smoking (OR = 2.87, PAR = 35.7%). This study was one of the first to demonstrate that psychological factors were more strongly related to MI risk than even hypertension and obesity, and using a worldwide perspective. Moreover, this study reported important sex differences in the impact of various CAD risk factors. With respect to increased ORs for MI, the risks associated with diabetes and hypertension were greater for women than for men, though alcohol consumption and regular exercise appeared to be more beneficial to women [53]. With respect to PAR for MI, smoking was associated with a much higher PAR for MI in men (42.7%) than in women (14.8%), while hypertension (29.0% vs. 14.9%) and psychological factors (45.0% vs. 28.8%) were related to a higher PAR for women compared to men. However,

[#]The metabolic syndrome reflects a constellation of metabolic risk factors including high blood pressure (> 90th percentile for age and sex), elevated fasting glucose (≥ 110 mg/dL), high triglycerides (≥ 110 mg/dL), and low HDL cholesterol (≤ 40 mg/dL). It is diagnosed when an individual has ≥ 3 of the above risk factors, though rates are comparable between men (24%) and women (23.4%) [2].

[*]PAR = Risk of the disease of the total population minus the risk in the unexposed group.

similar PARs were noted for both men and women for abnormal lipids (49.5% vs. 47.1%) and obesity (19.7% vs. 18.7%) [53]. Taken together, all nine risk factors (current smoking, diabetes, hypertension, obesity, fruit and vegetable consumption, regular exercise, alcohol consumption, abnormal lipids, and psychological factors) accounted for 90% of the total PAR for MI in men compared to 94% in women, highlighting the importance of including psychological factors when assessing global CAD risk.

In the INTERHEART Study, a composite score including several psychological variables was used to quantify psychological risk. Most research to date evaluating the impact of psychological factors on CAD has assessed single psychological variables. The most heavily researched of these include various negative mood states such as clinical and sub-clinical levels of depression and anxiety, and both state and trait measures of anger and hostility [54-56]. The following sections will review evidence of sex differences in both rates of each negative mood state, and their relative impact on CAD outcomes.

Sex Differences in Psychological Risk Factors for CAD

Depression

The psychological risk factor that has received the most attention and demonstrated the most robust link to the development and progression of CAD is depression [57-63]. Over the last two decades, several studies have documented a disproportionately high rate of depressive symptomatology and/or clinical depression (i.e. major depressive disorder (MDD)) among patients with established CAD [64, 65] and patients who have suffered from an acute MI [59, 66-68]. The prevalence of depressive symptomatology is estimated to be between 40 and 65% in patients who have recently suffered an acute MI [63]. MDD affects approximately 18% of post-MI patients [69, 70] and 18% of patients with no history of MI but with documented CAD [65]. Compared to the point (12-month) prevalence of depression in the general population (6.6%) [71], the rate of depression in CAD patients is substantially elevated.

Not only is depression common in patients with CAD, but there is evidence linking depression to the development and progression of CAD [72, 73]. A review [57] has identified at least 11 etiologic studies conducted in initially healthy individuals showing evidence of a link between depression and future development of CAD that was independent of more 'traditional' risk factors such as hypertension and smoking. However, the strongest and most extensive evidence linking depression to CAD comes from studies that measured depression following an acute MI, and evaluated the prognostic impact of depression on post-MI outcomes. In general, these studies have identified depression as an independent predictor of prognosis and/or mortality (including fatal MI, cardiac and all-cause mortality) [58-60, 62, 74-81]. However, some studies have failed to find significant associations between depression and post-MI outcomes [82-84]. Nonetheless, taken together, these findings suggest a relatively robust association between depression and CAD.

Though depression has been associated with increased cardiovascular risk in both men and women [85], a review of literature reveals a number of important sex differences in both the rates and impact of depression in CAD patients. Not only is depression more common in women than in men in the general population [71], it is also more common among women with CAD

[86, 87]. For example, significantly more women (47%) than men (26%) become depressed following an MI [87] and this may be particularly true for women under the age of 60 years [88]. Depression has also been shown to be more common in women than in men with heart failure [86], unstable angina [89] and following coronary artery bypass graft (CABG) surgery [90]. Although it is easy to understand why people may become depressed after a major cardiac event such an MI or CABG surgery, it may be surprising to learn that depression is more common in women suspected of having CAD. A recent study reported that among 2,262 patients referred for exercise stress testing (a common diagnostic test for CAD), 33% of women (vs. only 24% of men) met criteria for one or more depressive disorder [91]. This data suggests that depression may be more common among women, even prior to confirming a diagnosis of CAD.

Not only is depression more common in women with CAD, there is evidence to suggest that depression may contribute to worse CAD outcomes in women relative to men. For example, women who are diagnosed as depressed prior to undergoing CABG surgery had a worse functional status and quality of life six-months post-CABG compared to men [92]. Moreover, in a study assessing the impact of depression post-CABG, more depressed women (44%) than depressed men (20%) experienced a significant cardiac event or died in the 12-months following their surgery. Higher mortality rates have also been observed in depressed women (8.3%) relative to depressed men (7.0%), again highlighting the potential toxic combination of being female and depressed in this population.

Anxiety

Anxiety disorders (e.g. panic disorder, generalised anxiety disorder, social phobia) are the most common mental disorders in North America, with prevalence rates exceeding those of even mood (depressive) disorders [93]. Like depression, rates of both sub-clinical and clinical levels of anxiety are disproportionately high among patients with CAD [94]. The prevalence of anxious symptomatology is estimated to be between 16 and 40% in patients who have suffered a recent cardiac event [95-97] and may be as high as 63% in patients suffering from heart failure [98]. Levels of clinical anxiety (i.e. anxiety disorders) are also quite high, with rates of panic disorder ranging from 10 to 50% in cardiac outpatients [99]. More importantly, high levels of anxiety have been linked to worse cardiac outcomes, including increased risk of arrhythmias, MI and sudden cardiac death [66, 94, 100]. For example, cardiac events were more common and occurred earlier in post-MI patients who were highly anxious, compared to those who were not [101]. Higher anxiety scores post-MI have also been associated with a nearly five-fold increased risk of ischemic and/or arrhythmic complications [94]. In addition, there is evidence to suggest that anxiety may be a stronger risk factor for incident CAD than other negative mood states such as depression and anger. In a recent prospective study assessing the unique contributions of various negative mood states on incident CAD in over 1,300 men in the Normative Aging Study, only anxiety (and not depression or anger) was associated with increased incidence of CAD over a 20-year period [102]. However, it is noteworthy that the association between anxiety and cardiac outcomes may be less robust than that for depression, as many studies have failed to find significant associations between elevated anxiety levels and increased cardiac morbidity and mortality [84, 103]. Moreover, some studies have even reported positive associations between high anxiety levels and CAD outcomes, such as the severity of coronary plaques [104, 105].

Anxiety has been shown to be elevated in CAD patients of both sexes [94, 106] but similar to depression, women with CAD appear to exhibit higher levels of anxiety than men with CAD [106], particularly following an MI [107-109]. For example, one study assessing levels of anxiety in the first 72 hours following an acute MI found that women reported significantly higher levels of both state and trait anxiety (on the Spielberger State-Trait Anxiety Inventory (STAI)) than men, particularly 60-72 hours after the infarction [108]. A similar study assessing levels of anxiety within 72 hours post-MI also revealed higher anxiety scores (on the Brief Symptom Inventory) in women than in men, with 16% of women (vs. only 8% of men) reporting anxiety levels higher than observed in psychiatric patients [107]. Finally, women also appear to exhibit higher state and trait anxiety scores (on the STAI) both pre- and post-percutaneous transluminal coronary angioplasty (PTCA), with one study reporting anxiety levels in the range of psychiatric patients in 24% of women vs. only 16% of men [106].

Not only do women with CAD have higher rates of anxiety, but anxiety may contribute to greater morbidity and mortality among women. For example, one study reported that state anxiety and female gender predicted recurrent coronary syndromes in the first year following an acute MI [66]. Another study of women in the Framingham Study revealed positive associations between tension and anxiety and incident CAD in women [110]. Finally, high anxiety scores were found to predict total mortality to a slightly greater degree in women (OR = 1.27) than in men (OR = 1.22) in the Framingham Offspring Study [111]. Taken together, these findings are suggestive of a link between anxiety and increased cardiac risk in women relative to men. Given that women appear more likely to suffer from anxiety than men [112], assessments of anxiety levels and their impact on cardiac outcomes in women with CAD seems warranted.

Anger

Depression and anxiety both appear to be more prevalent among women with CAD. The available literature suggests these negative mood states may also be more detrimental to CAD outcomes in women relative to men. In contrast to depression and anxiety, anger has been considered an emotion disproportionately experienced by men [113]. This view may have been fostered by socialisation practices that accept and even encourage anger in men, but discourage anger in women [114, 115]. However, a review of the emotion literature reveals that despite these socialisation influences, women appear to experience anger to the same degree as men, as often, and for the same reasons [116-118]. However, where men and women appear to differ is in the way anger is expressed. Although women have been shown to be more emotionally expressive overall [119], previous research has shown that girls from a very young age may electively inhibit the expression of socially unacceptable emotions, namely anger [120, 121]. Although this has led to the assumption that women may be less likely to outwardly express their anger relative to men, this is only partially supported by the literature. For example, a group of middle-aged working women from the Framingham Study reported being more likely to suppress anger expression relative to middle-aged working men [122]. Other studies, however, have reported greater levels of anger suppression in men (e.g. greater anger-in scores on the Spielberger Anger Expression Scale) [123-125] or failed to report any significant sex differences in anger expression [126, 127].

Explaining Sex Differences in Anger Expression: Impact of Gender Role Expectancies

A number of hypotheses have been put forth to explain the apparent inconsistencies with regard to anger expression in men vs. women. In contrast to the experience of anger, which may be considered a psychological phenomenon, the expression of anger is considered more of a psychosocial phenomenon, highly influenced by social norms and gender role expectancies [114, 128]. Several studies assessing sex differences in anger expression have found evidence of social mediators that may be important to understanding the complexities of anger expression in women. For example, one study found that when social expectations about expressing different emotions, including anger, were experimentally manipulated to be comparable for men and women, no differences were observed in emotion ratings (including anger ratings) between men and women [128]. This suggests that when gender role expectancies are removed, men and women report similar levels of emotions that may otherwise be considered "socially unacceptable" for one's sex. Another study that measured anger expression, according to the amount of hot sauce delivered to an insulting confederate, found that women expressed less anger (i.e. delivered less hot sauce) than men, but only when the insulting confederate was present [129]. This finding suggests that women may be less likely to express anger when they fear negative appraisal or retaliation from an aggressor. Finally, a study conducted in our laboratory assessed anger in response to being personally harassed or while witnessing the harassment of a close female friend [130]. Given that women are socialised for protective roles [114, 121], we hypothesised that feeling angry or standing up to the aggressor of a close friend would cause less distress than feeling angry in self-defence, by giving women a socially acceptable outlet for feeling and expressing anger. Our results revealed that women reported feeling equally angry under both harassment conditions, but that women who were personally harassed also reported experiencing increased levels of guilt and depression. Moreover, women who were personally harassed exhibited significantly greater physiological responses during harassment (e.g. heart rate and blood pressure increases) relative to women who were only witnesses to the harassment of their friend. We concluded that women may feel social pressure to deny their anger if a "socially acceptable" reason to feel angry is lacking and that negative emotions (i.e. guilt and depression) felt as a result of these pressures may lead to heightened physiological responses that may, over time, be harmful to women's health. Taken together, this data suggests that the social environment is crucial to understanding sex differences related to the experience and expression of anger.

Impact of Anger on CAD

Both anger and trait hostility, the latter of which appears to be more common in men [118, 126], have been linked with the development and progression of CAD [131-136]. Anger and hostility have been associated with increased risk for ischemia, life-threatening arrhythmias, MI and even death [133, 134, 137-139]. It has been estimated that as many as 36,000 (2.4% of 1.5) heart attacks are precipitated by anger every year in the US [140]. Also, individuals who exhibit high levels of trait hostility may have a 1.3- to 5-fold increased risk of cardiac death compared to low-hostile individuals [133, 139]. Although a discussion of mechanisms is beyond the scope of this chapter, they include anger-related increases in sympathetic nervous system activity, which may lead to sinus tachycardia, increased blood pressure, reduced blood flow to the heart and myocardial electrical instability contributing to arrhythmias [137].

Sex Differences in Impact of Anger and Hostility on CAD

Though the anger/hostility-CAD association is quite robust, the majority of studies have been conducted exclusively using male cohorts [139] or have included relatively few women [133]. However, a review of the recent literature suggests that anger and hostility may be just as important to both CAD risk and outcome in women as it is in men. For example, data from the WISE Study revealed that women with high anger-out scores had a worse CAD risk factor profile relative to women without high anger-out scores [141]. Specifically, high anger-out women had a more than four-fold increased risk of having low HDL levels, high LDL levels, and a higher BMI, independent of age, menopausal status and socioeconomic status. A related report, also using WISE Study data, found that women with higher hostility scores (measured using the Cook Medley Hostility Scale (CMHS)), had worse three to six year cardiac event-free survival and were at higher risk for cardiac events than women with low hostility scores [135]. High hostility has also been found to be associated with increased risk for MI [142] and recurrent cardiac events [143] in post-menopausal women with CAD. For example, one study found that high scores on hostile affect (a subscale of the CMHS) was associated with a 20% increased risk for MI in a sample of 277 post-menopausal women [142]. Though few studies have directly compared the cardiovascular impact of anger/hostility in men vs. women, one study reported that in patients at high risk for CAD, high hostility was associated with an increased risk of carotid artery lesions (atherosclerosis) in high-risk women, but not men [144]. Moreover, these findings were independent of age, education, BMI, smoking history, drinking history and metabolic index. Although fewer in number, the available data suggests that anger/hostility may be just as important to cardiovascular disease risk and outcome in women as in men.

Conclusion

In this review, we have highlighted the unique presentation of CAD in women and discussed the inherent challenges faced by medical professionals when it comes to diagnosing CAD in women. We have also reviewed the major sex differences in both biological and psychological risk factors for CAD and the differential impact of these risk factors on CAD outcome in men vs. women.

Key Points

- ❑ Clearly, important sex differences exist at each level of the disease process and future research is needed to further clarify the pathogenesis of CAD in women.
- ❑ Recent work emanating from the WISE Study suggests that we may be looking at the wrong risk factors for CAD in women [145]. Women undergoing revascularisation procedures appear to have a higher prevalence of biological risk factors for CAD, yet their degree of disease severity is comparable to men.
- ❑ The extent to which biological risk factors may be less relevant for women is not known, but findings to date suggest novel risk factors need to be explored.
- ❑ Recent evidence of sex-specific cardiac biomarkers for CAD [146] and a higher prevalence of non-endothelial-dependent microvascular dysfunction in women compared to men [147] are promising avenues for future research.
- ❑ More research is also needed to better understand the differential impact of psychological risk factors in women relative to men. The fact that psychological distress is more prevalent

among women than men suggests that the risks associated with psychological factors may be particularly relevant to women.

- The relative paucity of research on the psychological vs. biological risk factors for CAD suggests an urgent need for greater research in this area.

Acknowledgements

This chapter was supported by an operating grant from the Canadian Institutes of Health Research (CIHR) (MOP 79445) and salary awards from the Fonds de la Recherche en Santé du Québec (FRSQ).

References

1. Heart and Stroke Foundation of Canada, 2003, "The Growing Burden of Heart Disease and Stroke in Canada 2003", Heart and Stroke Foundation of Canada, Ottawa, Ontario.
2. AHA, 2006, *Heart Disease and Stroke Statistics: 2006 Update*, American Heart Association, Dallas, Texas, USA.
3. CDC, CfDCaP, 2002, "Recent Trends in Mortality Rates for Four Major Cancers, by Sex and Race/Ethnicity: United States, 1990-1998", *Morbidity and Mortality Weekly Report 2002*, 51, pp. 49-53.
4. Statistics Canada, 2004, *Canadian Vital Statistics, Death Database 2002*.
5. Cooper, R., Cutler, J., Desvigne-Nickens P. et al., 2000, "Trends and Disparities in Coronary Heart Disease, Stroke and Other Cardiovascular Diseases in the United States", Findings of the National Conference on Cardiovascular Disease Prevention, *Circulation*, 102, pp. 3137-3147.
6. Hurst, W., 2002, *The Heart, Arteries and Veins*, 10th Edn., McGraw-Hill, New York.
7. Wenger, N.K., 1999, "Women, Myocardial Infarction and Coronary Revascularization: Concordant and Discordant Clinical Trial and Registry Data", *Cardiology in Review*, 7, pp. 117-120.
8. Douglas, P.S. and Ginsburg, G.S., 1996, "The Evaluation of Chest Pain in Women", *N. Engl. J. Med.*, 334, pp. 1311-1315.
9. Mosca, L., Appel, L.J., Benjamin, E.J. et al., 2004, "Evidence-based Guidelines for Cardiovascular Disease Prevention in Women", *J. Am. Coll. Cardiol.*, 43, pp. 900-921.
10. Shaw, L.J., Merz, C.N.B., Pepine C.J., et al., 2006, "Insights from the NHLBI-sponsored Women's Ischemia Syndrome Evaluation (WISE) Study: Part I: Gender Differences in Traditional and Novel Risk Factors, Symptom Evaluation, and Gender-optimized Diagnostic Strategies", *Journal of the American College of Cardiology*, 47, pp. 4S-20S.
11. Eastwood, J. and Doering, L.V., 2005, "Gender Differences in Coronary Artery Disease", *Journal of Cardiovascular Nursing*, 20, pp. 340-351.
12. Mieres, J.H., Shaw, L.J., Arai, A. et al., 2005, "Role of Non-invasive Testing in the Clinical Evaluation of Women with Suspected Coronary Artery Disease", Consensus Statement from the Cardiac Imaging Committee, Council on Clinical Cardiology and the Cardiovascular Imaging and Intervention Committee, Council on Cardiovascular Radiology and Intervention, American Heart Association, *Circulation*, 111, pp. 682-696.
13. Mosca, L., Grundy, S.M., Judelson, D. et al., 1999, "Guide to Preventive Cardiology for Women: AHA/ACC Scientific Statement Consensus Panel Statement", *Circulation*, 99, pp. 2480-2484.
14. McSweeney, J.C., Cody, M., O'Sullivan, P. et al., 2003, "Women's Early Warning Symptoms of Acute Myocardial Infarction", *Circulation*, 108, pp. 2619-2623.
15. Mieres, J.H., Rosman, D.R. and Shaw, L.J., 2004, "The Clinical Role of Stress Myocardial Perfusion Imaging in Women with Suspected Coronary Artery Disease", *Curr. Cardiology Rep.*, 6, pp. 27-31.

16. AHA, 2005, *Heart Disease and Stroke Statistics: 2005 Update*, American Heart Association, Dallas, Texas.
17. Hachamovitch, R., Berman, D.S., Kiat, H. et al., 1996, "Effective Risk Stratification Using Exercise Myocardial Perfusion SPECT in Women: Gender-related Differences in Prognostic Nuclear Testing", *J. Am. Coll. Cardiol.*, 28, pp. 34-44.
18. Pepine, C.J., 2004, "Ischemic Heart Disease in Women: Facts and Wishful Thinking", *J. Am. Coll. Cardiol.*, 43, pp. 1727-1730.
19. Rosengren, A., Wallentin, L., Gitt, K.A. et al., 2004, "Sex, Age and Clinical Presentation of Acute Coronary Syndromes", *Euro. Heart J.*, 25, pp. 663-670.
20. Bergelson, B.A. and Tommaso, C.L., 1995, "Gender Differences in Clinical Evaluation and Triage in Coronary Artery Disease", *Chest*, 108, pp. 1510-1513.
21. Roger, V.L., Farkouh, M.E., Weston, S.A. et al., 2000, "Sex Differences in Evaluation and Outcome of Unstable Angina", *JAMA*, 283, pp. 646-652.
22. Sheifer, S.E., Manolio, T.A. and Gersh, B.J., 2001, "Unrecognized Myocardial Infarction", *Ann. Int. Med.*, 135, pp. 801-811.
23. Anand, S.S., Xie, C.C., Mehta, S. et al., 2005, "Differences in the Management and Prognosis of Women and Men Who Suffer from Acute Coronary Syndromes", *J. Am. Coll. Cardiol.*, 46, p. 1845.
24. Hochman, J.S., Tamis, J.E., Thompson, T.D. et al., 1999, "Sex, Clinical Presentation and Outcome in Patients with Acute Coronary Syndromes", *N. Engl. J. Med.*, 341, pp. 226-232.
25. Mosca, L., Ferris, A., Fabunmi, R. et al., 2004, "Tracking Women's Awareness of Heart Disease: An American Heart Association National Study", *Circulation*, 109, pp. 573-579.
26. McGinn, A.P., Rosamond, W.D., Goff, J.D.C. et al., 2005, "Trends in Prehospital Delay Time and Use of Emergency Medical Services for Acute Myocardial Infarction: Experience in 4 US Communities from 1987-2000", *Am. Heart. J.*, 150, p. 392.
27. Sheifer, S.E., Rathore, S.S., Gersh, B.J. et al., 2000, "Time to Presentation with Acute Myocardial Infarction in the Elderly: Associations with Race, Sex and Socioeconomic Characteristics", *Circulation*, 102, pp. 1651-1656.
28. Mosca, L., Collins, P., Herrington, D.M. et al., 2001, "Hormone Replacement Therapy and Cardiovascular Disease: A Statement for Healthcare Professionals from the American Heart Association", *Circulation*, 104, pp. 499-503.
29. Merz, C.N.B., Johnson, B.D., Sharaf, B. et al., 2003, "Hypoestrogenemia of Hypothalamic Origin and Coronary Artery Disease in Premenopausal Women: A Report from the NHLBI-sponsored WISE Study", *J. Am. Coll. Cardiol.*, 41, pp. 413-419.
30. Milavetz, D.L., Hayes, S.N., Weston, S.A. et al., 2000, "Sex Differences in Left Ventricular Geometry in Aortic Stenosis: Impact on Outcome", *Chest 2000*, 117, pp. 1094-1099.
31. Sheifer, S.E., Canos, M.R., Weinfurt, K.P. et al., 2000, "Sex Differences in Coronary Artery Size Assessed by Intravascular Ultrasound", *Am. Heart J.*, 139, pp. 649-653.
32. Fisher, L.D., Kennedy, J.W., Davis, K.B. et al., 1982, "Association of Sex, Physical Size and Operative Mortality After Coronary Artery Bypass in the Coronary Artery Surgery Study (CASS)", *J. Thorac. Cardiovasc. Surg.*, 84, pp. 334-341.
33. Wilson, P.W.F., D'Agostino, R.B., Levy, D. et al., 1998, "Prediction of Coronary Heart Disease Using Risk Factor Categories", *Circulation*, 97, pp. 1837-1847.
34. Mieres, J.H. and Shaw, L.J., 2003, "Stress Myocardial Perfusion Imaging in the Diagnosis and Prognosis of Women with Suspected Coronary Artery Disease", *Cardiology in Review*, 11, pp. 330-336.
35. Wolf-Maier, K., Cooper, R.S., Banegas, J.R. et al., 2003, "Hypertension Prevalence and Blood Pressure Levels in 6 European Countries, Canada and the United States", *JAMA*, 289, pp. 2363-2369.

36. National Heart Lung and Blood Institute, 2003, "The Seventh Report of the Joint National Committee on Prevention, Detection, Evaluation and Treatment of High Blood Pressure", National Institutes of Health.
37. CDC, 1994, "Surveillance for Selected Tobacco-use Behaviors: United States, 1900-1994", In *CDC Surveillance Summaries* (November 18), *Morbidity and Mortality Weekly Report*.
38. CDC, 2005, "Cigarette Smoking Among Adults: United States, 2004", *Morbidity and Mortality Weekly Report 2005*, 54, pp. 1121-1124.
39. CDC, CfDCaP, 2006, "Use of Cigarettes and Other Tobacco Products Among Students Aged 13-15 Years Worldwide, 1999-2005", *MMWR Morbidity and Mortality Weekly Report 2006*, 55, pp. 553-556.
40. Hirsch, G.A. and Meagher, D.M., 1984, "Women and Coronary Artery Disease: A Review of the Literature", *Health Care for Women International*, 5, pp. 299-306.
41. CDC, CfDCaP, 2004, "The Health Consequences of Smoking: 2004 Executive Summary", *A Report of the Surgeon General*, pp. 1-20.
42. Manolio, T.A., Pearson, T.A., Wenger, N.K. et al., 1992, "Cholesterol and Heart Disease in Older Persons and Women", Review of an NHLBI Workshop, *Ann. Epid.*, 2, pp. 161-176.
43. Bass, K.M., Newschaffer, C.J., Klag, M.J. et al., 1993, "Plasma Lipoprotein Levels as Predictors of Cardiovascular Death in Women", *Arch. Int. Med.*, 153, pp. 2209-2216.
44. CDC, 2005, "General Information and National Estimates on Diabetes in the United States", *www.cdc.gov/od/oc/media/ pressrel/fs051026.htm*
45. CDC, 2001, "Diabetes and Women's Health Across the Life Stages: A Public Health Perspective", *www.cdc.gov/diabetes/ pubs/pdf/women.pdf*
46. Wolf, A.M. and Colditz, G.A., 1998, "Current Estimates of the Economic Cost of Obesity in the United States", *Obesity Research*, 6, pp. 97-106.
47. Katzmarzyk, P.T., 2002, "The Canadian Obesity Epidemic, 1985-1998", *CMAJ*, 166, pp. 1039-1040.
48. Lamon-Fava, S., Wilson, P.W.F. and Schaefer, E.J., 1996, "Impact of Body Mass Index on Coronary Heart Disease Risk Factors in Men and Women: The Framingham Offspring Study", *Arteriosclerosis, Thrombosis and Vascular Biology*, 16, pp. 1509-1515.
49. Poehlman, E.T., 2002, "Menopause, Energy Expenditure and Body Composition", *Acta Obstetricia et Gynecologica Scandinavica*, 81, pp. 603-611.
50. CDC, 2006, "Overweight and Obesity: Contributing Factors", *www.cdc.gov/nccdphp/dnpa/obesity/ contributing_factors.htm*
51. Janssen, I., Katzmarzyk, P.T. and Ross, R., 2002, "Body Mass Index, Waist Circumference and Health Risk: Evidence in Support of Current National Institutes of Health Guidelines", *Arch. Int. Med.*, 162, pp. 2074-2079.
52. Katzmarzyk, P.T. and Craig, C.L., 2006, "Independent Effects of Waist Circumference and Physical Activity on All-cause Mortality in Canadian Women", *Applied Physiology, Nutrition and Metabolism*, 31, pp. 271-276.
53. Yusuf, S., Hawken, S., Ounpuu, S. et al., 2004, "Effect of Potentially Modifiable Risk Factors Associated with Myocardial Infarction in 52 Countries (The INTERHEART Study): Case-control Study", *Lancet*, 364, pp. 937-952.
54. Rozanski, A., Blumenthal, J.A. and Kaplan, J., 1999, "Impact of Psychological Factors on the Pathogenesis of Cardiovascular Disease and Implications for Therapy", *Circulation*, 99, pp. 2192-2217.
55. Rozanski, A., Blumenthal, J.A., Davidson, K.W. et al., 2005, "The Epidemiology, Pathophysiology and Management of Psychosocial Risk Factors in Cardiac Practice: The Emerging Field of Behavioral Cardiology", *J. Am. Coll. Cardiol.*, 45, pp. 637-651.

56. Suls, J. and Bunde, J., 2005, "Anger, Anxiety and Depression as Risk Factors for Cardiovascular Disease: The Problems and Implications of Overlapping Affective Dispositions", *Psychol. Bull.*, 131, pp. 260-300.
57. Frasure-Smith, N. and Lesperance, F., 2005, "Reflections on Depression as a Cardiac Risk Factor", *Psychosom. Med.*, 67 Suppl., 1, pp. S19-25.
58. Frasure-Smith, N., Lesperance, F. and Talajic, M., 1995, "Depression and 18-month Prognosis After Myocardial Infarction", *Circulation*, 91, pp. 999-1005.
59. Frasure-Smith, N., Lesperance, F. and Talajic, M., 1993, "Depression Following Myocardial Infarction: Impact on 6-month Survival", *JAMA*, 270, pp. 1819-1825.
60. Lesperance, F., Frasure-Smith, N., Talajic, M. et al., 2002, "Five-year Risk of Cardiac Mortality in Relation to Initial Severity and One-year Changes in Depression Symptoms After Myocardial Infarction", *Circulation*, 105, pp. 1049-1053.
61. Penninx, B.W.J.H., Beekman, A.T.F., Honig, A. et al., 2001, "Depression and Cardiac Mortality: Results From a Community-Based Longitudinal Study", *Arch. Gen. Psychiatry.*, 58, pp. 221-227.
62. Carney, R.M., Blumenthal, J.A., Catellier, D. et al., 2003, "Depression as a Risk Factor for Mortality After Acute Myocardial Infarction", *Am. J. Cardiol.*, 92, pp. 1277-1281.
63. Carney, R.M., Freedland, K.E., Rich, M.W. et al., 1995, "Depression as a Risk Factor for Cardiac Events in Established Coronary Artery Disease", *Ann. Behav. Med.*, 17, pp. 142-149.
64. Barefoot, J.C., Brummett, B.H., Helms, M.J. et al., 2000, "Depressive Symptoms and Survival of Patients with Coronary Artery Disease", *Psychosom. Med.*, 62, pp. 790-795.
65. Carney, R.M., Rich, M.W., Tevelde, A. et al., 1987, "Major Depressive Disorder in Coronary Artery Disease", *Am. J. Cardiol.*, 60, pp. 1273-1275.
66. Frasure-Smith, N., Lesperance, F. and Talajic, M., 1995, "The Impact of Negative Emotions on Prognosis Following Myocardial Infarction: Is it More than Depression?" *Health Psychol.*, 14, pp. 388-398.
67. Lane, D., Carroll, D., Ring, C. et al., 2002, "In-hospital Symptoms of Depression Do Not Predict Mortality Three Years After Myocardial Infarction", *Psychosom. Med.*, 63, pp. 221-230.
68. Steeds, R., Bickerton, D., Smith, M. et al., 2004, "Assessment of Depression Following Acute Myocardial Infarction Using the Beck Depression Inventory", *Heart*, 90, pp. 217-218.
69. Schleifer, S.J., Macari-Hinson, M.M., Coyle, D.A. et al., 1989, "The Nature and Course of Depression Following Myocardial Infarction", *Arch. Int. Med.*, 149, pp. 1785-1789.
70. Bush, D.E., Ziegelstein, R.C., Tayback, M. et al., 2001, "Even Minimal Symptoms of Depression Increase Mortality Risk After Acute Myocardial Infarction", *Am. J. Cardiol.*, 88, pp. 337-341.
71. Kessler, R.C., Berglund, P., Demler, O. et al., 2003, "The Epidemiology of Major Depressive Disorder: Results from the National Comorbidity Survey Replication (NCS-R)", *JAMA*, 289, pp. 3095-3105.
72. Barefoot, J.C., Helms, M.J., Mark, D.B. et al., 1996, "Depression and Long-term Mortality Risk in Patients with Coronary Artery Disease", *Am. J. Cardiol.*, 78, pp. 613-617.
73. Anda, R., Williamson, D., Jones, D. et al., 1993, "Depressed Affect, Hopelessness and the Risk of Ischemic Heart Disease in a Cohort of U.S. Adults", *Epidemiology*, 4, pp. 285-294.
74. Ahern, D.K., Gorkin, L., Anderson, J.L. et al., 1990, "Biobehavioral Variables and Mortality or Cardiac Arrest in the Cardiac Arrhythmia Pilot Study (CAPS)", *Am. J. Cardiol.*, 66, pp. 59-62.
75. Strik, J.J.M.H., Denollet, J., Lousberg, R. et al., 2003, "Comparing Symptoms of Depression and Anxiety as Predictors of Cardiac Events and Increased Health Care Consumption After Myocardial Infarction", *J. Am. Coll. Cardiol.*, 42, pp. 1801-1807.
76. Welin, C., Lappas, G. and Wilhelmsen, L., 2000, "Independent Importance of Psychosocial Factors for Prognosis After Myocardial Infarction", *Journal of Internal Medicine*, 247, pp. 629-639.

77. Lauzon, C., Beck, C.A., Huynh, T. et al., 2003, "Depression and Prognosis Following Hospital Admission Because of Acute Myocardial Infarction", *CMAJ*, 168, pp. 547-552.
78. Shiotani, I., Sato, H., Kinjo, K. et al., 2002, "Depressive Symptoms Predict 12-month Prognosis in Elderly Patients with Acute Myocardial Infarction", *Journal of Cardiovascular Risk*, 9, pp. 153-160.
79. Ladwig, K., Kieser, M., Konig, J. et al., 1991, "Affective Disorders and Survival After Acute Myocardial Infarction: Results from the Post-infarction Late Potential Study", *Euro. Heart J.*, 12, pp. 959-964.
80. Kaufmann, M.W., Fitzgibbons, J.P., Sussman, E.J. et al., 1999, "Relation Between Myocardial Infarction, Depression, Hostility and Death", *Am. Heart J.*, 138, pp. 549-554.
81. Irvine, J., Basinski, A., Baker, B. et al., 1999, "Depression and Risk of Sudden Cardiac Death After Acute Myocardial Infarction: Testing for the Confounding Effects of Fatigue", *Psychosom. Med.* 61, pp. 729-737.
82. Lane, D., Carroll, D., Ring, C. et al., 2002, "In-hospital Symptoms of Depression Do Not Predict Mortality 3 Years After Myocardial Infarction", *Int. J. Epidemiol.*, 31, pp. 1179-1182.
83. Lane, D., Carroll, D., Ring, C. et al., 2001, "Mortality and Quality of Life 12 Months After Myocardial Infarction: Effects of Depression and Anxiety", *Psychosom. Med.*, 63, pp. 221-230.
84. Mayou, R.A., Gill, D., Thompson, D.R. et al., 2000, "Depression and Anxiety as Predictors of Outcome After Myocardial Infarction", *Psychosom. Med.*, 62, pp. 212-219.
85. Barefoot, J.C. and Schroll, M., 1996, "Symptoms of Depression, Acute Myocardial Infarction and Total Mortality in a Community Sample", *Circulation*, 93, pp. 1976-1980.
86. Gottlieb, S.S., Khatta, M., Friedmann, E. et al., 2004, "The Influence of Age, Gender and Race on the Prevalence of Depression in Heart Failure Patients", *J. Am. Coll. Cardiol.*, 43, pp. 1542-1549.
87. Frasure-Smith, N., Lesperance, F., Juneau, M. et al., 1999, "Gender, Depression and One-Year Prognosis After Myocardial Infarction", *Psychosom. Med.*, 61, pp. 26-37.
88. Mallik, S., Spertus, J.A., Reid, K.J. et al., 2006, "Depressive Symptoms After Acute Myocardial Infarction: Evidence for Highest Rates in Younger Women", *Arch. Int. Med.*, 166, pp. 876-883.
89. DeVon, H.A. and Zerwic, J.J., 2003, "The Symptoms of Unstable Angina: Do Women and Men Differ?" *Nursing Research*, 52, pp. 108-118.
90. Connerney, I., Shapiro, P.A., McLaughlin, J.S. et al., 2001, "Relation Between Depression After Coronary Artery Bypass Surgery and 12-month Outcome: A Prospective Study", *Lancet*, 358, pp. 1766.
91. Stébenne, P.R., Bacon, S.L., Pelletier, R. et al., 2006, "Sex Differences in the Prevalence of Psychiatric Disorders in 2,262 Patients Referred for Nuclear Stress Testing", *Psychosom. Med.*, 68, p. A-53.
92. Mallik, S., Krumholz, H.M., Lin, Z.Q. et al., 2005, "Patients with Depressive Symptoms Have Lower Health Status Benefits After Coronary Artery Bypass Surgery", *Circulation*, 111, pp. 271-277.
93. Kessler, R.C., Chiu, W.T., Demler, O. et al., 2005, "Prevalence, Severity and Comorbidity of 12-Month DSM-IV Disorders in the National Comorbidity Survey Replication", *Arch. Gen. Psychiatry.*, 62, pp. 617-627.
94. Moser, D.K. and Dracup, K., 1996, "Is Anxiety Early After Myocardial Infarction Associated with Subsequent Ischemic and Arrhythmic Events?" *Psychosom. Med.*, 58, pp. 395-401.
95. Lane, D., Carroll, D., Ring, C. et al., 2002, "The Prevalence and Persistence of Depression and Anxiety Following Myocardial Infarction", *British Journal of Health Psychology*, 7, pp. 11-21.
96. Crowe, J.M., Runions, J., Ebbesen, L.S. et al., 1996, "Anxiety and Depression After Acute Myocardial Infarction", *Heart Lung*, 25, pp. 98-107.
97. Havik, O.E. and Maeland, J.G., 1990, "Patterns of Emotional Reactions After a Myocardial Infarction", *J. Psychosom. Res.*, 34, pp. 271-285.

98. Konstam, V., Moser, D.K. and De Jong, M.J., 2005, "Depression and Anxiety in Heart Failure", *Journal of Cardiac Failure*, 11, pp. 455-463.
99. Fleet, R., Lavoie, K. and Beitman, B.D., 2000, "Is Panic Disorder Associated with Coronary Artery Disease? A Critical Review of the Literature", *J. Psychosom. Res.*, 48, pp. 347-356.
100. Haines, A.P., Imeson, J.D. and Meade, T.W., 1987, "Phobic Anxiety and Ischaemic Heart Disease", *British Medicine Journal*, 295, pp. 297-299.
101. Benninghoven, D., Kaduk, A., Wiegand, U. et al., 2006, "Influence of Anxiety on the Course of Heart Disease After Acute Myocardial Infarction: Risk Factor or Protective Function?" *Psychotherapy and Psychosomatics*, 75, pp. 56-61.
102. Kubzansky, L.D., Cole, S.R., Kawachi, I. et al., 2006, "Shared and Unique Contributions of Anger, Anxiety and Depression to Coronary Heart Disease: A Prospective Study in the Normative Aging Study", *Ann. Behav. Med.*, 31, pp. 21-29.
103. Lane, D., Carroll, D., Ring, C. et al., 2000, "Do Depression and Anxiety Predict Recurrent Coronary Events 12 Months After Myocardial Infarction?" *Quarterly Journal of Medicine*, 93, pp. 739-744.
104. Bacon, S.L., Ring, C., Carroll, D. et al., 2001, "Psychological Distress and Anger in Patients with Differing Degrees of Coronary Artery Disease (CAD)", *Psychosom. Med.*, 63, p. 174.
105. Blumenthal, J.A., Thompson, L.W., Williams, R.B.J. et al., 1979, "Anxiety-proneness and Coronary Heart Disease", *J. Psychosom. Res.*, 23, pp. 17-21.
106. Astin, F., Jones, K. and Thompson, D.R., 2005, "Prevalence and Patterns of Anxiety and Depression in Patients Undergoing Elective Percutaneous Transluminal Coronary Angioplasty", *Heart and Lung: The Journal of Acute and Critical Care*, 34, pp. 393-401.
107. Moser, D.K., Dracup, K., McKinley, S. et al., 2003, "An International Perspective on Gender Differences in Anxiety Early After Acute Myocardial Infarction", *Psychosom. Med.*, 65, pp. 511-516.
108. An, K., De Jong, M.J., Riegel, B.J. et al., 2004, "A Cross-sectional Examination of Changes in Anxiety Early After Acute Myocardial Infarction", *Heart and Lung: The Journal of Acute and Critical Care*, 33, pp. 75-82.
109. Uuskula, M., 1996, "Psychological Differences Between Young Male and Female Survivors of Myocardial Infarction", *Psychotherapy and Psychosomatics*, 65, pp. 327-330.
110. Eaker, E.D., Pinsky, J., Castelli, W.P., 1992, "Myocardial Infarction and Coronary Death Among Women: Psychosocial Predictors from a 20-year Follow-up of Women in the Framingham Study", *Am. J. Epidemiol.*, 135, pp. 854-864.
111. Eaker, E.D., Sullivan, L.M., Kelly-Hayes, M. et al., 2005, "Tension and Anxiety and the Prediction of the 10-Year Incidence of Coronary Heart Disease, Atrial Fibrillation and Total Mortality: The Framingham Offspring Study", *Psychosom. Med.*, 67, pp. 692-696.
112. Kessler, R.C., Chiu, W.T., Jin, R. et al., 2006, "The Epidemiology of Panic Attacks, Panic Disorder and Agoraphobia in the National Comorbidity Survey Replication", *Arch. Gen. Psychiatry*, 63, pp. 415-424.
113. Shields, S.A., 1987, "Women, Men and the Dilemma of Emotion", In *Sex and Gender*, P. Shaver and C. Hendrick (Eds.), Sage, Newbury Park, California, pp. 229-250.
114. Brody, L.R., 1985, "Gender Differences in Emotional Development: A Review of Theories and Research", *J. Pers. Assess.*, 53, pp. 102-149.
115. Kopper, B.A. and Epperson, D.L., 1996, "The Experience and Expression of Anger: Relationships with Gender, Gender Role Socialization, Depression and Mental Health Functioning", *Journal of Counselling Psychology*, 43, pp. 158-165.
116. Lerner, H.G., 1985, *The Dance of Anger*, Academic Press, New York.
117. Mirowsky, J. and Ross, C.E., 1995, "Sex Differences in Distress: Real or Artifact?" *American Sociological Review*, 60, pp. 449-468.

118. Stoney, C.M. and Engbreston, T.O., 1994, "Anger and Hostility: Potential Mediators of the Gender Difference in Coronary Artery Disease", In *Anger, Hostility and the Heart*, T. Smith and A.W. Seigman (Eds.), Lawrence Erlbaum, New York, pp. 215-237.
119. Kring, A.M. and Gordon, A.H., 1998, "Sex Differences in Emotion: Expression, Experience and Physiology", *Journal of Personality and Social Psychology*, 74, pp. 686-703.
120. Birnbaum, D.A., Nosanchuk, T.A. and Croll, W.L., 1980, "Children's Stereotypes About Sex Differences in Emotionality", *Sex Roles*, 6, pp. 435-443.
121. Gordon, S.L., 1989, "The Socialization of Children's Emotions: Emotion Culture, Competence and Exposure", In *Children's Understanding of Emotion*, C. Saarni and P. Harris (Eds.), Cambridge Univeristy Press, New York, pp. 319-349.
122. Haynes, S.G. and Feinleib, M., 1980, "Women, Work and Coronary Artery Disease: Prospective Findings from the Framingham Heart Study", *Am. J. Pub. Health*, 70, pp. 133-141.
123. Matthews, K.A., Manuck, S.B., Stoney, C.M. et al., 1988, "Familial Aggregation of Behaviors Associated with Risk for Coronary Heart Disease-I: Blood Pressure and Heart Rate Responses to Physiological and Exercise Stress", *Psychosom. Med.*, 50, pp. 341-352.
124. Siegel, J.M., 1985, "The Measurement of Anger as a Multidimensional Construct", In *Anger and Hostility in Cardiovascular and Behavioral Disorders*, M.A. Chesney and R.H. Rosenman (Eds.), McGraw-Hill, New York, pp. 59-82.
125. Spielberger, C.D., Johnson, E.H., Russell, S.F. et al., 1985, "The Experience and Expression of Anger: Contruction and Validation of an Anger Expression Scale", In *Anger and Hostility in Cardiovascular and Behavioral Disorders*, M.A. Chesney and R.H. Rosenman (Eds.), McGraw-Hill, New York, pp. 5-30.
126. Engbreston, T.O. and Matthews, K.A., 1992, "Dimensions of Hostility in Men, Women and Boys: Relationships to Personality and Cardiovascular Responses to Stress", *Psychosom. Med.*, 54, pp. 311-323.
127. Balswick, J. and Avertt, C.P., 1977, "Differences in Expressiveness: Gender, Interpersonal Orientation and Perceived Parental Expressiveness as Contributing Factors", *Journal of Marriage and Family*, 39, pp. 121-127.
128. Grossman, M. and Wood, W., 1993, "Sex Differences in Intensity of Emotional Experience: A Social Role Interpretation", *Journal of Personality and Social Psychology*, 65, pp. 1010-1022.
129. Evers, C., Fischer, A.H., Rodriquez-Mosquera, P.M. et al., 2005, "Anger and Social Appraisal: A "Spicy" Sex Difference?" *Emotion*, 5, pp. 258-266.
130. Lavoie, K.L., Miller, S.B., Conway, M. et al., 2001, "Anger, Negative Emotions and Cardiovascular Reactivity During Interpersonal Conflict in Women", *J. Psychosom. Res.*, 51, pp. 503-512.
131. Smith, T.W., Glazer, K., Ruiz, J.M. et al., 2004, "Hostility, Anger, Aggressiveness and Coronary Heart Disease: An Interpersonal Perspective on Personality, Emotion and Health", *J. Personality*, 72, pp. 1217-1270.
132. Angerer, P., Siebert, U., Kothny, W. et al., 2000, "Impact of Social Support, Cynical Hostility and Anger Expression on Progression of Coronary Atherosclerosis", *J. Am. Coll. Cardiol.*, 36, pp. 1781-1788.
133. Boyle, S.H., Williams, R.B., Mark, D.B. et al., 2004, "Hostility as a Predictor of Survival in Patients with Coronary Artery Disease", *Psychosom. Med.*, 66, pp. 629-632.
134. Mittleman, M.A., Maclure, M., Sherwood, J.B. et al., 1995, "Triggering of Acute Myocardial-Infarction Onset by Episodes of Anger", *Circulation*, 92, pp. 1720-1725.
135. Olson, M.B., Krantz, D.S., Kelsey, S.F. et al., 2005, "Hostility Scores Are Associated with Increased Risk of Cardiovascular Events in Women Undergoing Coronary Angiography: A Report from the NHLBI-Sponsored WISE Study", *Psychosom. Med.*, 67, pp. 546-552.

136. Kawachi, I., Sparrow, D., Spiro, A. III et al., 1996, "A Prospective Study of Anger and Coronary Heart Disease: The Normative Aging Study", *Circulation*, 94, pp. 2090-2095.
137. Verrier, R.L. and Mittleman, M.A., 1996, "Life-threatening Cardiovascular Consequences of Anger in Patients with Coronary Heart Disease", *Cardiol. Clin.*, 14, pp. 289-307.
138. Helmers, K.F., Krantz, D.S., Merz, C.N.B. et al., 1995, "Defensive Hostility: Relationship to Multiple Markers of Cardiac Ischemia in Patients with Coronary Disease", *Health Psychol.*, 14, pp. 202-209.
139. Matthews, K.A., Gump, B.B., Harris, K.F. et al., 2004, "Hostile Behaviors Predict Cardiovascular Mortality Among Men Enrolled in the Multiple Risk Factor Intervention Trial", *Circulation*, 109, pp. 66-70.
140. Verrier, R.L. and Mittelman, M.A., 1997, "Cardiovascular Consequences of Anger and Other Stress States", *Baillieres Clin. Neurol.*, 6, pp. 245-259.
141. Rutledge, T., Reis, S.E., Olson, M. et al., 2001, "Psychosocial Variables Are Associated with Atherosclerosis Risk Factors Among Women with Chest Pain: The WISE Study", *Psychosom. Med.*, 63, pp. 282-288.
142. Lahad, A., Heckbert, S.R., Koepsell, T.D. et al., 1997, "Hostility, Aggression and the Risk of Nonfatal Myocardial Infarction in Post-menopausal Women", *Journal of Psychosomatic Research*, 43, pp. 183-195.
143. Chaput, L.A., Adams, S.H., Simon, J.A. et al., 2002, "Hostility Predicts Recurrent Events Among Post-menopausal Women with Coronary Heart Disease", *Am. J. Epidemiol.*, 126, pp. 1092-1096.
144. Knox, S.S., Weidner, G., Adelman, A. et al., 2004, "Hostility and Physiological Risk in the National Heart, Lung, and Blood Institute Family Heart Study", *Arch. Int. Med.*, 164, pp. 2442-2447.
145. Jacobs, A.K., 2006, "Women, Ischemic Heart Disease, Revascularization and the Gender Gap: What Are We Missing?" *J. Am. Coll. Cardiol.*, 47, pp. 63S-65S.
146. Wiviott, S.D., Cannon, C.P., Morrow, D.A. et al., 2004, "Differential Expression of Cardiac Biomarkers by Gender in Patients with Unstable Angina/Non-ST-Elevation Myocardial Infarction: A Treat Angina with Aggrastat and determine Cost of Therapy with an Invasive or Conservative Strategy-Thrombolysis in Myocardial Infarction (TACTICS-TIMI) 18 Substudy", *Circulation*, 109, pp. 580-586.
147. Merz, C.N.B., Shaw, L.J., Reis, S.E. et al., 2006, "Insights from the NHLBI-Sponsored Women's Ischemia Syndrome Evaluation (WISE) Study-Part II: Gender Differences in Presentation, Diagnosis and Outcome with Regard to Gender-based Pathophysiology of Atherosclerosis and Macrovascular and Microvascular Coronary Disease", *J. Am. Coll. Cardiol.*, 47, pp. S21-S29.

The AHA-Syndrome and Cardiovascular Diseases
Editors: Swati Y. Bhave and Sunil Saini
Copyright © 2010 Anamaya Publishers, New Delhi, India

14. Psychosocial Factors and Risk for Coronary Heart Disease

Janice E. Williams
P.O. Box 3168, LaGrange, Georgia 30241, USA

Abstract: The present chapter focusses on the role of four psychosocial factors in coronary heart disease (CHD) – depression, anger/hostility, socioeconomic status (SES), and social support/social isolation. It summarises selected research studies that are representative of investigations in this field. For each psychosocial factor, a description of the putative mechanisms linking it to CHD is provided.

Keywords: Psychosocial risk factors, Coronary heart disease.

Introduction

Cardiovascular disease (CVD) is the number one killer of people in the industrialised world and a rapidly growing epidemic in developing countries [1]. Coronary heart disease (CHD), expressed as angina pectoris, myocardial infarction (MI), sudden cardiac death, or congestive heart failure, is one of the clinical manifestations of CVD. Traditional CHD risk factors include: age, cigarette smoking, physical inactivity, diabetes mellitus, elevated lipids (cholesterol, triglycerides) and high blood pressure levels. There are also several emerging or novel CHD risk factors, including biologic entities, such as non-specific markers of inflammation (e.g., C-reactive protein, fibrinogen) and serum homocysteine concentrations, as well as psychosocial entities, such as depression, anger/hostility, anxiety, socioeconomic status (SES), and social support/social isolation. Although negative studies do exist [2, 3], preponderant evidence from large, epidemiologic studies has demonstrated that psychosocial factors have a strong predictive value for incident CHD – a risk that is often on par with that of the traditional CHD risk factors. Further, research has shown that the presence of these factors in the aftermath of a major CHD event can adversely affect its clinical course.

Depression

The research evidence implicating depression as a factor in the onset and course of CHD is compelling. Results of two meta-analyses of prospective cohort studies that were published between 1993 and 2000 support a significant role for depression in the development of CHD [4, 5]. Rugulies [4] reviewed 11 studies, three of which had samples with and without CHD at baseline. They reported that depression (clinical depression or depressed mood) conferred a relative risk of 1.64 for CHD among all studies combined, and relative risks of 2.69 and 1.49 among studies in which the exposure was clinical depression and depressed mood, respectively. Wulsin and Singal [5] also reported that depression conferred a relative of 1.64 for incident CHD – all studies had samples without CHD at baseline, seven of which overlapped with those in the Rugulies review [4].

More recent findings have supported and extended the conclusions of previously published meta-analyses. In a sample of community-dwelling elderly men and women with and without CHD at baseline, prospective analyses showed that, compared to their nondepressed counterparts, depressed men had a 66% greater risk for fatal and nonfatal CHD and were at two and a half times the risk for cardiovascular mortality [6]. The risk for total mortality was twice as great in depressed men and 43% higher in depressed women. In another population-based cohort of elderly men and women without CHD at baseline, prospective analyses indicated that depressed participants, relative to their nondepressed counterparts, were at twice the risk for any cardiac event and at three times the risk for the ischemic subtype [7]. In related findings, depression was associated with 50% and 32% increases in risk for CVD death and all-cause mortality, respectively, among older postmenopausal women without CVD at baseline [8] and with a 43% greater likelihood of cardiac arrest in a sample of middle-aged men and women with and without existing CHD [9].

Depression and CHD frequently exist as co-morbid conditions. In turn, depression has strong implications for clinical outcomes among people with CHD. Two recent reviews provide the aggregate results of prospective cohort studies on this topic [10, 11]. van Melle et al. [10] conducted a meta-analysis of 22 studies published up to 2003 and reported that depression in patients with MI substantially increased their chances of future adverse events. More specifically, within two years of the initial MI, depressed patients were at more than twice the risk for all-cause mortality and cardiac mortality relative to their nondepressed counterparts. In a meta-analysis of 20 studies published between 1988 and 2003, Barth et al. [11] reported that CHD patients with depressive symptoms or clinical depression were more likely than their nondepressed counterparts to die of cardiovascular- or all-causes. In short- and medium-term follow-up, CHD patients with depressive symptoms had more than twice the likelihood of death; in long-term follow-up, their odds were 78% higher. Also, in long-term follow-up, CHD patients with clinical depression were nearly three times as likely to die as their nondepressed counterparts.

Potential Mechanisms

Behavioural

The precise mechanism by which depression influences CHD remains unclear. One hypothesis is behavioural in emphasis and suggests that depressed individuals are likely to engage in deleterious health behaviours that place them at increased risk for CHD [12-21]. Further, noncompliance with treatment regimens might explain the association between depression and recurrent events among people with CHD [22].

Depression and CHD risk factors have been shown to be associated with one another. In cross-sectional analyses, cigarette smoking was positively associated with depression among participants in the first National Health and Nutrition Examination Survey (NHANES) [12], the Wisconsin Longitudinal Study [13], and the Women's Ischemia Syndrome Evaluation Study (WISE) [14]. Longitudinal data analyses from the NHANES I Epidemiologic Follow-Up Study demonstrated that depressed smokers were substantially less likely than their nondepressed counterparts to quit smoking [12]. Further, in a five-year prospective cohort study, participants with a history of clinical depression at baseline were three times as likely to progress to daily smoking as their counterparts without depression [15]. Conversely, participants with a history of smoking at baseline had a 90% greater likelihood of developing major depression compared to their peers without such a history.

Depression is also positively associated with hypertension, diabetes, and obesity – components of the metabolic syndrome. Results from the NHANES I Epidemiologic Follow-Up Study indicated that the presence of negative affect (depressive symptoms and anxiety) at baseline was associated with an increased risk for developing hypertension over 22 years of follow-up [16]. During five years of follow-up in the Coronary Artery Risk Development in Young Adults (CARDIA) Study, black participants with high depression scores at baseline were nearly three times as likely to develop hypertension as their counterparts with low scores; the odds in black participants with moderate depression scores were 2.31 [17]. Results of a recent meta-analysis of 10 studies published between 1980 and 2005 revealed that depression was more prevalent in people with Type II diabetes than in those without the disease [18]. Among participants in the Atherosclerosis Risk in Communities (ARIC) Study, the presence of depressive symptoms was associated with a 38% increase in the risk for incident diabetes [18]. Finally, in cross-sectional analyses, obese men and women were 41% more likely to be depressed than their counterparts of normal body weight [19]. In another report, body mass index was found to be positively associated with depression in women [20].

Direct, Pathophysiological

Direct, pathophysiological mechanisms involving hemodynamic and neurohormonal processes of the sympathetic adrenomedullary system and of the hypothalamic-pituitary adrenocortical (HPA) axis have been hypothesised to explain the depression-CHD association [23]. Further, depression has been shown to be associated with increased platelet activation [24], endothelial dysfunction [25], and alterations in cardiac autonomic tone [26] – each of which has been implicated in the development of acute coronary syndromes and/or the pathogenesis of atherosclerosis. Increased depression has also been shown to be associated with higher levels of proinflammatory cytokines, such as IL-1β [27], IL-6 [27-29], tumor necrosis factor (TNF)-α [28, 30] and IL-8 [30], and with higher levels of C-reactive protein, a non-specific marker of inflammation [31].

Anger/Hostility

Anger/hostility is another psychosocial factor that has received widespread research attention for its impact on CHD. Most large-scale, epidemiologic studies have shown a positive association between anger/hostility and CHD onset, although negative findings have been reported [2, 3]. The risk of a major CHD event associated with anger/hostility has been substantial, with several studies showing an effect that is independent of the established risk factors, and similar in magnitude to that observed for the traditional risk factors.

A number of studies have supported a positive association between anger/hostility and atherosclerosis, the underlying vascular disorder in CHD. Null findings have also been reported [32, 33]. Positive results were reported of Finnish men in whom high cynical distrust and high anger control independently predicted the progression of carotid intima media thickness (IMT), a subclinical manifestation of atherosclerosis [34]. In a United States sample of untreated hypertensive men, trait anger, anger temperament, and anger out were positively associated with carotid IMT, independent of the established risk factors [35]. Among postmenopausal women, anger in and hostile attitudes predicted carotid IMT prospectively, independent of the traditional risk factors [36]. Additional research revealed a positive association between hostility and the development of subclinical vascular disease in young adult men and women [37]. Further, among middle-aged women, researchers reported a positive association between baseline trait anger and carotid IMT progression over a three-year period – an association that was mediated by the metabolic syndrome [38].

Results of a meta-analysis of 45 studies published by the mid-1990s indicated that anger/hostility has positive predictive value for CHD events, independent of the established risk factors [39]. More recently, long-term follow-up studies have been consistent with previous findings, showing that high anger/hostility at baseline influences the onset of major CHD events. Across nine years of follow-up in the Kuopio Ischemic Heart Disease Risk Factor Study, high-hostile men were at 2.18 times the risk for MI compared to their low-hostile counterparts [40]. After multivariate adjustment, the traditional risk factors accounted for the relationship. Among men followed for an average of seven years in the Veterans Administrative Normative Aging Study, a near three-fold increase in CHD risk (nonfatal MI, fatal CHD and angina pectoris) was observed among participants who reported high anger control compared to those who reported low anger control [41]. During 16 years of follow-up in the Multiple Risk Factor Intervention Trial, men with high hostility scores had a 61% greater likelihood of CVD death compared to their counterparts with low scores [42]. Hostility also predicted recurrent events such that high-hostile men who had a nonfatal event during the trial, subsequently, were five times as likely to die of CVD as their low-hostile counterparts who did not have an event during the trial. In longer-term follow-up (range = 32 to 48 years, median = 36 years), high-hostile men in the Johns Hopkins Precursors Study had three times the risk for premature CVD (onset before age 55) compared to men with low hostility [43]. Further, results from the Atherosclerosis Risk in Communities (ARIC) Study, a large-scale epidemiologic investigation of CVD in middle-aged men and women supported a positive relationship between trait anger and incident CHD among individuals with normal blood pressure levels [44].

Potential Mechanisms

Behavioural

The behavioural hypothesis is similar to that which has been advanced to explain the causal link between depression and CHD. Indeed, studies have shown significant associations between anger/hostility and CHD risk factors. A recent meta-analysis of 27 studies published between 1991 and 2003 revealed that hostility scores on the Cook-Medley Hostility Scale were associated with insulin resistance, the lipid ratio, body mass index (BMI), waist-to-hip ratio, triglycerides, glucose, alcohol consumption, SES, and cigarette smoking [45]. A study that was not included in this review also has supportive results, i.e. in prospective analyses from the University of North Carolina Alumni Heart Study, hostility measured during the college years predicted CHD risk factors up to 30 years forward [46]. In addition to negative emotional and social life assessments, higher levels of hostility as a young adult were associated with a greater likelihood of drinking alcohol and smoking cigarettes in later life. Further, among women enrolled in the WISE Study, anger out scores were positively associated with LDL-cholesterol level and BMI, and negatively associated with HDL-cholesterol level [14]. A review of the literature on anger and blood pressure concluded that anger is positively associated with systolic blood pressure levels [47]. In addition, results from the CARDIA Study indicated that, compared to their counterparts in the lowest hostility quartile, participants in the highest quartile were 84% more likely to develop hypertension over 15-years of follow-up [48].

Direct, Pathophysiological

The biological mechanisms invoked to explain the positive association between anger/hostility and CHD involve the activity of the sympathetic adrenomedullary system and of the HPA axis. Compared with their low-hostile peers in stressful situations and to their high- and low-hostile peers in nonstressful situations, high-hostile persons in stressful situations have been observed to exhibit greater blood pressure and heart rate reactivity, and increased catecholamine and cortisol secretions [49]. High anger/hostility has also been associated with increased platelet reactivity [50]. In addition, angry/hostile individuals have been shown to have heightened levels of proinflammatory cytokines, such as IL-1α, IL-1β, IL-8 [30], IL-6 [28, 29] and TNF-α [28, 51], and elevated C-reactive protein [31] and serum homocysteine levels [52]. In one report, the investigators failed to find an independent association between hostility and IL-6 or TNF-α [28]. Rather, they observed positive associations of IL-6 and TNF-α levels with hostility in the presence of low depression, and less positive to no association in the presence of moderate and high depression, respectively.

Socioeconomic Status

SES is a well-known predictor of health status in the industrialised world, particularly in countries with wide disparities in wealth [53]. Repeatedly, studies have shown a graded, inverse association between SES and CHD outcomes, after controlling for potential confounders. This pattern is present for individual- and neighbourhood-level SES [54-59], as well as for measures of life-course SES [60]. However, the current SES differential in CHD, CHD mortality in particular, is a relatively recent phenomenon that can be understood within the context of an epidemiologic transition. Prior to the 1950s, CHD mortality in industrialised nations was more common among individuals in the upper SES strata [61]. Since the 1950s, it has been more prevalent among less affluent people – an inequality that has been exacerbated by substantially greater declines among the more affluent [62].

The SES disparity in CHD has long been documented at the individual level [53]. Recent findings from large-scale, epidemiologic studies of middle-aged [54] and young adults [55] continue to support previous findings. Analyses from the ARIC Study demonstrated a significant linear trend in the relationship of personal income to prevalent CHD among both blacks and whites, adjusting for the traditional CHD risk factors [54]. For education, the trend was significant in whites, but not in blacks. For occupational category, the trend was significant in men, but not in women. Also, results from the CARDIA Study showed that SES (as measured by personal education, parental education, and financial hardship) was inversely associated with CVD risk at baseline in women and with a cumulative multifactor CVD risk index in women and in white men during a 10-year follow-up period [55].

Using group-level wealth, income, education, and occupational status as indicators, studies have demonstrated that the SES disparity in CHD exists at the neighbourhood level as well. In ARIC analyses, residents of low-SES neighbourhoods were more likely to have prevalent CHD and a greater burden of CVD risk factors compared to residents of high-SES neighbourhoods, although some estimates were attenuated after adjustment for individual-level SES indicators [56]. Also, counterintuitive results were observed among black men residing in disadvantaged communities in one southern United States city, i.e. in these communities, as the social indicators declined the CHD prevalence decreased. In prospective ARIC analyses with a median of 9.1 years of follow-up, residents of low-SES neighbourhoods were at significantly increased risk for incident CHD, controlling for personal income, education, and occupation [57]. Another notable finding was that low-SES individuals residing in the lowest SES neighbourhoods were at considerably higher risk for incident CHD compared with high-SES individuals residing in the highest SES neighbourhoods – three times the risk among whites and two and a half among blacks. Similar findings have been reported among elderly members of the Cardiovascular Health Study, among whom the relationship between individual and neighbourhood-level SES and subclinical CVD was investigated [58]. Subclinical CVD prevalence was inversely associated with education, income, and neighbourhood SES indicators in models adjusted for demographic and behavioural risk factors. After further adjustment for biomedical factors, the odds of disease remained elevated, but were statistically significant only in the association with income. Finally, analyses among Swedish men and women also demonstrated that living in low-SES neighbourhoods was associated with increased CHD incidence and case fatality, adjusting for demographic and individual-level SES indicators [59].

Potential Mechanisms

There are several possible mechanisms linking SES to CHD. The association may be mediated by loss of the ability to cope with the stresses and strains of life, and by accompanying negative emotions, such as hopelessness, depression, and anger/hostility [63]. Indeed, studies document that low SES is associated with increased exposure to psychosocial stress and with elevated levels of hostility and depression [64, 65]. Other potential explanations include the notion that people with chronic disease may 'drift' into lower SES strata as a result of their illness [66] and, conversely, the notion that people in lower SES strata more frequently engage in deleterious health behaviours that place them at greater risk for CHD [56]. People with low SES may be less likely than their higher SES counterparts to subscribe to the prevailing guidelines for disease prevention and health promotion, owing either to the failure of public information campaigns to reach their communities, to their reduced consumption of health information, or to their lower levels of health literacy.

Social Support/Social Isolation

The link between health and social support (and its variants – social isolation, social integration, and social participation) is well established. Lack of social support has strong predictive value for CHD onset. A recent review of studies published before 2005 indicated that people with low social support have up to twice the risk for CHD events compared to their counterparts with high social support [67]. Moreover, the lack of social ties is independently associated with poor survival following a major event. In a 10-year follow-up study, Swedish men and women with MI who had low social support were nearly three times as likely to die of cardiac causes as their peers with high social support [68]. In a seven-year follow-up study, Swiss men with MI who did not have partners were at more than three times the risk for death compared to their counterparts with partners [69]. Further, the results of a study conducted in the United Kingdom revealed that low social support among patients undergoing coronary artery bypass grafting was associated with continued breathlessness following the procedure [70].

Potential Mechanisms

The mechanism linking social support to health promotion and disease prevention remains unclear. Social ties may buffer people from the damaging effects of psychological stress by inhibiting its negative emotional and physiological sequelae. The presence of close social networks may also promote better compliance with medical regimens, adoption of healthier lifestyles, and greater access to social and medical resources. Alternatively, low social support may be associated with CHD through its synergism with other psychosocial risk factors for CHD, such as low SES [66], depression [66], and hostility [71].

Summary

A preponderance of evidence from large, epidemiologic studies has demonstrated that psychosocial factors, such as depression, anger/hostility, SES, and social support have strong predictive value for incident CHD. The presence of these factors in the aftermath of a major event can adversely affect the clinical course of disease, predisposing people to recurrent CHD events, cardiac mortality, and all-cause mortality. Although the precise mechanisms by which these factors are associated with CHD are unknown, there are several putative behavioural and physiological pathways.

Conclusion

The research on psychosocial risk factors for CHD underscores the importance of positive affect, adaptive coping resources, and a supportive environment for positive health outcomes. In the 21st century when diseases of lifestyle predominate, systematic attention to the role of psychological and social risk factors in CHD onset and prevention is prudent.

References

1. Reddy, K.S. and Yusuf, S., 1998, "Emerging Epidemic of Cardiovascular Disease in Developing Countries", *Circulation*, 97, pp. 596-601.
2. Hearn, M.D., Murray, D.M. and Luepker, R.V., 1989, "Hostility, Coronary Heart Disease and Total Mortality: A 33-year Follow-up Study of University Students", *J. Behav. Med.*, 12, pp. 105-121.

3. Maruta, T., Hamburgen, M.E., Jennings, C.A., Offord, K.P., Colligan, R.C., Frye, R.L. and Malinchoc, M., 1993, "Keeping Hostility in Perspective: Coronary Heart Disease and the Hostility Scale on the Minnesota Multiphasic Personality Inventory", *Mayo. Clin. Proc.*, 68, pp. 109-114.
4. Rugulies, R., 2002, "Depression as a Predictor for Coronary Heart Disease: A Review and Meta-analysis", *Am. J. Prev. Med.*, 23, pp. 51-61.
5. Wulsin, L.R. and Singal, B.M., 2003, "Do Depressive Symptoms Increase the Risk for the Onset of Coronary Disease? A Systematic Quantitative Review", *Psychosom. Med.*, 65, pp. 201-210.
6. Marzari, C., Maggi, S., Manzato, E., Destro, C., Noale, M., Bianchi, D., Minicuci, N., Farchi, G., Baldereschi, M., Di Carlo, A., Crepaldi G. and the Italian Longitudinal Study on Aging Working Group, 2005, "Depressive Symptoms and Development of Coronary Heart Disease Events: The Italian Longitudinal Study on Aging", *J. Gerontology*, 60A, pp. 85-92.
7. Bremmer, M.A., Hoogendijk, W.J.G., Deg, D.J.H., Schoevers, R.A., Schalk, B.W.M. and Beekman, A.T.F., 2006, "Depression in Older Age is a Risk Factor for First Ischemic Cardiac Events", *Am. J. Geriatr. Psychiatry*, 14, pp. 523-530.
8. Wassertheil-Smoller, S., Shumaker, S., Ockene, J., Talavera, G.A., Greenland, P., Cochrane, B., Robbins, J., Aragaki, A. and Dunbar-Jacob, J., 2004, "Depression and Cardiovascular Sequelae in Postmenopausal Women: The Women's Health Initiative (WHI)", *Arch. Intern. Med.*, 164, pp. 289-298.
9. Empana, J.P., Jouven, X., Lemaitre, R.N., Sotoodehnia, N., Rea, T., Raghunathan, T.E., Simon, G. and Siscovick, D.S., 2006, "Clinical Depression and Risk of Out-of-hospital Cardiac Arrest", *Arch. Intern. Med.*, 166, pp. 195-200.
10. van Melle, J.P., de Jonge, P., Spijkerman, T.A., Tijssen, J.G., Ormel, J., van Veldhuisen, D.J., van den Brink, R.H. and van den Berg, M.P., 2004, "Prognostic Association of Depression Following Myocardial Infarction with Mortality and Cardiovascular Events: A Meta-analysis", *Psychosom. Med.*, 66, pp. 814-822.
11. Barth, J., Schumacher, M. and Herrmann-Lingen, C., 2004, "Depression as a Risk Factor for Mortality in Patients with Coronary Heart Disease: A Meta-analysis", *Psychosom. Med.*, 66, pp. 802-813.
12. Anda, R.F., Williamson, D.F., Escobedo, L.G., Mast, E.E., Giovino, G.A. and Remington, P.L., 1990, "Depression and the Dynamics of Smoking: A National Perspective", *JAMA*, 264, pp. 1541-1545.
13. Johnson, E.O. and Breslau, N., 2006, "Is the Association of Smoking and Depression a Recent Phenomenon?" *Nicotine Tob. Res.*, 8, pp. 257-262.
14. Rutledge, T., Reis, S.E., Olson, M., Owens, J., Kelsey, S.F., Pepine, C.J., Reichek, N., Rogers, W.J., Merz, N.B., Sopko, G., Cornell, C.E. and Matthews, K.A., 2001, "Psychosocial Variables are Associated with Atherosclerosis Risk Factors Among Women with Chest Pain: The WISE Study", *Psychosom. Med.*, 63, pp. 282-288.
15. Breslau, N., Peterson, E.L., Schultz, L.R., Chilcoat, H.D. and Andreski, P., 1998, "Major Depression and Stages of Smoking: A Longitudinal Investigation", *Arch. Gen. Psychiatry*, 55, pp. 161-166.
16. Jonas, B.S. and Lando, J.F., 2000, "Negative Affect as a Prospective Risk Factor for Hypertension", *Psychosom. Med.*, 62, pp. 188-196.
17. Davidson, K., Jonas, B.S., Dixon, K.E. and Markovitz, J.H., 2000, "Do Depression Symptoms Predict Early Hypertension Incidence in Young Adults in the CARDIA Study?" *Arch. Intern. Med.*, 160, pp. 1495-1500.
18. Ali, S., Stone, M.A., Peters, J.L., Davies, M.J. and Khunti, K., 2006, "The Prevalence of Co-morbid Depression in Adults with Type 2 Diabetes: A Systematic Review and Meta-analysis", *Diabet. Med.*, 23, pp. 1165-1173.
19. Golden, S.H., Williams, J.E., Ford, D.E., Yeh, H.C., Sanford, C.P., Nieto, F.J. and Brancati, F.L., 2004, "Depressive Symptoms and the Risk of Type 2 Diabetes: The Atherosclerosis Risk in Communities Study", *Diabetes Care*, 27, pp. 429-435.

20. Johnston, E., Johnson, S., McLeod, P. and Johnston, M., 2004, "The Relation of Body Mass Index to Depressive Symptoms", *Canadian J. Public Health*, 95, pp. 179-183.
21. Carpenter, K.M., Hasin, D.S., Allison, D.B. and Faith, M.S., 2000, "Relationships Between Obesity and DSM-IV Major Depressive Disorder, Suicide Ideation and Suicide Attempts: Results from a General Population Study", *Am. J. Public Health*, 90, pp. 251-257.
22. Ziegelstein, R.C., Fauerbach, J.A., Stevens, S.S., Romanelli, J., Richter, D.P. and Bush, D.E., 2000, "Patients with Depression are Less Likely to Follow Recommendations to Reduce Cardiac Risk During Recovery from a Myocardial Infarction", *Arch. Intern. Med.*, 160, pp. 1818-1823.
23. Joynt, K.E., Whellan, D.J. and O'Connor, C.M., 2003, "Depression and Cardiovascular Disease: Mechanisms of Interaction", *Biol. Psychiatry*, 54, pp. 248-261.
24. Musselman, D.L., Marzec, U., Davidoff, M., Manatunga, A.K., Gao, F., Reemsnyder, A., Duggirala, S., Larsen, H., Taylor, R.W., Hanson, S. and Nemeroff, C.B., 2002, "Platelet Activation and Secretion in Patients with Major Depression, Thoracic Aortic Atherosclerosis or Renal Dialysis Treatment", *Depress. Anxiety*, 15, pp. 91-101.
25. Sherwood, A., Hinderliter, A.L., Watkins, L.L., Waugh, R.A. and Blumenthal, J.A., 2005, "Impaired Endothelial Function in Coronary Heart Disease Patients with Depressive Symptomatology", *J. Am. Coll. Cardiol.*, 46, pp. 656-659.
26. Gorman, J.M. and Sloan, R.P., 2000, "Heart Rate Variability in Depressive and Anxiety Disorders", *Am. Heart J.*, 140 (4 Suppl), pp. 77-83.
27. Appels, A., Bär, F.W., Bär, J., Bruggeman, C. and de Baets, M., 2000, "Inflammation, Depressive Symptomatology and Coronary Artery Disease", *Psychosom. Med.*, 62, pp. 601-605.
28. Miller, G.E., Freedland, K.E., Carney, R.M., Stetler, C.A. and Banks, W.A., 2003, "Cynical Hostility, Depressive Symptoms and the Expression of Inflammatory Risk Markers for Coronary Artery Disease", *J. Behav. Med.*, 26, pp. 501-515.
29. Suarez, E.C., 2003, "Plasma Interleukin-6 is Associated with Psychological Coronary Risk Factors: Moderation by Use of Multivitamin Supplements", *Brain, Behavior and Immunity*, 17, pp. 296-303.
30. Suarez, E.C., Lewis, J.G., Krishnan, R.R. and Young, K.H., 2004, "Enhanced Expression of Cytokines and Chemokines by Blood Monocytes to *in vitro* Lipopolysaccharide Stimulation are Associated with Hostility and Severity of Depressive Symptoms in Healthy Women", *Psychoneuroendocrinology*, 29, pp. 1119-1128.
31. Suarez, E.C., 2004, "C-reactive Protein is Associated with Psychological Risk Factors of Cardiovascular Disease in Apparently Healthy Adults", *Psychosom. Med.*, 66, pp. 684-691.
32. Helmer, D.C., Ragland, D.R. and Syme, S.L., 1991, "Hostility and Coronary Artery Disease", *Am. J. Epidemiol.*, 133, pp. 112-122.
33. O'Malley, P.G., Jones, D.L., Feurerstein, I.M. and Taylor, A.J., 2000, "Lack of Correlation Between Psychological Factors and Subclinical Coronary Artery Disease", *New England Journal of Med.*, 343, pp. 1298-1304.
34. Julkunen, J., Salonen, R., Kaplan, G.A., Chesney, M.A. and Salonen, J.T., 1994, "Hostility and the Progression of Carotid Atherosclerosis", *Psychosom. Med.*, 56, pp. 519-25.
35. Bleil, M.E., McCaffery, J.M., Muldoon, M.F., Sutton-Tyrrell, K. and Manuck, S.B., 2004, "Anger-related Personality Traits and Carotid Artery Atherosclerosis in Untreated Hypertensive Men", *Psychosom. Med.*, 66, pp. 633-639.
36. Matthews, K.A., Owens, J.F., Kuller, L.H., Sutton-Tyrrell, K. and Jansen-McWilliams, L., 1998, "Are Hostility and Anxiety Associated with Carotid Atherosclerosis in Healthy Postmenopausal Women?" *Psychosom. Med.*, 60, pp. 633-638.
37. Iribarren, C., Sidney, S., Bild, D.E., Liu, K., Markovitz, J.H., Roseman, J.M. and Matthews, K., 2000, "Association of Hostility with Coronary Artery Calcification in Young Adults: The CARDIA Study", *JAMA*, 283, pp. 2546-2551.

38. Räikkönen, K., Matthews, K.A., Sutton-Tyrrell, K. and Kuller, L.H., 2004, "Trait Anger and the Metabolic Syndrome Predict Progression of Carotid Atherosclerosis in Healthy Middle-aged Women", *Psychosom. Med.*, 66, pp. 903-908.
39. Miller, T.Q., Smith, T.W., Turner, C.W., Guijarro, M.L. and Hallet, A.J., 1996, "A Meta-analytic Review of Research on Hostility and Physical Health", *Psychol. Bull.*, 119, pp. 322-348.
40. Everson, S.A., Kauhanen, J., Kaplan, G.A., Goldberg, D.E., Julkunen, J., Tuomilehto, J. and Salonen J.T., 1997, "Hostility and Increased Risk of Mortality and Acute Myocardial Infarction: The Mediating Role of Behavioral Risk Factors", *Am. J. Epidemiol.*, 146, pp. 142-152.
41. Kawachi, I., Sparrow, D., Spiro, III, A., Vokonas, P. and Weiss, S.T., 1996, "A Prospective Study of Anger and Coronary Heart Disease", *Circulation*, 94, pp. 2090-2095.
42. Matthews, K.A., Gump, B.B., Harris, K.F., Haney, T.L. and Barefoot, J.C., 2004, "Hostile Behaviors Predict Cardiovascular Mortality Among Men Enrolled in the Multiple Risk Factor Intervention Trial", *Circulation*, 109, pp. 66-70.
43. Chang, P.P., Ford, D.E., Meoni, L.A., Wang, N.Y. and Klag, M.J., 2002, "Anger in Young Men and Subsequent Premature Cardiovascular Disease: The Precursors Study", *Arch. Intern. Med.*, 162, pp. 901-906.
44. Williams, J.E., Paton, C.C., Siegler, I.C., Eigenbrodt, M.L., Nieto, F.J. and Tyroler, H.A., 2000, "Anger Proneness Predicts Incident Coronary Heart Disease Risk: Prospective Analysis from the Atherosclerosis Risk in Communities (ARIC) Study", *Circulation*, 101, pp. 2034-2039.
45. Bunde, J. and Suls, J., 2006, "A Quantitative Analysis of the Relationship Between the Cook-Medley Hostility Scale and Traditional Coronary Artery Disease Risk Factors", *Health Psych.*, 25, pp. 493-500.
46. Siegler, I.C., Costa, P.T., Brummett, B.H., Helms, M.J., Barefoot, J.C., Williams, R.B., Dahlstrom, W.G., Kaplan, B.H., Vitaliano, P.P., Nichaman, M.Z., Day, R.S. and Rimer, B.K., 2003, "Patterns of Change in Hostility from College to Midlife in the UNC Alumni Heart Study Predict High-risk Status", *Psychosom. Med.*, 65, pp. 738-745.
47. Schum, J.L., Jorgensen, R.S., Verhaeghen, P., Sauro, M. and Thibodeau, R., 2003, "Trait Anger, Anger Expression and Ambulatory Blood Pressure", *J. Behav. Med.*, 26, pp. 395-415.
48. Yan, L.L., Liu, K., Matthews, K.A., Daviglus, M.L., Ferguson, T.F. and Kiefe, C.I., 2003, "Psychosocial Factors and Risk of Hypertension: The Coronary Artery Risk Development in Young Adults (CARDIA) Study", *JAMA*, 290, pp. 2138-2148.
49. Suarez, E.C., Kuhn, C.M., Schanberg, S.M., Williams Jr., R.B. and Zimmerman, E.A., 1998, "Neuroendocrine, Cardiovascular and Emotional Responses of Hostile Men: The Role of Interpersonal Challenge", *Psychosom. Med.*, 60, pp. 78-88.
50. Markovitz, J.H., Matthews, K.A., Kiss, J. and Smitherman, T.C., 1996, "Effects of Hostility on Platelet Reactivity to Psychological Stress in Coronary Heart Disease Patients and in Healthy Controls", *Psychosom. Med.*, 58, pp. 143-149.
51. Suarez, E.C., Lewis, J.G. and Kuhn, C., 2002, "The Relation of Aggression, Hostility and Anger to Lipopolysaccharide-stimulated Tumor Necrosis Factor (TNF)-α by Blood Monocytes from Normal Men", *Brain Behav. Immun.*, 16, pp. 675-684.
52. Panagiotakos, D.B., Pitsavos, C., Chrysohoou, C., Tsetsekou, E., Papageorgiou, C., Christodoulou, G. and Stefanadis, C., 2004, "Increased Plasma Homocysteine Concentrations in Healthy People with Hostile Behavior: The Attica Study", *Med. Sci. Monit.*, 10, pp. CR457-462.
53. Lehman, E.W., 1967, "Social Class and Coronary Heart Disease: A Sociological Assessment of the Medical Literature", *J. Chronic. Dis.*, 20, pp. 381-391.
54. Diez-Rouz, A.V., Nieto, F.J., Tyroler, H.A., Crum, L.D. and Szklo, M., 1995, "Social Inequalities and Atherosclerosis", *Am. J. Epidemiol.*, 141, pp. 960-972.

55. Karlamangla, A.S., Singer, B.H., Williams, D.R., Schwartz, J.E., Matthews, K.A., Kiefe, C.I. and Seeman, T.E., 2005, "Impact of Socioeconomic Status on Longitudinal Accumulation of Cardiovascular Risk in Young Adults: The CARDIA Study (USA)", *Soc. Sci. Med.*, 60, pp. 999-1015.
56. Diez-Rouz, A.V., Nieto, F.J., Muntaner, C., Tyroler, H.A., Comstock, G.W., Shahar, E., Cooper, L.S., Watson, R.L. and Szklo, M., 1997, "Neighborhood Environments and Coronary Heart Disease: A Multilevel Analysis", *Am. J. Epidemiol.*, 146, pp. 48-63.
57. Diez-Rouz, A.V., Merkin, S.S., Arnett, D., Chambless, L., Massing, M., Nieto, F.J., Sorlie, P., Szklo, M., Tyroler, H.A. and Watson, R.L., 2001, "Neighborhood of Residence and Incidence of Coronary Heart Disease", *N. Engl. J. Med.*, 345, pp. 99-106.
58. Nordstrom, C.K., Diez-Rouz, A.V., Jackson, S.A. and Gardin, J.M., 2004, "The Association of Personal and Neighbourhood Socioeconomic Indicators with Subclinical Cardiovascular Disease in an Elderly Cohort: The Cardiovascular Health Study", *Soc. Sci. Med.*, 59, pp. 2139-2147.
59. Winkleby, M., Sundquist, K. and Cubbin, C., 2007, "Inequities in CHD Incidence and Case Fatality by Neighbourhood Deprivation", *American Journal of Preventive Medicine*, 32, pp. 97-106.
60. Pollitt, R.A., Rose, K.M. and Kaufman, J.S., 2005, "Evaluating the Evidence for Models of Life Course Socioeconomic Factors and Cardiovascular Outcomes: A Systematic Review", *BMC Public Health*, Review, 5, p. 7.
61. Susser, M.W., Watson, W. and Hopper, K., 1985, *Sociology in Medicine*, 3rd Edn., Oxford University Press, New York, pp. 213-275.
62. Pappas, G., Queen, S., Hadden, W. and Fisher, G., 1993, "The Increasing Disparity in Mortality Between Socioeconomic Groups in the United States, 1960 and 1986", *N. Engl. J. Med.*, 329, pp. 103-109.
63. Gallo, L.C. and Matthews, K.A., 2003, "Understanding the Association Between Socioeconomic Status and Physical Health: Do Negative Emotions Play a Role?" *Psychological Bulletin*, 129, pp. 10-51.
64. Turner, R.J., Wheaton, B. and Lloyd, D.A., 1995, "The Epidemiology of Social Stress", *American Sociological Review*, 60, pp. 104-125.
65. Haukkala, A., 2002, "Socio-economic Differences in Hostility Measures: A Population Based Study", *Psychology and Health*, 17, pp. 191-202.
66. Liberatos, P., Link, B.G. and Kelsey, J.L., 1988, "The Measurement of Social Class in Epidemiology", *Epidemiol. Rev.*, 10, pp. 87-121.
67. Lett, H.S., Blumenthal, J.A., Babyak, M.A., Strauman, T.J., Robins, C. and Sherwood, A., 2005, "Social Support and Coronary Heart Disease: Epidemiologic Evidence and Implications for Treatment", *Psychosom. Med.*, 67, pp. 869-878.
68. Welin, C., Lappas, G. and Wilhelmsen, L., 2000, "Independent Importance of Psychosocial Factors for Prognosis After Myocardial Infarction", *J. Intern. Med.*, 247, pp. 629-639.
69. Pfiffner, D. and Hoffman, A., 2004, "Psychosocial Predictors of Death for Low-risk Patients After a First Myocardial Infarction: A Seven-year Follow-up Study", *J. Cardiopulmonary Rehabilitation*, 24, pp. 87-93.
70. Lindsay, G.M., Smith, L.N., Hanlon, P. and Wheatley, D.J., 2001, "The Influence of General Health Status and Social Support on Symptomatic Outcome Following Coronary Artery Bypass Grafting", *Heart*, 85, pp. 80-86.
71. Angerer, P., Siebert, U., Kothny, W., Mühlbauer, D., Mudra, H. and von Schacky, C., 2000, "Impact of Social Support, Cynical Hostility and Anger Expression on Progression of Coronary Atherosclerosis", *J. American College of Cardiology*, 36, pp. 1781-1788.

The AHA-Syndrome and Cardiovascular Diseases
Editors: Swati Y. Bhave and Sunil Saini
Copyright © 2010 Anamaya Publishers, New Delhi, India

15. Workplace Stressors, Hypertension and Cardiovascular Disease: Epidemiology, Prevention and Management

Paul A. Landsbergis[1] and Peter L. Schnall[2]

[1]Department of Environmental and Occupational Health Sciences, State University of New York-Downstate Medical Center, Brooklyn, New York, USA

[2]Division of Occupational and Environmental Medicine, Department of Medicine, University of California Irvine, California, USA

Abstract: Research has linked individual behaviours, such as smoking and sedentary behaviour, as well as social factors, such as social class, work organisation and work-related psychosocial stressors, to hypertension and cardiovascular disease (CVD). Increased CVD risk has been associated with job characteristics, such as long work hours and shift work, and work-related psychosocial stressors, such as "job strain" (a combination of high psychological work demands and low job decision latitude, or job control), "effort-reward imbalance", job insecurity, and "threat-avoidant" vigilant work. Job stressors may increase the risk of hypertension and CVD through a variety of mechanisms including, possibly, by promoting negative affect, such as anger, hostility, anxiety and depression. A number of public health strategies are needed to address the burgeoning pandemic of CVD, including worksite surveillance, development of the field of occupational cardiology, integration of health promotion with occupational health approaches, and job redesign.

Keywords: Work-related psychosocial stressors, Hypertension, Cardiovascular diseases.

Introduction

Cardiovascular disease (CVD) is the major cause of morbidity and mortality in the industrialised world, and is projected to become the most common cause of death worldwide early in the 21st century [1, 2]. Epidemiologic evidence supports the conclusion that CVD and hypertension are epidemics of recent historical origin, developing concurrently with industrialisation and urbanisation, and now increasing in the context of economic globalisation. Modern medicine focusses on individual risk factors for hypertension and CVD, often ignoring the important role that social factors, such as social class, work organisation, and work-related psychosocial stressors, play in the etiology of essential hypertension and CVD. Social factors need to be fully integrated into models of disease etiology.

The Social-Historical Context

In 2003, CVD caused 29.2% of all global deaths. Also, 80% of all CVD deaths worldwide took place in developing, low and middle-income countries [1]. In India, CVD mortality in the working-age population (age 30-59 years) was 211 (per 100,000) for men and 139 for women in 2000, much higher than developed countries, such as the US, and higher than other developing countries, such as China and Brazil [3]. The prevalence of hypertension in India increased from 1-3% in 1950 to 10-30% in 2000 [4]. The prevalence of type II diabetes has more than doubled in India's urban areas in the past 20 years [5].

Modern cardiology has identified a number of individual risk factors for CVD [6]. However, many cases of CVD do not occur in "high risk" individuals [7]. For example, in the Multiple Risk Factor Intervention Trial, more than 30% of the coronary heart disease (CHD) deaths due to systolic blood pressure (BP) > 110 mm Hg were in the group with 'normal' systolic BP (110-139 mm Hg) [8]. Essential hypertension, one of the most important 'standard' risk factors for CVD, is itself an unexplained disease (hence the name 'essential'). Thus, much remains to be learned about the etiology of CVD.

Based primarily on studies of non-industrialised populations [9, 10], CVD and hypertension appear to be epidemics of recent historical origin [11, 12]. A major cross-cultural study found virtually no rise in BP with age and no hypertension among hunter-gatherers, herders or traditional family farmers [12]. In contrast, men and women in urban industrial societies have steady rises of BP with age and hypertension is common [11, 12].

Social Patterning of CVD: Social Class and Working Conditions

An extensive body of evidence has documented that lower socioeconomic status (SES) [13] and work stressors [14, 15] are important risk factors for hypertension and CVD. One explanation for the social class gradient in CVD is greater exposure to unhealthy working conditions among lower SES groups. For example, job control was "the biggest factor contributing to the socioeconomic gradient in CHD risk across civil service employment grade", in the British Whitehall Study [16, 17].

Current Economic and Workplace Trends

Current economic and workplace trends, resulting in part from economic globalisation, may be having dramatic effects on workers' health, especially lower SES workers [18, 19]. These trends include offshoring, outsourcing, downsizing, contingent and temporary work, new management systems such as "lean production", which contribute to intensification of work [20] and, in the US, stagnant or falling real income. Concurrently, substantial changes in job characteristics have been occurring. In Europe, "time constraints" (workload demands) increased between 1977-96 [21] and in the US, increases between 1977-97 were reported for "never enough time to get everything done on my job" (from 40 to 60%) [22]. European surveys in 2005 showed continuing increases in work intensity and job demands, but no change or slight declines in job control or autonomy [23, 24], suggesting an increase in the prevalence of job strain. American workers' average weekly work hours are now the longest in the developed world [25], working in jobs that are more stressful than in the past.

These trends may be affecting the working conditions of lower SES workers more severely. For example, the prevalence of "hectic plus monotonous work" in Sweden increased from 8.6 to 11.% from 1992-2000 for the whole workforce. However, for manual workers, the prevalence increased from 12.6 to 20% [26].

CVD Mortality and Incidence Trends

Despite large declines in CVD mortality over the past 40 years in the US [27], there has been little or no decline in CVD *incidence* in the past 20 years [28-31]. While smoking prevalence and cholesterol levels have declined, there have been increases in diabetes [32], overweight [33] and hypertension [34] and increasing recognition that psychosocial stressors may be contributing to these trends [35]. Given the stable incidence rates, combined with the aging of the population, the prevalence of CVD has increased dramatically in the US.

The higher CVD mortality among men and women in lower SES groups, e.g. manual workers, began to appear in the 1950-60s [36, 37]. The gap between higher and lower SES has risen progressively [38, 39]. In the US, men from counties with the lowest (vs. highest) SES had a 30% greater risk of CVD mortality in 1969-70. However, this disparity increased to 80% by 1997-98 [40]. The disparity between higher and lower SES in CVD incidence is also increasing [41, 42]. Increases in work stressors and income inequality produced by economic globalisation may be playing a role in maintaining incidence rates for CVD and promoting the pandemic of CVD worldwide.

Work Organisation and CVD

Work Hours and Schedules

Research studies suggest that a modest association (RR $\approx$ 1.4) between shift work and heart disease exists [43]. Four comprehensive reviews of research on long work hours (overtime work) point to a wide variety of health effects, including work accidents and injuries, musculoskeletal disorders, fatigue, psychological symptoms, health behaviours, cardiovascular risk factors (such as high BP) and CVD [44-47].

Studies, beginning in 1958, have suggested that long working hours may increase risk of heart disease [48-53]. The impact of overtime on health may be greater for workers in stressful jobs, such as professional drivers [54], shift workers [47] and older workers [45, 55].

Work-Related Psychosocial Stressors

Various models of work stressors have been investigated over the past 30 years [56-59]. The most highly studied construct is "job strain", i.e. work which combines high psychological job demands with low job decision latitude or job control [14]. The "effort-reward" model defines stressful job conditions as a "mismatch between high workload [high demand] and low control over long-term rewards" [60]. Low reward includes low "esteem reward" (respect and support), low income and low "status control" (poor promotion prospects, job insecurity and status inconsistency). Other studies have examined "threat-avoidant" vigilant work, i.e. work that involves continuously maintaining a high level of vigilance in order to avoid disaster, such as loss of human life [58]. This is a feature of a number of occupations at high risk for CVD, e.g. truck drivers, air traffic controllers, and sea pilots. Researchers have been investigating the health effects of job insecurity and 'downsizing' [61].

Job Strain and CVD

Out of the 34 studies of job strain and CVD, published between 1981 and 2002, 18 studies showed significant positive associations [59]. An additional three studies had mixed positive and null results. In many of the studies, the design of the studies tended to bias the results toward the null (i.e., produce either weaker or non-significant associations). Men showed strong, consistent evidence of an association between exposure to job strain and CVD [59].

Effort-Reward Imbalance and CVD

A number of studies among men [60, 62-67] have found significant positive associations between exposure to effort-reward imbalance and CVD. For example, a study of Finnish industrial workers found that those in the top one-third of effort-reward imbalance had an increased risk of 2.42 of death due to heart disease compared to the bottom one-third over a follow-up period of 25.6 years, controlling for other CVD risk factors [67].

Threat-Avoidant Vigilant Work and CVD

Only a few epidemiologic studies have specifically examined aspects of threat-avoidant vigilant activity and CVD outcomes [50, 68-70]. The strongest evidence for this risk factor comes from studies of single occupations, where professional drivers, particularly urban transport operators, emerge as the occupation with the most consistent evidence of elevated risk of CHD [71, 72] and hypertension [73].

Downsizing and CVD

Workforce reductions ('downsizing') were associated with a doubling of the risk of CVD mortality [61] among Finnish public employees, mediated in part by increased levels of physical work demands and job insecurity, and decreased levels of skill discretion and participation [74].

Synergism with Low SES

Among men, the impact of job strain on CVD is more consistent and stronger among blue-collar workers [75, 76], with risk ratios as high as 10.0 [77], than among men in jobs with higher SES. A similar interaction with SES was observed for effort-reward imbalance in the Whitehall II Study [78]. An interaction between job strain and low SES was also observed for BP among New York City men [79] and Framingham men and women [80].

Population Attributable Risk of Psychosocial Work Stressors

The population attributable risk (PAR%) of CVD due to psychosocial work stressors may be substantial. Karasek and Theorell estimated a prevalence of exposure of 15-25% in Sweden and a resulting PAR% of 7-16% for men [14]. In Denmark, the PAR% for monotonous high paced work (a conservative proxy measure for job strain) was estimated at 6% for men and 14% for women [57]. However, few studies have examined the combined or synergistic effect of workplace stressors, which would increase estimates of the proportion of CVD due to work. One Swedish study [66] did find that the combined effects of exposure to job strain and to effort-reward imbalance upon CVD were much stronger than the separate effects of each model.

Work Organisation and Hypertension

Effect of BP Measurement Techniques

Is the increased risk of CVD due to job strain mediated by increased BP? Few studies of job strain and casual clinic BP have shown significant associations [56, 58], with the exception of a very large study (n = 8395) [81]. However, strong evidence of an association is found in studies where BP is measured by an ambulatory (portable) monitor [58]. This difference in findings may be explained, in part, by the imprecision and possible biases of taking 'casual' BP measurements. For example, relaxation can occur when people are away from work resulting in lower BP. There are also various atypical psychosocial stimuli present in a clinic that can affect BP, such as anxiety due to seeing a doctor. An alternative method of BP measurement is ambulatory (ABP) monitoring, in which a person wears an automatic monitor on his or her arm throughout the workday [82]. Compared to casual BP measurements, ABP monitoring provides a more reliable measure of BP, since there is no observer bias and the number of readings is increased. It is also a more valid measure of average BP, since BP is measured during a person's normal daily activities and exposure to the daily stressors that influence persistent increases in BP. ABP is also a better predictor than casual clinic BP of target organ damage, such as increases in the size of the heart's left ventricle [83] and CVD [84].

Long Work Hours and BP

Two Japanese studies found evidence linking overtime work and BP among men working more than 55 h per week [55, 85], although other studies found no association [86] or an inverse relation [87]. Only Hayashi et al. [85] measured BP by averaging multiple readings at work using ABP monitoring methods. A recent US study analysed self-reported data from the California Health Information Survey and found that employees working more than 50 h per week had a 29% increased risk of developing hypertension (OR = 1.29, 95% CI: 1.10-1.52) compared to those working 11-39 h per week [88].

Job Strain and BP

As of 2000, of the 10 cross-sectional studies of job strain (or its components) and ABP among men, many indicated significant positive associations with work ABP [58]. In the five studies where measurements were also made outside of work, job strain was associated with non-work systolic ABP. Of the six cross-sectional studies of job strain and ABP among women, four indicated a significant positive association with work systolic ABP [89]. Work systolic ABP in workers facing job strain is typically 4-8 mm Hg higher than those without job strain.

The only long-term prospective study of job stressors and ABP, the New York City Work Site BP Study (WSBPS), began in 1985. At the first round of data collection (Time 1), men employed in "high strain" jobs were at increased risk of hypertension (OR = 2.7), had increased left ventricular mass index (7.3 g/m^2) [90] and had higher levels of work (6.7 mm Hg systolic, 2.7 mm Hg diastolic), home and sleep ABP, controlling for potential risk factors [91, 92].

By adding a second round of data collection three years later (Time 2), it was possible to construct a measure of repeated or cumulative exposure to job strain. The chronically exposed group exhibited an 11-12 mm Hg higher systolic and 6-9 mm Hg higher diastolic work ABP than the group unexposed at both times. These effect sizes are substantial, more than twice the difference between African-Americans and whites in this sample and more than the estimated effect of aging 25 years or gaining 50 pounds in weight [93]. Finally, those men reporting job strain at Time 1 but no job strain at Time 2 exhibited a decrease in systolic ABP of 5.3 mm Hg at work and 4.7 mm Hg at home ($p < 0.05$) [93].

Effort-Reward Imbalance and BP

Studies of high effort/low reward at work have shown significant positive associations with systolic ABP [94], hypertension in men [95], or in men and women [96], and with a co-manifestation of hypertension and high LDL-cholesterol in men [97].

Threat-Avoidant Vigilant Work and BP

In a study of San Francisco transit operators, experts' ratings of objective stressors, i.e. job barriers and time pressure, were each significantly associated with high BP (i.e. 'hypertension', defined as ≥ 160/95 mm Hg casual BP and/or currently taking antihypertensive medication) after taking into account age, gender and seniority [73].

Other Mechanisms By Which Work Organisation Can Lead to CVD

Job Strain

Job strain (or its components) have been associated with smoking intensity and cessation [98-101], body mass index (BMI) [102], skinfold thickness [103] and sedentary behaviour [98, 104]. However, null studies also exist. Job strain was associated with decreased heart rate variability (HRV) in one study [105]. Hypertension has been found to contribute to atherosclerosis [106]. In addition, low decision latitude is associated with high plasma fibrinogen, suggesting a link with coagulation and, thus, atherosclerosis [107, 108]. Progression of coronary atherosclerosis over time has been associated with low job decision latitude [109, 110], high demands and low economic rewards at work [65], job strain in men [111] and job strain in women but not men [112].

Effort-Reward Imbalance

Effort-reward imbalance was associated with BMI among Finnish factory workers [67], the co-manifestation of behavioural risk factors: BMI ≥ 25, smoking, heavy alcohol consumption and physical inactivity among Finnish public employees [113] and incident type 2 diabetes among men (but not women) in the British Whitehall Study [114]. Effort-reward imbalance was associated with LDL/HDL cholesterol ratio in several studies [96, 115] and with the combined occurrence of hypertension and hyperlipidemia [97].

Long Work Hours

Overtime was associated with unhealthy weight gain in two studies, increased alcohol use in two of three studies, and increased smoking in one of two studies, but not leisure-time physical activity or drug abuse [47]. One [116] of two [87, 116] Japanese studies found an association between work hours and adult onset diabetes.

Social Psychological Mechanisms

Modern medical science has tended to view behavioural/psychological factors in isolation, ignoring their relationship to objective stressors in the work environment and elsewhere. Affect, behaviour and personality can be seen as outcomes of social conditions and may act as mediators of the effects of social stressors on CVD risk. Further research is needed on the hypothesis that job stressors may increase the risk of hypertension and CVD, in part, by shaping personality or increasing negative affect, such as anger, hostility, anxiety or depression [14, 117].

Hypertension

Little evidence exists for "hypertensive personality" [118]. Hypertension has been associated with internalised aggression [119] and anxiety [120, 121], although other studies have failed to find these associations [120-122]. Methodological problems have plagued studies of this association [123]. Another limitation is the lack of a model, which predicts specific interactions or mediation between work stressors and personality characteristics in the development of hypertension, e.g. in one study, suppressed anger was associated with hypertension in male hourly workers only among those reporting job stress [124]. Other studies have shown that asymptomatic participants with hypertension [125], as well as those with normal BP with a family history of hypertension [126], express fewer emotions and have a non-complaining attitude [14]. Theorell hypothesises that such personality characteristics may result, in part, from a stressful work environment that "enforces a no complaining attitude and prevents development of active emotional coping" [126].

CVD

Job stressors may also increase the risk of CVD, in part, by influencing personality characteristics or negative affect. Many emotions "are responses to power and status differentials embedded within social situations" [127]. Positive associations have been found between job stressors and anxiety [128-130], burnout [131-133], depression [117, 128, 134, 135] and hostility [136, 137]. However, most studies of associations between affect and blood pressure/hypertension have been negative or only weakly positive.

Masked (Occult) Hypertension

ABP monitoring allows for the identification of *masked* (also known as *occult*) hypertension, i.e. elevated ABP while working or for 24 hours, but normal in an office setting [138, 139]. Masked hypertension is a rarely studied entity, but of major clinical and public health significance. People with masked hypertension have levels of target organ damage, such as left ventricular mass index [140, 141] or carotid plaque [140] or risk of CVD [84, 142] similar to diagnosed hypertensives and significantly higher than normotensives. People with masked hypertension and no previous diagnosis of hypertension, require counselling, possibly treatment, and workplace stressor assessment, but rarely receive these because their office BPs appear normal. The prevalence of masked hypertension among people in the general population with normal clinic BP is 10-30% [138, 139, 143].

Several studies have identified predictors of masked hypertension, including male gender [84, 144, 145], cigarette smoking [84, 144, 145], coffee [84], alcohol [145] and older age [145]. However, only three studies have examined work-related predictors of masked hypertension. In the WSBPS, masked hypertension was somewhat more common among workers exposed to job strain than those not exposed to job strain [138] – a prevalence ratio of 1.55 (95% CI: 0.82-2.91). Among women in Ohio, masked hypertension, based on systolic BP, was more common among blue-collar and clerical workers than among higher status white-collar workers. However, such a pattern was not observed for diastolic BP [143]. In unpublished data from a hospital in New York City, increased risk of masked hypertension was observed among workers exposed to job strain, effort reward imbalance and evening, night or rotating shiftwork Further research is needed to determine whether job strain or other job stressors increase the risk of masked hypertension.

Worksite Surveillance

Experts in Japan, Europe and the US have called for surveillance programmes at individual workplaces and monitoring at national and regional levels in order to identify the extent of work-stress related health problems and to provide baselines against which to evaluate efforts at amelioration [146]. Surveillance can be effectively conducted through teams consisting of physicians, psychologists, nurses, health educators, ergonomists, epidemiologists and labour union and management representatives.

First, the surveillance team needs to determine whether the occupation(s) being assessed are at high risk; whether workers are exposed to any physical, chemical, work schedule or psychosocial CVD risk factors at work; and have any of these been increasing over time [147]. Questionnaires, such as the Job Content Questionnaire [148], the Effort-Reward Imbalance Questionnaire [149] and the Occupational Stress Index [150] can be used to assess job characteristics and job stressors. Second, workplace screening should be conducted for biomedical CVD risk factors, including use of ABP monitoring methods to determine levels of BP at work and over a 24 h period [151]. Such surveillance can help to identify those individuals with masked hypertension as well as clusters of work-related hypertension within job titles, departments or workplaces and help target these groups for primary and secondary prevention programmes.

Occupational Cardiology

The development of the field of occupational cardiology is an essential component of efforts to identify and prevent work-related hypertension and CVD. Clinicians require familiarity with the work environment and an ability to take their patients' work histories and assess their work stressors, to evaluate their hypertension and CVD, including the presence of masked hypertension (at least 10 million cases estimated in the US) [152]. There is an urgent need to formulate and validate algorithms and guidelines for the diagnosis and management of work-related hypertension, relevant pre-pathologic conditions and CVD, including protocols on return-to-work for a patient following a heart attack to the same cardionoxious work environment.

Integration of Health Promotion and Occupational Health

Worksite health promotion, including efforts to promote exercise, healthy diet and smoking cessation, is an important component to combat the epidemic of CVD. Unfortunately, cardiac risk factor counselling in isolation often has poor efficacy, particularly among occupational groups with a heavy burden of exposure to work stressors. For example, Fisher and Belkic state: "despite devotion of substantial time and the use of state-of-the-art methods, our efforts applied systematically among professional drivers were, at best, only minimally effective, unless there was a concomitant amelioration in stressful working conditions" [153].

Many health promotion "programmes have emphasised risk-factor reduction strategies but have not integrated disease prevention and safety programmes with organisational policies to enhance the physical and social quality of the workplace" [154]. A number of researchers have recommended integrating workplace health promotion and occupational health, to develop complementary behavioural and environmental interventions [155, 156]. Integrated health promotion-occupational health programmes have shown positive results in a randomised controlled trial in the US [157] and a programme among Dutch manufacturing employees [158].

Job Redesign

The effectiveness of interventions to improve work organisation and job design, reduce job stressors, and create a more healthy work organisation have been documented [159-161]. For example, an intervention among Swedish civil servants included worker committees which developed and carried out action plans to reduce work stressors. A significant decrease in apolipoprotein B/AI ratio occurred in the intervention group, but not in the control group [162]. An intervention on a Stockholm bus line, designed to diminish time pressure and promote traffic flow, resulted in a significant decline in systolic BP (– 10.7 mm Hg) in the intervention group, greater than in the comparison group [– 4.3 mm Hg] [163]. A Swedish field study also showed that systolic BP, heart rate, epinephrine and self-reported tiredness increased significantly from the start to the end of a day shift at a traditional auto assembly line, but not at a more flexible work organisation with small autonomous groups having greater opportunities to influence the pace and content of their work [164].

A number of job redesign programmes in the US have examined other stress-related health outcomes and provide valuable guidance. These programmes have included efforts to reduce 'burnout' symptoms among state child protection agency employees through a labour-management committee and new technology [165], increase participation in decision-making through labour-management committees at an automobile manufacturer [166] and reduce work-related musculoskeletal disorders through job redesign at a meatpacking plant [167]. "Systems approaches" (emphasising primary prevention; integrating primary with secondary and tertiary prevention; including meaningful participation of targetted groups) appear to be the most effective in addressing the organisational and individual impacts of job stress [168].

Conclusions

It is important that the role of social mechanisms, such as social class, work organisation and work-related psychosocial stressors, in the etiology of essential hypertension and CVD, be integrated into medical models of disease etiology. Work-related stressors may increase the risk of hypertension and CVD through a variety of mechanisms, including possibly by promoting traditional risk factors (e.g. smoking and sedentary behaviour) or promoting negative affect, such as anger, hostility, anxiety and depression. A number of public health strategies that reflect our current broader understanding of the social etiology of CVD are needed to address the burgeoning pandemic of CVD, including worksite surveillance, development of the field of occupational cardiology, integration of health promotion with occupational health approaches, and job redesign.

Key Points

- CVD is the major cause of morbidity and mortality in the industrialised world. It is well on its way to becoming the most common cause of death worldwide early in the 21st century.
- CVD and hypertension are epidemics of recent historical origin, developing concurrently with industrialisation and urbanisation and now increasing in the context of globalisation.
- Research has linked hypertension and CVD to lower SES and work stressors, including long work hours, shift work, "job strain", "effort-reward imbalance", downsizing and "threat-avoidant" vigilant work.
- Job stressors may increase the risk of hypertension and CVD, in part, by shaping personality or increasing negative affect, such as anger, hostility, anxiety or depression.
- The role of social mechanisms in the etiology of illness is still poorly integrated into modern medicine.
- A number of public health strategies are needed to address the burgeoning pandemic of CVD, including worksite surveillance, development of the field of occupational cardiology, integration of health promotion with occupational health approaches and job redesign.

Acknowledgements

Some of the research findings in this chapter were supported in part by grants HL18232, HL30605, HL55165 and HL47540 from the National Heart, Lung and Blood Institute, Bethesda, MD and grant OH07577 from the National Institute for Occupational Safety and Health, Cincinnati, Ohio, USA.

References

1. WHO, 2004, *The Atlas of Heart Disease and Stroke*, World Health Organization, Geneva.
2. Graziano, J., 2004, "Global Burden of Cardiovascular Disease", In *Heart Disease*, D. Zipes, P. Libby, R. Bonow and E. Braunwald (Eds.), Elsevier, London, pp. 1-19.
3. Greenberg, H., Raymond, S. and Leeder, S., 2005, "Cardiovascular Disease and Global Health: Threat and Opportunity", *Health Affairs*, DOI 10.1377/hlthaff.W5.31.
4. Padmavati, S., 2002, "Prevention of Heart Disease in India in the Twenty-first Century: Need for a Concerted Effort", *Indian Heart Journal*, 54(1), pp. 99-102.
5. Ramachandran, A., Snehalatha, C., Latha, E., Vijay, V. and Viswanathan, M., 1997, "Rising Prevalence of NIDDM in an Urban Population in India", *Diabetologia*, 40(2), pp. 232-237.
6. Kannel, W.B., 1992, "The Framingham Experience", In *Coronary Heart Disease Epidemiology*, M. Marmot and P. Elliott (Eds.), Oxford University Press, Oxford, pp. 67-82.
7. Whelton, P.K., He, J. and Klag, M.J., 1994, "Blood Pressure in Westernized Populations", In *Textbook of Hypertension*, J.D. Swales (Ed.), Blackwell Scientific Publications, London, pp. 11-21.
8. Stamler, J., 1991, "Blood Pressure and High Blood Pressure: Aspects of Risk", *Hypertension*, 18 (Suppl. 1), pp. 95-107.

9. Carvalho, J.J.M., Baruzzi, R.G., Howard, P.F., Poulter, N., Alpers, M.P., Franco, L.J. et al., 1989, "Blood Pressure in Four Remote Populations in the INTERSALT Study", *Hypertension*, 14, pp. 238-246.
10. Cooper, R.S., Rotimi, C.N. and Ward, R., 1999, "The Puzzle of Hypertension in African-Americans", *Scientific American*.
11. Schnall, P.L. and Kern, R., 1981, "Hypertension in American Society: An Introduction to Historical Materialist Epidemiology", In *The Sociology of Health and Illness: Critical Perspectives*, P. Conrad and R. Kern (Eds.), St. Martin's Press, New York, pp. 97-122.
12. Waldron, I., Nowatarski, M., Freimer, M., Henry, J.P., Post, N. and Written, C., 1982, "Cross-cultural Variation in Blood Pressure: A Qualitative Analysis of the Relationship of Blood Pressure to Cultural Characteristics, Salt Consumption and Body Weight", *Social Science and Medicine*, 16, pp. 419-430.
13. Kaplan, G.A. and Keil, J.E., 1993, "Socioeconomic Factors and Cardiovascular Disease: A Review of the Literature", *Circulation*, 88 (4 Pt. 1), pp. 1973-98.
14. Karasek, R. and Theorell, T., 1990, *Healthy Work: Stress, Productivity, and the Reconstruction of Working Life*, Basic Books, New York.
15. Schnall, P., Belkic, K., Landsbergis, P.A. and Baker, D., 2000a, "The Workplace and Cardiovascular Disease", In *Occupational Medicine: State-of-the-Art Reviews*, Hanley and Belfus, Philadelphia.
16. Kawachi, I. and Marmot, M., 1998, "What Can We Learn from Studies of Occupational Class and Cardiovascular Disease?" *American Journal of Epidemiology*, 148, pp. 160-163.
17. Marmot, M.G., Bosma, H., Hemingway, H., Brunner, E. and Stansfeld, S., 1997, "Contribution of Job Control and Other Risk Factors to Social Variations in Coronary Heart Disease Incidence", *Lancet*, 350, pp. 235-239.
18. Cooper, C., 1996, "Working Hours and Health", *Work and Stress*, 10, pp. 1-4.
19. Tuchsen, F., 1993, "Working Hours and Ischaemic Heart Disease in Danish Men: A Four-year Cohort Study of Hospitalization", *International Journal of Epidemiology*, 22, pp. 215-221.
20. Landsbergis, P.A., Cahill, J. and Schnall, P., 1999, "The Impact of Lean Production and Related New Systems of Work Organization on Worker Health", *Journal of Occupational Health Psychology*, 4(2), pp. 108-130.
21. European Foundation, 1997b, *Time Constraints and Autonomy at Work in the European Union*, European Foundation for the Improvement of Living and Working Conditions, Dublin.
22. Bond, J.T., Galinsky, E. and Swanberg, J.E., 1998, *The 1997 National Study of the Changing Workforce*, Families and Work Institute, New York.
23. Paoli, P. and Merllié, D., 2001, *Third European Survey on Working Conditions*, European Foundation for the Improvement of Living and Working Conditions, Dublin.
24. European Foundation, 2006, "Fifteen Years of Working Conditions in the EU: Charting the Trends", Dublin, Ireland.
25. ILO, 2001, *Key Indicators of the Labour Market 2001-2002*, International Labour Office, Geneva.
26. Vogel, J., 2002, "Swedish Level of Living Survey Data", *Statistics Sweden*, Stockholm.
27. Liao, Y. and Cooper, R.S., 1995, "Continued Adverse Trends in Coronary Heart Disease Mortality Among Blacks, 1980-91", *Public Health Reports*, 110, pp. 572-579.
28. Rosamond, W.D., Chanbless, L.E., Folsom, A.R., Cooper, L.S., Conwill, D.E., Clegg, L. et al., 1998, "Trends in the Incidence of Myocardial Infarction and in Mortality Due to Coronary Heart Disease, 1987 to 1994", *The New England Journal of Medicine*, 339, p. 863.
29. Goldberg, R.J., Yarzebski, J., Lessard, D. and Gore, J.M., 1999, "A Two-decades (1975 to 1995) Long Experience in the Incidence, In-hospital and Long-term Case-fatality Rates of Acute Myocardial Infarction: A Community-wide Perspective", *Journal of the American College of Cardiology*, 33(6), pp. 1533-1539.

30. McGovern, P.G., Jacobs, Jr., D.R., Shahar, E., Arnett, D.K., Folsom, A.R., Blackburn, H. et al., 2001, "Trends in Acute Coronary Heart Disease Mortality, Morbidity, and Medical Care from 1985 Through 1997: The Minnesota Heart Survey", *Circulation*, 104, pp. 19-24.
31. Rosamond, W.D., Folsom, A.R., Chambless, L.E. and Wang, C.-H., 2001, "Coronary Heart Disease Trends in Four United States Communities: The Atherosclerosis Risk in Communities (ARIC) Study 1987-1996", *International Journal of Epidemiology*, 30, pp. S17-S22.
32. Harris, M.I., Flegal, K.M., Cowie, C.C., Eberhardt, M.S., Golstein, D.E., Little, R.R. et al., 1998, "Prevalence of Diabetes, Impaired Fasting Glucose, and Impaired Glucose Tolerance in US Adults: The Third National Health and Nutrition Examination Survey, 1988-1994", *Diabetes Care*, 21 (N4, April), pp. 518-524.
33. Kuczmarski, R.J., Flegal, K.M., Campbell, S.M. and Johnson, C.L., 1994, "Increasing Prevalence of Overweight Among US Adults", *JAMA*, 272, pp. 205-211.
34. Hajjar, I. and Kotchen, T., 2003, "Trends in Prevalence, Awareness, Treatment, and Control of Hypertension in the United States, 1988-2000", *JAMA*, 290(2).
35. Gornel, D.L., 1999, "Rates of Death from Coronary Heart Disease: Letter to the Editor", *New England Journal of Medicine*, 340(9), pp. 730-732.
36. Marmot, M., Rose, G., Shipley, M. et al., 1978, "Employment Grade and Coronary Heart Disease in British Civil Servants", *J. Epid. Commun. Health*, 32, pp. 244-249.
37. Wing, S., Dargent-Molina, P., Casper, M., Riggan, W., Hayes, C.G. and Tyroler, H.A., 1987, "Changing Association Between Community Structure and Ischaemic Heart Disease Mortality in the United States", *Lancet*, 2(8567), pp. 1067-1070.
38. Marmot, M. and Theorell, T., 1991, "Social Class and Cardiovascular Disease: The Contribution of Work", In *The Psychosocial Work Environment: Work Organization, Democratization and Health*, J.V. Johnson and G. Johansson (Eds.), Baywood Publishing Company, Amityville, New York, pp. 33-48.
39. Gonzalez, M.A., Artalejo, F.R. and Calero, J.R., 1998, "Relationship Between Socioeconomic Status and Ischaemic Heart Disease in Cohort and Case-control Studies: 1960-1993", *International Journal of Epidemiology*, 27(3), pp. 350-358.
40. Singh, G.K. and Siahpush, M., 2002, "Increasing Inequalities in All-cause and Cardiovascular Mortality Among US Adults Aged 25-64 years by Area Socioeconomic Status, 1969-1998", *International Journal of Epidemiology*, 31, pp. 600-613.
41. Hallqvist, J., Lundberg, M., Diderichsen, F. and Ahlbom, A., 1998, "Socioeconomic Differences in Risk of Myocardial Infarction 1971-1994 in Sweden: Time Trends, Relative Risks and Population Attributable Risks", *International Journal of Epidemiology*, 27, pp. 410-415.
42. Tuchsen, F. and Endahl, L.A., 1999, "Increasing Inequality in Ischaemic Heart Disease Morbidity Among Employed Men in Denmark 1981-1993: The Need for a New Preventive Policy", *International Journal of Epidemiology*, 28, pp. 640-644.
43. Steenland, K., 2000, "Shift Work, Long Hours and CVD: A Review", *Occupational Medicine: State-of-the-Art Reviews*, 15(1), pp. 7-17.
44. Spurgeon, A., Harrington, J.M. and Cooper, C.L., 1997, "Health and Safety Problems Associated with Long Working Hours: A Review of the Current Position", *Occup. Environ. Med.*, 54(6), pp. 367-375.
45. Sparks, K., Cooper, C., Fried, Y. and Shirom, A., 1997, "The Effects of Hours of Work on Health: A Meta-analytic Review", *Journal of Occupational and Organizational Psychology*, 70, pp. 391-408.
46. van der Hulst, M., 2003, "Long Workhours and Health", *Scandinavian Journal of Work Environment and Health*, 29(3), pp. 171-188.

47. Caruso, C., Hitchcock, E., Dick, R., Russo, J. and Schmit, J., 2004, "Overtime and Extended Work Shifts: Recent Findings on Illnesses, Injuries, and Health Behaviors", *NIOSH*, Report No. 2004, Cincinnati, Ohio, p. 143.
48. Russek, H.I. and Zohman, B.L., 1958, "Relative Significance of Heredity, Diet, and Occupational Stress in Coronary Heart Disease of Young Adults", *Am. J. Med. Sci.*, 235, pp. 266-275.
49. Theorell, T. and Rahe, R.H., 1972, "Behavior and Life Satisfactions of Swedish Subjects with Myocardial Infarction", *J. Chron. Dis.*, 25, pp. 139-147.
50. Alfredsson, L., Spetz, C. and Theorell, T., 1985, "Type of Occupation and Near-future Hospitalization for Myocardial Infarction and Some Other Diagnoses", *International Journal of Epidemiology*, 14, pp. 378-388.
51. Falger, P.R.J. and Schouten, E.G.W., 1992, "Exhaustion, Psychologic Stress in the Work Environment and Acute Myocardial Infarction in Adult Men", *Journal of Psychosomatic Research*, 36, pp. 777-786.
52. Liu, Y. and Tanaka, H., 2002, "Overtime Work, Insufficient Sleep, and Risk of Nonfatal Acute Myocardial Infarction in Japanese Men (The Fukuoka Heart Study Group)", *Occup. Environ. Med.*, 59, pp. 447-451.
53. Sokejima, S. and Kagamimori, S., 1998, "Working Hours as a Risk Factor for Acute Myocardial Infarction in Japan: Case-control Study", *BMJ*, 317, pp. 775-780.
54. Raggatt, P., 1991, "Work Stress Among Long-distance Coach Drivers: A Survey and Correlational Study", *Journal of Organizational Behavior*, 12, pp. 565-579.
55. Iwasaki, K., Sasaki, T., Oka, T. and Hisanaga, N., 1998, "Effect of Working Hours on Biological Functions Related to Cardiovascular System Among Salesmen in a Machinery Manufacturing Company", *Ind. Health*, 36, pp. 361-367.
56. Schnall, P.L., Landsbergis, P.A. and Baker, D., 1994, "Job Strain and Cardiovascular Disease", *Annual Review of Public Health*, 15, pp. 381-411.
57. Kristensen, T.S., Kronitzer, M. and Alfedsson, L., 1998, *Social Factors, Work, Stress and Cardiovascular Disease Prevention*, The European Heart Network, Brussels.
58. Belkic, K., Landsbergis, P.A., Schnall, P., Baker, D., Theorell, T., Siegrist, J. et al., 2000c, "Psychosocial Factors: Review of the Empirical Data Among Men", In *The Workplace and Cardiovascular Disease – Occupational Medicine: State of the Art Reviews*, P. Schnall, K. Belkic, P.A. Landsbergis and D. Baker (Eds.), Hanley and Belfus, Philadelphia, pp. 24-46.
59. Belkic, K., Landsbergis, P.A., Schnall, P. and Baker, D., 2004, "Is Job Strain a Major Source of Cardiovascular Disease Risk?" *Scandinavian Journal of Work Environment and Health*, 30(2), pp. 85-128.
60. Siegrist, J., Peter, R., Junge, A., Cremer, P. and Seidel, D., 1990, "Low Status Control, High Effort at Work and Ischaemic Heart Disease: Prospective Evidence from Blue Collar Men", *Social Science and Medicine*, 31, pp. 1127-1134.
61. Vahtera, J., Kivimaki, M., Pentti, J., Linna, A., Virtanen, M., Virtanen, P. et al., 2004, "Organisational Downsizing, Sickness Absence, and Mortality: 10-town Prospective Cohort Study", *BMJ*, 328(7439), p. 555.
62. Siegrist, J., 1996, "Adverse Health Effects of High-effort/Low-reward Conditions", *Journal of Occupational Health Psychology*, 1, pp. 27-41.
63. Bosma, H., Peter, R., Siegrist, J. and Marmot, M., 1998, "Two Alternative Job Stress Models and the Risk of Coronary Heart Disease", *American Journal of Public Health*, 88, pp. 68-74.
64. Lynch, J., Krause, N., Kaplan, G.A., Tuomilehto, J. and Salonen, J.T., 1997a, "Workplace Conditions, Socioeconomic Status, and the Risk of Mortality and Acute Myocardial Infarction: The Kuopio Ischemic Heart Disease Risk Factor Study", *American Journal of Public Health*, 87, pp. 617-622.

65. Lynch, J., Krause, N., Kaplan, G.A., Salonen, R. and Salonen, J.T., 1997b, "Workplace Demands, Economic Reward and Progression of Carotid Atherosclerosis", *Circulation*, 96(1), pp. 302-307.
66. Peter, R., Siegrist, J., Hallqvist, J., Reuterwall, C., Theorell, T. and The SHEEP Study Group, 2002, "Psychosocial Work Environment and Myocardial Infarction: Improving Risk Estimation by Combining Two Complementary Job Stress Models in the SHEEP Study", *J. Epidemiol. Community Health*, 56(4), pp. 294-300.
67. Kivimaki, M., Leino-Arjas, P., Luukkonen, R., Riihimaki, H., Vahtera, J. and Kirjonen, J., 2002, "Work Stress and Risk of Cardiovascular Mortality: Prospective Cohort Study of Industrial Employees", *BMJ*, 325, p. 857.
68. Menotti, A. and Seccareccia, F., 1985, "Pysical Activity at Work and Job Responsibility as Risk Factors for Fatal Coronary Heart Disease and Other Causes of Death", *Journal of Epidemiology and Community Health*, 39, pp. 325-329.
69. Murphy, L.R., 1991, "Job Dimensions Associated with Severe Disability Due to Cardiovascular Disease", *Journal of Clinical Epidemiology*, 44(2), pp. 155-166.
70. Suurnakki, T., Ilmarinen, J., Wagar, G., Jarvinen, E. and Landau, K., 1987, "Municipal Employees' Cardiovascular Diseases and Occupational Stress Factors in Finland", *Int. Arch. Occup. Environ. Health*, 59(2), pp. 107-114.
71. Belkic, K., Emdad, R. and Theorell, T., 1998, "Occupational Profile and Cardiac Risk: Possible Mechanisms and Implications for Professional Drivers", *International Journal of Occupational Medicine and Environmental Health*, 11, pp. 37-57.
72. Tuchsen, F., 2000, "High-risk Occupations for Cardiovascular Disease", In *The Workplace and Cardiovascular Disease*, P. Schnall, K. Belkic, P.A. Landsbergis and D. Baker (Eds.), Hanley and Belfus, Philadelphia, pp. 57-60.
73. Greiner, B., Krause, N., Ragland, D. and Fisher, J., 2004, "Occupational Stressors and Hypertension: A Multi-method Study Using Observer-based Job Analysis and Self-reports in Urban Transit Operators", *Social Science and Medicine*, 59, pp. 1081-1094.
74. Kivimaki, M., Vahtera, J., Pentti, J. and Ferrie, J.E., 2000, "Factors Underlying the Effect of Organisational Downsizing on Health of Employees: Longitudinal Cohort Study", *BMJ*, 320(7240), pp. 971-975.
75. Johnson, J.V. and Hall, E.M., 1988, "Job Strain, Workplace Social Support, and Cardiovascular Disease: A Cross-sectional Study of a Random Sample of the Swedish Working Population", *American Journal of Public Health*, 78(10), pp. 1336-1342.
76. Theorell, T., Tsutsumi, A., Hallqvist, J., Reuterwall, C., Hogstedt, C., Fredlund, P. et al., 1998, "Decision Latitude, Job Strain and Myocardical Infarction: A Study of Working Men in Stockholm", *American Journal of Public Health*, 88, pp. 382-388.
77. Hallqvist, J., Diderichsen, F., Theorell, T., Reuterwall, C. and Ahlbom, A., 1998, "Is the Effect of Job Strain on Myocardial Infarction Due to Interaction Between High Psychological Demands and Low Decision Latitude? Results from Stockholm Heart Epidemiology Program (SHEEP)", *Social Science and Medicine*, The SHEEP Study Group, 46(11), pp. 1405-1415.
78. Kuper, H., Singh-Manouz, A., Siegrist, J. and Marmot, M., 2002, "When Reciprocity Fails: Effort-reward Imbalance in Relation to Coronary Heart Disease and Health Functioning in the Whitehall II Study", *Occupational and Environmental Medicine*, 59, pp. 777-784.
79. Landsbergis, P.A., Schnall, P., Pickering, T., Warren, K. and Schwartz, J., 2003, "Lower Socioeconomic Status Among Men in Relation to the Association Between Job Strain and Blood Pressure", *Scandinavian Journal of Work, Environment and Health*, 29(3), pp. 206-215.
80. Landsbergis, P.A., Schnall, P., Chace, R., Sullivan, L. and D'Agostino, R., 2005, "Psychosocial Job Stressors and Cardiovascular Disease in the Framingham Offspring Study: A Prospective Analysis (Poster)", *4th ICOH Conference on Work Environment and Cardiovascular Disease*, California.

81. Guimont, C., Brisson, C., Dagenais, G., Milot, A., Vézina, M., Mâsse, B. et al., 2006, "Effects of Job Strain on Blood Pressure: A Prospective Study of Male and Female White-Collar Workers", *American Journal of Public Health*, 96(8), pp. 1436-1443.
82. Pickering, T., Shimbo, D. and Haas, D., 2006, "Ambulatory Blood Pressure Monitoring", *The New England Journal of Medicine*, 354, pp. 2368-2374.
83. Verdecchia, P., Clement, D., Fagard, R., Palatini, P. and Parati, G., 1999, "Task force III: Target-organ Damage, Morbidity and Mortality", *Blood Pressure Monitoring*, 4, pp. 303-317.
84. Pierdomenico, S., Lapenna, D., Bucci, A., Di Tommaso, R., Di Mascio, R., Manente, B. et al., 2005, "Cardiovascular Outcome in Treated Hypertensive Patients with Responder, Masked, False Resistant, and True Resistant Hypertension", *American Journal of Hypertension*, 18, pp. 1422-1428.
85. Hayashi, T., Kobayashi, Y., Yamaoka, K. and Yano, E., 1996, "Effect of Overtime Work on 24-hour Ambulatory Blood Pressure", *J. Occup. Environ. Med.*, 38(10), pp. 1007-1011.
86. Park, J., Kim, Y., Cho, Y., Woo, K., Chung, H., Iwasaki, K. et al., 2001, "Regular Overtime and Cardiovascular Functions", *Industrial Health*, 39(3), pp. 244-249.
87. Nakanishi, N., Yoshida, H., Nagano, K., Kawashimo, H., Nakamura, K. and Tatara, K., 2001, "Long Working Hours and Risk for Hypertension in Japanese Male White Collar Workers", *J. Epidemiol. Community Health*, 55(5), pp. 316-322.
88. Yang, H., Schnall, P., Jauregui, M., Su, T. and Baker, D., 2006, "Work Hours and Self-reported Hypertension Among Working People in California", *Hypertension*, 48, DOI:10.1161/01.HYP.0000 238327.41911.52.
89. Brisson, C., 2000, "Women, Work and Cardiovascular Disease", In *The Workplace and Cardiovascular Disease – Occupational Medicine: State-of-the-art Reviews*, P. Schnall, K. Belkic, P.A. Landsbergis and D. Baker (Eds.), Hanley and Belfus, Philadelphia, pp. 49-57.
90. Schnall, P.L., Pieper, C., Schwartz, J.E., Karasek, R.A., Schlussel, Y., Devereux, R.B. et al., 1990, "The Relationship Between 'Job Strain', Workplace Diastolic Blood Pressure, and Left Ventricular Mass Index", Results of a Case-control Study (Published Erratum Appears in *JAMA* 1992 March 4, 267(9), p. 1209), *JAMA*, 263(14), pp. 1929-1935.
91. Landsbergis, P.A., Schnall, P.L., Warren, K., Pickering, T.G. and Schwartz, J.E., 1994, "Association Between Ambulatory Blood Pressure and Alternative Formulations of Job Strain", *Scandinavian Journal of Work, Environment and Health*, 20(5), pp. 349-363.
92. Schnall, P.L., Schwartz, J.E., Landsbergis, P.A., Warren, K. and Pickering, T.G., 1992b, "Relation Between Job Strain, Alcohol, and Ambulatory Blood Pressure", *Hypertension*, 19, pp. 488-494.
93. Schnall, P.L., Landsbergis, P.A., Schwartz, J., Warren, K. and Pickering, T.G., 1998a, "A Longitudinal Study of Job Strain and Ambulatory Blood Pressure: Results from a Three-year Follow-up", *Psychosomatic Medicine*, 60, pp. 697-706.
94. Vrijkotte, T.G., van Doornen, L.J. and de Geus, E.J., 2000, "Effects of Work Stress on Ambulatory Blood Pressure, Heart Rate, and Heart Rate Variability", *Hypertension*, 35(4), pp. 880-886.
95. Peter, R. and Siegrist, J., 1997, "Chronic Work Stress, Sickness Absence, and Hypertension in Middle Managers: General or Specific Sociological Explanations?" *Social Science and Medicine*, 45, pp. 1111-1120.
96. Peter, R., Alfredsson, L., Hammar, N., Siegrist, J., Theorell, T. and Westerholm, P., 1998, "High Effort, Low Reward, and Cardiovascular Risk Factors in Employed Swedish Men and Women: Baseline Results from the WOLF Study", *Journal of Epidemiology and Community Health*, 52(9), pp. 540-547.
97. Siegrist, J., Peter, R., Georg, W., Cremer, P. and Seidel, D., 1991, "Psychosocial and Biobehavioral Characteristics of Hypertensive Men with Elevated Atherogenic Lipids", *Atherosclerosis*, 86, pp. 211-218.

98. Hellerstedt, W.L. and Jeffery, R.W., 1997, "The Association of Job Strain and Health Behaviours in Men and Women", *International Journal of Epidemiology*, 26(3), pp. 575-583.
99. Kawakami, N., Haratani, T. and Araki, S., 1998, "Job Strain and Arterial Blood Pressure, Serum Cholesterol, and Smoking as Risk Factors for Coronary Heart Disease in Japan", *International Archives of Occupational and Environmental Health*, 71(6), pp. 429-432.
100. Green, K.L. and Johnson, J.V., 1990, "The Effects of Psychosocial Work Organization on Patterns of Cigarette Smoking Among Male Chemical Plant Employees", *American Journal of Public Health*, 80, pp. 1368-1371.
101. Landsbergis, P.A., Schnall, P.L., Deitz, D.K., Warren, K., Pickering, T.G. and Schwartz, J.E., 1998, "Job Strain and Health Behaviors: Results of a Prospective Study", *American Journal of Health Promotion*, 12(4), pp. 237-245.
102. Netterstrom, B., Kristensen, T.S., Damsgaard, M.T., Olsen, O. and Sjol, A., 1991, "Job Strain and Cardiovascular Risk Factors: A Cross Sectional Study of Employed Danish Men and Women", *British Journal of Industrial Medicine*, 48(10), pp. 684-689.
103. Georges, E., Wear, M.L. and Mueller, W.H., 1992, "Body Fat Distribution and Job Stress in Mexican-American Men of the Hispanic Health and Nutrition Examination Survey", *American Journal of Human Biology*, 4, pp. 657-667.
104. Johansson, G., Johnson, J.V. and Hall, E.M., 1991, "Smoking and Sedentary Behavior as Related to Work Organization", *Social Science and Medicine*, 32, pp. 837-846.
105. Collins, S.M., Karasek, R.A. and Costas, K., 2005, "Job Strain and Autonomic Indices of Cardiovascular Disease Risk", *American Journal of Industrial Medicine*, 48, pp. 182-193.
106. Steptoe, A. and Marmot, M., 2000, "Atherogenesis, Coagulation and Stress Mechanisms", *Occupational Medicine: State of the Art Reviews*, 15(1), pp. 136-138.
107. Markowe, H.L., Marmot, M.G., Shipley, M.J., Bulpitt, C.H., Meade, T.W., Stirling, Y. et al., 1985, "Fibrinogen: A Possible Link Between Social Class and Coronary Heart Disease", *British Medical Journal*, 291, pp. 1312-1314.
108. Brunner, E.J., Smith, G.D., Marmot, M.G., Canner, R., Beksinska, M. and O'Brien, J., 1996, "Childhood Social Circumstances and Psychosocial and Behavioral Factors as Determinants of Plasma Fibrinogen", *Lancet*, 347, pp. 1008-1013.
109. Langosch, W., Brodner, B. and Borcherding, M., 1983, "Psychosocial and Vocational Longterm Outcomes of Cardiac Rehabilitation with Postinfarction Patients Under the Age of Forty", *Psychosomatic Medicine*, 40, pp. 115-128.
110. Muntaner, C., Nieto, F.J., Cooper, L., Meyer, J., Szklo, M. and Tyroler, H.A., 1998, "Work Organization and Artherosclerosis: Findings from the ARIC Study: Atherosclerosis Risk in Communities", *Am. J. Prev. Med.*, 14, pp. 9-18.
111. Hintsanen, M., Kivimaki, M., Elovainio, M., Pulkki-Raback, L., Keskivaara, P., Juonala, M. et al., 2005, "Job Strain and Early Atherosclerosis: The Cardiovascular Risk in Young Finns Study", *Psychosomatic Medicine*, 67(5), pp. 740-747.
112. Rosvall, M., Ostergren, P.-O., Hedblad, B., Isacsson, S.-O., Janzon, L. and Berglund, G., 2002, "Work-related Psychosocial Factors and Carotid Atherosclerosis", *International Journal of Epidemiology*, 31(6), pp. 1169-1178.
113. Kouvonen, A., Kivimäki, M., Virtanen, M., Heponiemi, T., Elovainio, M., Pentti, J. et al., 2006, "Effort-reward Imbalance at Work and the Co-occurrence of Lifestyle Risk Factors: Cross-sectional Survey in a Sample of 36,127 Public Sector Employees", *BMC Public Health*, 6, p. 24, doi:10.1186/1471-2458-6-24.
114. Kumari, M., Head, J. and Marmot, M., 2004, "Prospective Study of Social and Other Risk Factors for Incidence of Type 2 Diabetes in the Whitehall II Study", *Arch. Intern. Med.*, 164, pp. 1873-1880.

115. Siegrist, J., Matschinger, H., Cremer, P. and Seidel, D., 1988, "Atherogenic Risk in Men Suffering from Occupational Stress", *Atherosclerosis*, 69, pp. 211-218.
116. Kawakami, N., Araki, S., Takatsuka, N., Shimizu, H. and Ishibashi, H., 1999, "Overtime, Psychosocial Working Conditions and Occurrence of Non-insulin Dependent Diabetes Mellitus in Japanese Men", *J. Epidemiol. Community Health*, 53(6), pp. 359-363.
117. Karasek, R.A., 1979, "Job Demands, Job Decision Latitude and Mental Strain: Implications for Job Redesign", *Administrative Science Quarterly*, 24, pp. 285-308.
118. Shapiro, A.P., 1988, "Psychological Factors in Hypertension: An Overview", *American Heart Journal*, 116, pp. 632-637.
119. Perini, C., Muller, F.B., Rauchfleisch, U., Battegay, R., Hobi, V. and Buhler, F.R., 1990, "Psychosomatic Factors in Borderline Hypertensive Subjects and Offspring of Hypertensive Parents", *Hypertension*, 16, pp. 627-634.
120. Markovitz, J., Matthews, K.A., Kannel, W.B., Cobb, J.L. and D'Agostino, J.B., 1993, "Psychological Predictors of Hypertension in the Framingham Study: Is There Tension in Hypertension?", *JAMA*, 270(20), pp. 2439-2443.
121. Jonas, B.S., Franks, P. and Ingram, D.D., 1997, "Are Symptoms of Anxiety and Depression Risk Factors for Hypertension? Longitudinal Evidence from the National Health and Nutrition Examination Survey I: Epidemiologic Follow-up Study", *Archives of Family Medicine*, 6, pp. 43-51.
122. Sparrow, D., Garvey, A.J., Rosner, B. and Thomas, H.E., 1982, "Factors in Predicting Blood Pressure Change", *Circulation*, 65, pp. 789-794.
123. Friedman, R., Landsbergis, P.A., Schnall, P.L., Pieper, C., Gerin, W., Pickering, T.G. et al., 2001, "Psychological Variables in Hypertension: Relationship to Casual or Ambulatory Blood Pressure in Men", *Psychosomatic Medicine*, 63, pp. 19-31.
124. Cottington, E.M., Matthews, K.A., Talbott, E. and Kuller, L.H., 1986, "Occupational Stress, Suppressed Anger and Hypertension", *Psychosomatic Medicine*, 48, pp. 249-260.
125. Knox, S., Svensson, J., Waller, D. and Theorell, T., 1988, "Emotional Coping and the Psychophysiological Substrates of Elevated Blood Pressure", *Behavioral Medicine*, 2, pp. 52-58.
126. Theorell, T., 1990, "Family History of Hypertension: An Individual Trait Interacting with Spontaneously Occuring Job Stressors", *Scandinavian Journal of Work, Environment and Health*, 16 Suppl. 1, pp. 74-79.
127. Kubzansky, L.D., Kawachi, I., Weiss, S. and Sparrow, D., 1998, "Anxiety and Coronary Heart Disease: A Synthesis of Epdemiological, Psychological, and Experimental Evidence", *Annals of Behavioral Medicine*, 20(2), pp. 47-58.
128. Stansfeld, S.A., North, F.M., White, I. and Marmot, M.G., 1995, "Work Characteristics and Psychiatric Disorder in Civil Servants in London", *Journal of Epidemiology and Community Health*, 49, pp. 48-53.
129. Bourbonnais, R., Brisson, C., Moisan, J. and Vezina, M., 1996, "Job Strain and Psychological Distress in White-collar Workers", *Scandinavian Journal of Work, Environment and Health*, 22, pp. 139-145.
130. Bourbonnais, R., Comeau, M. and Vezina, M., 1999, "Job Strain and Evolution of Mental Health Among Nurses", *Journal of Occupational Health Psychology*, 4, pp. 95-107.
131. Landsbergis, P.A., 1988, "Occupational Stress Faced by Health Care Workers: A Test of the Job Demand-control Model", *J. Organizational Beh.*, 9, pp. 217-239.
132. Borritz, M., Bültmann, U., Rugulies, R., Christensen, K., Villadsen, E. and Kristensen, T., 2005, "Psychosocial Work Environment Factors as Predictors for Burnout: Prospective Findings from Three-year Follow-up of the PUMA Study", *Journal of Occupational and Environmental Medicine*, 47(10), pp. 1015-1025.

133. Ahola, K., Honkonen, T., Kivimaki, M., Virtanen, M., Isometsa, E., Aromaa, A. et al., 2006, "Contribution of Burnout to the Association Between Job Strain and Depression: The Health 2000 Study", *Journal of Occupational and Environmental Medicine*, 48(10), pp. 1023-1030.
134. Lennon, M.C., 1987, "Sex Differences in Distress: The Impact of Gender and Work Roles", *J. Health Soc. Beh.*, 28, pp. 290-305.
135. Mausner-Dorsch, H. and Eaton, W., 2000, "Psychosocial Work Environment and Depression: Epidemiologic Assessment of the Demand-control Model", *American Journal of Public Health*, 90, pp. 1765-1770.
136. Bosma, H., Stansfeld, S.A. and Marmot, M.G., 1998a, "Job Control, Personal Characteristics, and Heart Disease", *Journal of Occupational Health Psychology*, 3(4), pp. 402-409.
137. Landsbergis, P.A,. Schnall, P.L., Deitz, D., Friedman, R. and Pickering, T., 1992, "The Patterning of Psychological Attributes and Distress by "Job Strain" and Social Support in a Sample of Working Men", *Journal of Behavioral Medicine*, 15(4), pp. 379-405.
138. Belkic, K.B., Schnall, P.L., Landsbergis, P.A., Schwartz, J.E., Gerber, L., Baker, D. et al., 2001, "Hypertension at the Workplace: An Occult Disease? The Need for Work Site Surveillance", *Advances in Psychosomatic Medicine*, 22, pp. 116-138.
139. Landsbergis, P., Schnall, P., Belkic, K., Schwartz, J., Baker, D. and Pickering, T., 2008 (in press), "Work Conditions and Masked (Hidden) Hypertension – Insights Into the Global Epidemic of Hypertension", *Scandinavian Journal of Work, Environment and Health*, Suppl. 5.
140. Liu, J.E., Roman, M.J., Pini, R., Schwartz, J.E., Pickering, T.G. and Devereux, R.B., 1999, "Cardiac and Arterial Target Organ Damage in Adults with Elevated Ambulatory and Normal Office Blood Pressure" (see comments), *Ann. Intern. Med.*, 131(8), pp. 564-572.
141. Sega, R., Trocino, G., Lanzarotti, A. et al., 2001, "Alterations of Cardiac Structure in Patients with Isolated Office, Ambulatory or Home Hypertension: Data from the General Population – Pressione Arteriose Monitorate E Loro Associazioni (PAMELA) Study, *Circulation*, 104(12), pp. 1385-1392.
142. Bobrie, G., Chatellier, G., Genes, N., Clerson, P., Vaur, L., Vaisse, B. et al., 2004, "Cardiovascular Prognosis of "Masked Hypertension" Detected by Blood Pressure Self-measurement in Elderly Treated Hypertensive Patients", *JAMA*, 291, pp. 1342-1349.
143. Gallo, L.C., Bogart, L.M., Vranceanu, A.M. and Walt, L.C., 2004, "Job Characteristics, Occupational Status, and Ambulatory Cardiovascular Activity in Women", *Ann. Behav. Med.*, 28(1), pp. 62-73.
144. Wing, L., Brown, M., Beilin, L. et al., 2002, "Reverse White-coat Hypertension in Older Hypertensives", *Journal of Hypertension*, 20(4), pp. 639-644.
145. Selenta, C., Hogan, B.E. and Linden, W., 2000, "How Often Do Office Blood Pressure Measurements Fail to Identify True Hypertension? An Exploration of White-coat Normotension", *Arch. Fam. Med.*, 9(6), pp. 533-540.
146. The Tokyo Declaration, 1998, *Journal of the Tokyo Medical University*, 56(6), pp. 760-767.
147. Belkic, K., Schnall, P. and Ugljesic, M., 2000a, "Cardiovascular Evaluation of the Worker and Workplace: A Practical Guide for Clinicians", *Occupational Medicine: State of the Art Reviews*, 15(1), pp. 213-222.
148. Karasek, R.A., Gordon, G., Pietrokovsky, C., Frese, M., Pieper, C., Schwartz, J. et al., 1985, *Job Content Instrument: Questionnaire and User's Guide*, University of Southern California/University of Massachusetts, Los Angeles/Lowell.
149. Siegrist, J. and Peter, R., 1996, *Measuring Effort-reward Imbalance at Work: Guidelines*, University of Dusseldorf, Dusseldorf.
150. Belkic, K., Savic, C., Theorell, T. and Cizinsky, S., 1995a, "Work Stressors and Cardiovascular Risk: Assessment for Clinical Practice: Part I", National Institute for Psychosocial Factors and Health, Stockholm, Section for Stress Research, Karolinska Institute, WHO Psychosocial Center, Report No. 256.

151. Schnall, P. and Belkic, K., 2000b, "Point Estimates of Blood Pressure at the Worksite", *Occupational Medicine: State-of-the-Art Reviews*, 15(1), pp. 203-208.
152. Pickering, T., Davidson, K., Gerin, W. and Schwartz, J., 2002, "Masked Hypertension", *Hypertension*, 40, pp. 795-796.
153. Fisher, J. and Belkic, K., 2000, "A Public Health Approach in Clinical Practice", In *The Workplace and Cardiovascular Disease – Occupational Medicine: State of the Art Reviews*, P. Schnall, K. Belkic, P.A. Landsbergis and D. Baker (Eds.), Hanley and Belfus, Philadelphia, pp. 245-256.
154. Stokols, D., Pelletier, K.R. and Fielding, J.E., 1995, "Integration of Medical Care and Work Site Health Promotion", *JAMA*, 273(14), pp. 1136-1142.
155. Heaney, C.A. and Goetzel, R.Z., 1997, "A Review of Health-related Outcomes of Multi-component Worksite Health Promotion Programs", *American Journal of Health Promotion*, 11, pp. 290-308.
156. Dejoy, D.M. and Southern, D.J., 1993, "An Integrative Perspective on Work Site Health Promotion", *Journal of Occupational Medicine*, 35(12), pp. 1221-1230.
157. Sorensen, G., Stoddard, A., Ockene, J.K., Hunt, M.K. and Youngstrom, R., 1996, "Worker Participation in an Integrated Health Promotion/health Protection Program: Results from the WellWorks Project", *Health Education Quarterly*, 23, pp. 191-203.
158. Maes, S., Verhoeven, C., Kittel, F. and Scholten, H., 1998, "Effects of a Dutch Work Site Wellness-health Program: The Brabantia Project", *Am. J. Public Health*, 88(7), pp. 1037-1041.
159. Murphy, L., Hurrell, J., Sauter, S. and Keita, G.E., 1995, "Job Stress Interventions", *American Psychological Association*, Washington, D.C.
160. ILO, 1992, *Conditions of Work Digest: Preventing Stress at Work*, International Labour Office, Geneva.
161. Landsbergis, P.A., Schurman, S.J., Israel, B.A., Schnall, P.L., Hugentobler, M.K., Cahill, J. et al., 1993, "Job Stress and Heart Disease: Evidence and Strategies for Prevention", *New Solutions*, Summer, pp. 42-58.
162. Orth-Gomer, K., Eriksson, I., Moser, V., Theorell, T. and Fredlund, P., 1994, "Lipid Lowering Through Work Stress Reduction", *International J. of Behavioral Medicine*, 1(3), pp. 204-214.
163. Rydstedt, L.W., Johansson, G. and Evans, G.W., 1998, "The Human Side of the Road: Improving the Working Conditions of Urban Bus Drivers", *Journal of Occupational Health Psychology*, 3, pp. 161-171.
164. Melin, B., Lundberg, U., Soderlund, J. and Granqvist, M., 1999, "Psychophysiological Stress Reactions of Male and Female Assembly Workers: A Comparison Between Two Different Forms of Work Organization", *Journal of Organizational Behavior*, 20, pp. 47-61.
165. Cahill, J. and Feldman, L.H., 1993, "Computers in Child Welfare: Planning for a More Serviceable Work Environment", *Child Welfare*, 72, pp. 3-12.
166. Israel, B.A., Schurman, S.J. and House, J.S., 1989, "Action Research on Occupational Stress: Involving Workers as Researchers", *International Journal of Health Services*, 19, pp. 135-155.
167. Smith, M. and Zehel, D., 1992, "A Stress Reduction Intervention Programme for Meat Processors Emphasizing Job Design and Work Organization", *Conditions of Work Digest*, 11(2), pp. 204-213.
168. LaMontagne, A., Keegel, T., Louie, A., Ostry, A. and Landsbergis, P., 2007, "A Systematic Review of the Job Stress Intervention Evaluation Literature: 1990-2005", *International Journal of Occupational and Environmental Health*, 13, pp. 268-280.

The AHA-Syndrome and Cardiovascular Diseases
Editors: Swati Y. Bhave and Sunil Saini
Copyright © 2010 Anamaya Publishers, New Delhi, India

16. Early Risk Factors for Coronary Artery Disease

Ana García-León and Gustavo Adolfo Reyes del Paso
Department of Psychology, University of Jaen, Campus Las Lagunillas, s/n, 23071 Jaen, Spain

Abstract: This chapter reviews some early risk factors for coronary heart disease (CHD) whose actuation in a long temporal period, usually more than 10 years, increases the probability of developing cardiac events. Specifically, we review the effects of anger on cardiovascular reactivity (CVR) in relation to harassment, active coping, competition and interpersonal interaction (anger can also act as an acute risk factor); socioeconomic and educational status; isolation and social support; and obesity-diet. These early conditions accelerate the progression of the atherosclerosis process, promoting the development of a severe coronary artery disease (CAD). The paper also reviews the evidence of the possible mediating mechanisms by which these factors increase the risk of CHD and cardiac events, as the increases in cardiovascular and catecholamine reactivity, augmented circulating lipids, reduced autonomic regulation, and rise in pro-inflammatory markers etc.

Keywords: Anger, Cardiovascular reactivity, Active coping, Harassment, Competition, Rumination, Cardiovascular recovery, Socioeconomic status, Social support, Obesity, Diet.

Introduction

Cardiovascular diseases are a multidimensional process in which different risk factors interact with each other and present in each patient a unique idiosyncratic combination. To understand these interactions of factors we need the multiple analysis levels perspective of the bio-psycho-social model. A method to distinguish psychosocial factors involved in coronary heart disease (CHD) is a temporal perspective based on the duration of the risk factors and their temporal proximity to the occurrence of the coronary events [1]: background risk conditions (e.g. socioeconomic status), chronic (more than 10 years, e.g. hostility), episodic (from several months to two years, e.g. depression) and acute psychosocial factors (that triggers cardiac events within one hour, e.g. acute anger). In this chapter we analyse some heterogeneous early risk factors for CHD that comprised both chronic and background factors.

Anger and Cardiovascular Reactivity

Anger, hostility and aggression may be considered as single elements of a wider construct. Hostility can be defined as a lasting cognitive disposition (e.g. cynicism, hostile attributions, dominance or suspicion). Anger refers to the temporal experience of subjective feelings of annoyance, irritation or rage (e.g. anger coping styles: express or suppress anger). Lastly, aggression can be considered as the behaviour (e.g. physical or verbal) that occurs when we are annoyed.

Epidemiological evidence supports individual differences in anger and hostility as risk factors for coronary artery disease (CAD) and all-cause mortality. Cardiovascular reactivity is the main proposed mechanism linking these psychosocial risk factors and CAD [2].

Anger and hostility have been related to CAD and cardiovascular reactivity (CVR) using different self-report measures of this construct as Cook-Medley Hostility Scale (Ho), Buss-Durkee Hostility Inventory (BDHI), Spielberger Anger Expression Scale (AX), and Buss and Perry's Aggression Questionnaire (AQ) [3, 4]. However, there are some studies in which anger and/or hostility are not associated with CAD or CVR [5, 6]. These are some reasons, which explain why the results are inconsistent.

(i) When instruments that assess different facets of anger/hostility are used, it is not usually distinguished among these different components and their consequences on CAD and CVR.
(ii) Effects of different types of tasks, and their combination with anger, on CVR assessment are often ignored.
(iii) Most of the studies have investigated heightened CVR of hostile individuals, ignoring both other important physiological parameters as cardiovascular recovery and other psychological processes as worry or rumination, which may be especially relevant for these individuals in respect to their relationship with CAD.

Differential Components of Anger/Hostility

It has been suggested that different interpersonal styles could reflect differing mechanisms linking these traits with health [2]. For example, the hostile dominance associated with verbal aggressiveness and anger-out scales suggests that these traits might influence health through a pattern of "moving against" people. In an adversarial and controlling cycle, people high in hostile dominance are likely to make frequent effortful attempts to influence others, often eliciting equally unfriendly resistance. Efforts to influence and control others evoke increases in blood pressure (BP) and heart rate (HR) and this reactivity could contribute to cardiovascular disease. In contrast, the hostile submissiveness associated with hostility and anger-in scales suggest a pattern of "moving away" in which a less confident and assertive individual may engage in chronic vigilance to detect potential mistreatment he or she cannot otherwise easily manage. This weariness could lead to low levels of social support. Vigilance and low social support have also been associated with heightened CVR.

Other psychologists are examining whether coping skills affect cardiovascular health [7]. They have examined people's anger expression on a continuum that ranges from people who always express their anger to those who always suppress their anger. Those in the middle of the scale have flexible coping skills. Compared with flexible copers, people who always vent or suppress their anger have significantly greater rises in BP levels of homocysteine (an amino acid that is a risk factor for heart disease). It seems that people with more rigid style are physiologically a little bit different, with health-damaging consequences.

Burns, Evon and Strain-Saloum [8] have found that anger repressors show a pattern of self-report and physiological responses to provocation distinct from low and high anger expressors; specifically, self-report and physiology may be dissociated in repressors. Not only assessment techniques need to be sensitive enough to reliably differentiate repressors from low expressors, but repressors may deny angry feelings altogether or at least claim that anger poses no problems for them. Furthermore, future work is needed to examine explicitly the distinctions between anger/hostility repressors, who may deny strong anger to themselves and others to defend a positive self-concept, from defensive but angry/hostile individuals, who may seek social approval from people who they resent or distrust.

Lastly, in the laboratory, individuals may use different strategies for expressing anger than in unobserved "real-life" interactions. This may be problematic, given that a portion of the effects of anger-related traits on CVR may be a function of the cardiovascular demands of managing the expression of emotion. Neither survey nor laboratory studies permit an evaluation of the degree to which hostility influences the frequency of exposure to negative interactions and concomitant cardiovascular activation during the course of everyday events.

Anger/Hostility and Type of Task/Situation

In respect to the different tasks associated with heightened CVR, most research on specific cardiovascular stressors during the last few decades has addressed the distinction between active and passive coping.

Active Coping

It refers to the mental or physical effort exerted to achieve actual or perceived control over the outcome of a situation. It is also related to perceptions of task difficulty, task predictability and self-efficacy. The cardiovascular response pattern produced during active coping is predominantly characterised by β-adrenergic stimulation. Analysis of some psychophysiological research findings indicates that experimental tasks most effective in stimulating a strong increase in cardiovascular activity do not involve the performance of familiar mental or sensorimotor operations, such as basic arithmetic, pressing a key in reaction time tasks or playing video games. Gendolla and Krüsken [9] have found that mood state and task difficulty interact during task performance to determine autonomic reactivity with respect to active coping. It seems that the effect of task difficulty depends on the instrumentality of behaviour: it is more powerful when the behaviour leads to anticipate change in the environment (e.g. punishment avoidance) than when it leads to no such outcomes. Likewise, in accordance with the theoretical predictions about the role of ego involvement in active coping, high ego involvement increases the performance-related reactivity of systolic BP (SBP), diastolic BP (DBP), heart rate (HR) and also the number of unspecific skin conductance responses (SCR) when task difficulty is unfixed (do your best). On the contrary, ego involvement has no impact on autonomic reactivity when task difficulty is easy [10].

Passive Coping

Such tasks, on the other hand, are those in which subjects are not allowed to exert control over the outcome of a situation. Such tasks have been reported to induce a vascular response pattern, fundamentally reflecting α-adrenergic influences.

However, the differentiation between active and passive coping is always relative, because, by definition, any laboratory task always requires some kind of active effort, regardless of the experimenter's manipulation of the outcome. Moreover, there is a substantial variability among active coping tasks in terms of psychological responses and concomitant haemodynamic response patterns. Indeed, there is evidence that some properties of active coping tasks differentially induce CVR. This is the case, e.g. with active coping stressors that involve competition and social interaction [11]. Competition provokes increases in BP and HR and a significant shortening of the pre-ejection period, an index of enhanced β-adrenergic influences on the heart. Participants with high scores in competitiveness and desire to win usually show higher BP reactions and greater shortening of the pre-ejection period to competition than those with low scores in these characteristics [12]. On the other hand, manipulations involving the social environment have been shown to affect the magnitude of cardiovascular responses to laboratory challenges. Social interaction, apart from a specific task, may also alter cardiovascular activity. Cardiovascular responding is enhanced by efforts to influence the opinions of others or by social conflict. These findings and the fact that daily stressors are often social ones, suggest that assessments of CVR should include social challenges along with cognitive or psychomotor tasks [13].

Finally, a number of studies document a relationship between anger/hostility and elevated CVR to laboratory stressors, particularly those involving interpersonal conflict or provocation [8, 14]. Although different kind of situations have been proposed in the literature to provoke both the state of anger and CVR, typical laboratory manipulations have been based on interpersonal challenge situations involving either frustration, harassment or both.

Frustration

It is related to the blocking of goal achievement and can include distraction, interruptions or total failure caused by inability to solve the task or insufficient time for its completion. Frustration alone does not usually produce increases in CVR. Berkowitz [15] suggested that frustration would exert weak effects on CVR because the most important feelings experienced during situations of intense frustration may be loss of control and helplessness rather than anger. In this sense, frustration could produce aggressive inclinations only to the extent that stimuli used were aversive and, therefore, give rise to negative affects. Besides, the relation between frustration and anger/aggression also depends on the anger and/or aggression having instrumental value.

Harassment

It is related to interpersonal situations that include verbal attacks (e.g. insult, rudeness or sarcasm) or threats of physical danger (e.g. electric shocks). Laboratory studies show that in comparison with individuals with low hostility scores, those with high hostility scores rate negative interpersonal experiences in the laboratory (e.g. harassment) as significantly more anger-inducing, irritation-inducing and tension-inducing [16]. Harassment also seems to be associated with an increase of sympathetic activation and vagal withdrawal under conditions characterised by active coping, competition and negative interpersonal interaction [11, 17], especially in subjects with high scores in hostility [18-20].

Other relevant social stressors that evoke heightened reactivity among hostile participants include evaluative public speaking, recall and discussion of past anger-inducing events, current events discussions or debates and watching anger-inducing films [21, 22]. But not all studies have supported the relationship between hostility and CVR. Some negative results may be attributable to the fact that hostile participants respond to less compelling stressors with decreased task engagement. So, recent theory and research suggest that impaired physiological recovery from social stressors among hostile people might be at least as important as heightened reactivity. Stress-related thoughts and emotions are not limited to those occasions when a stressor is physically present. For most people, relatively little time is spent "in the heat of the moment". However, the greater portion of a lifetime can be spent in anticipation of future stressors and recovery from past stressors. The cumulative effects of these stress-related episodes of heightened CVR may contribute to the development of CHD through a number of pathophysiological mechanisms [16]. Since CVR captures only the magnitude of response to an acute stressor during its presentation, future studies should assess all dimensions of the cardiovascular response to stress, also focussing on the cumulative duration of responding in hostile subjects.

Anger/Hostility, Cardiovascular Recovery and Rumination

Most cardiovascular laboratory experiments on anger have been focussed on CVR, rather than on prolonged cardiovascular activation. However, in 13 out of 15 studies revisited by Brosschot and Thayer [23], they found that a lack of opportunity to counteract after being harassed slows cardiovascular recovery. An analysis of some of these studies suggests that the perceived ability to counter-react in a preferred manner and not actual performance of this behaviour, speeds cardiovascular recovery.

Brosschot and Thayer [24] and others investigators [25] argue that due to the lack of response opportunity, angered individuals would tend to ruminate over the frustration/harassment situation and that this angry perseverative thinking (maintaining the cognitive representation of anger situation) could be the direct cause both of an increase in negative affect (e.g. anger or anxiety) and of their prolonged higher cardiovascular activation. A difficulty in untangling the causality between cognition, affect and physiological response is that they may be reciprocally determined: increased autonomic arousal may prolong anger and vice versa; and the prolonged anger may promote ruminative thoughts and vice versa. These constructs would operate as a "feed-forward" process and would continue to precipitate the process until a distraction occurs to displace the angry thoughts.

It has been demonstrated that continued rumination about an angering situation prolongs cardiovascular responses to these situations [26-28]. Stressor tasks with an emotional component (harassment) were associated with BP elevations during directed rumination and with delayed recovery. All these effects were independent of the original reactivity the task evoked. If a distracting task was given to participants immediately following the stressor, they showed significantly lower BP levels later. The distractor prevented the participants from ruminating and decreased angry mood. This allowed the almost complete BP [29] or HR recovery [30]. In short, the results of these studies suggest that the emotional nature of a cardiovascular stressor may play a critical role in the duration of the psychophysiological response, providing support for a psychological rather than physiological explanation for the delayed recovery following emotional tasks.

Hostile individuals may be especially prone to anger reactions, because they usually perceive or even induce many more angering situations and at the same time be more easily and more intensely angered. This hostile predisposition may, thus, serve to maintain the body's physiological stress reaction as is apparent in the slow recovery. This slower recovery, in turn, can be seen as a potential pathway for hostility's negative long-term effect on health [31]. The crucial pathogenic property, therefore, in perseverative cognition, is not due to its acute, short-term effects on any given system (i.e. intensity or amplitude), but rather is due to its duration and the inadequate autonomic emotional regulation associated with it. An individual's response may ultimately affect at least one of several pathophysiological pathways that can lead to CAD. These may include atherosclerotic progression, decreased heart rate variability (HRV), elevated BP or HR, increased platelet activation and myocardial ischemia.

Socio-Economic Status (SES)

Measured by income, professional occupation or education, SES is strongly associated with cardiovascular risk. The first studies on the relation between SES and CHD held a threshold view that asserts that SES has a negative influence when it was above the poverty line. However, more than in terms of a threshold, the evidence from several studies shows the existence of a social gradient in the relationships between SES and cardiovascular diseases [32]. Health improves and mortality decreases at each higher socioeconomic level, showing an influence of the relative position of the person in society.

The Whitehall studies in Britain, in which SES was measured by the grade of employment, were the first to show reliable evidence of this social gradient. The difference in age-adjusted mortality was three-fold between highest and lowest grades. Adjustment for classical risk factors only reduces this ratio by 30% [33]. The mortality after acute myocardial infraction (MI) was also associated strongly and inversely to income [34]. The gradient that link SES and cardiovascular morbidity-mortality have been observed in many countries and populations, including those that met the subsistence needs of its members and provide publicly medical coverage.

It can be concluded that the inequity in the distribution of medical care has a limited role in contributing to the social gradient in CHD. Some health-related behaviours are related to SES. For example, in the Whitehall Study, SES was associated to smoking, physical exercise in the leisure time, prevalence of obesity and some diet factors. The other possibility is that the relationships between SES and CHD could result from the greater levels of chronic stress in individuals with lower SES. There is a lineal relation between SES and the prevalence of perceived financial strain, stressful life events, low self-esteem and fatalism [35], factors reliably associated to cardiovascular diseases [36]. On the contrary, higher income is associated to more happiness and self-confidence. In the Whitehall II Study, lower professional grades reported lower control over their work, felt less satisfied with their work conditions and had more frequency of stressful life events and financial problems. Those with the higher grades were mostly involved in hobbies and their social support pattern was more positive. Finally, those with lower grades had higher scores on hostility and they reported believing it was not possible to reduce the risk of heart attack [33]. Hence, it can be concluded that three psychosocial mechanisms could be acting: job strain, low social support and low control. Several studies have found an inverse relationship between SES and depressive symptoms, hostility, social isolation and job strain. Also, these same factors appear to explain the increase in cardiovascular morbidity and mortality (especially from premature CVD) in Eastern European countries with political changes occurring there, as shown, e.g. in the LiVicordia Study [37].

High-density lipoprotein (HDL) increases linearly with each higher social status [38]. Reports have found that SES is associated with inflammatory markers. Specifically low SES was associated with significant elevated levels of IL-6, C-reactive protein (CRP) and tumour necrosis factor (TNF)-α compared to high SES [39].

Education, as an element of SES, seems to be a very important factor. Some prospective studies have shown that education level is negatively associated with all causes of cardiovascular mortality. Independent of other risk factors, the education level can predict sudden cardiac death in survivals from MI. Both education and income substantially and independently affect mortality after an acute MI, indicating that each indicator has specific effects on mortality and that these indicators are not interchangeable [40]. In the CARDIA study, evidence was obtained to show that education was inversely associated with coronary artery calcium, an indicator of subclinical atherosclerosis [41].

As possible mediating mechanisms, education can affect health by increasing knowledge of the risk factors and then promoting health behaviours and auto-regulation. Also, it can increase the access to medical care and stress control strategies. Low educational level is associated to lower social support. Men with low educational levels were more socially isolated and experienced more stress than men with higher educational levels. The former are twice more likely to die from subsequent cardiac events after a MI than the latter [42]. Education level was also inversely associated to levels of inflammatory markers as the CRP, even after controlling for clinical risk factors [43].

Social Support

Social support is a multidimensional construct with three major dimensions: structure (features of own social network), functional support (tangible social support act) and subjective perception of support (perceived subjective adequacy of social support available or received). It is also usual to distinguish between emotional (have someone to talk about personal matters and express comfort and concern for one's well-being), instrumental (help with task, provide transportation, money etc.) and belongingness (the sense of being part of a group with which one shares values and interests).

There is evidence for a reliable relation between social support and total morbidity and mortality, especially from cardiovascular disorders. On the contrary, social isolation predicts mortality. Using relatively simple measures of the structure of social support (marital status, number of close friends and relatives, participations in group activities) it has been possible to predict mortality risk in several studies across regions and countries, often between 10 and 20 years after evaluations [44].

Epidemiological evidence suggests that social support plays a relevant role in the development and progression of CHD [45]. Several prospective studies (some with a follow-up up to 15 years) have shown that individuals with low social support were at 50% greater risk of severe CHD and have about three times higher incidence of MI than those with higher social support [35, 44, 45]. Further, this association remains significant after controlling for standard risk factors. Several longitudinal, community-based studies have examined the effects of social isolation on mortality risk. These studies show that social isolation or lack of social support is associated with increased mortality risk. The relative risk associated with isolation is over two-fold after controlling for other variables [44]. A review of the relation between social support and CAD event showed, after controlling for other risk factors, that low social support confers a risk of 1.5 to 2 in both healthy populations and in patients with established CHD [46].

After a MI, patients with high social support have fewer re-hospitalisations and survive longer than patients who are more socially isolated. Follow-up studies show that patients who live alone, lack social support, are not married, have no confidant, nor participate in community activities, have two- to three-fold mortality risk in the five years following the MI [35, 45]. After controlling for age, severity of the MI and co-morbidities, patients reporting no sources of emotional support had a three-fold higher risk of mortality than those reporting to have one or more sources [44].

Receiving social support while performing a stress-evoking task can reduce CVR. Importantly, the support provided by women is significantly more effective in reducing CVR than the support provided by men [47]. But not only human support, even the comfort provided by pets can attenuate home BP and rennin reactivity to mental stress [48]. Analysis of the accumulated evidence of the relation between social support and cardiovascular and neuroendocrine reactivity suggests that availability of social support attenuates sympathetic-adrenergic mechanisms (individuals with low social support had higher noradrenaline and epinephrine levels) and could also attenuate cortisol response [45].

Regarding the progression of the atherosclerosis process and the onset of new cardiovascular events, social support influences coronary artery atherosclerosis and occlusion. In patients undergoing coronary angiography, less coronary atherosclerosis was seen among people who had friends to help them [44].

Some moderators of the effects of social support on CHD are gender, age and personality. Epidemiological evidence suggests that deficits in social support such as social isolation, single-married, bereavement-widowhood etc. have a more deleterious effect in men than in women [47]. The effect of social support on health may be particularly important for older people and the studies summarised in the meta-analysis of Uchino, Cacioppo and Kiecolt-Glaser [45] are consistent with the notion that social support may moderate the changes in the cardiovascular system and in the general decline in physical health occurring with the aging process. For example, individuals low in social support were characterised by age-related increases in BP, whereas those with high social support were characterised by low and comparable BP across all ages. There is an age-related dysregulation of pro-inflammatory cytokines, particularly IL-6 and negative emotions can modulate this increase [49]. In the elderly, when biological vulnerability is at the greatest point and energy lower, largest deleterious consequences of negative emotions are likely to occur, especially when smaller social support networks are available. Finally, as personality is concerned, high cynicism individuals do not benefit from social support [50].

As regards to possible mediating mechanisms in the relation between social support and CHD, health-related behaviours do not appear to be the major pathway, the effects of social support remains after controlling for the traditional risks factors. Social support is positively associated with medication use and compliance, SES and coping resources. At psychological levels, it is negatively associated to perceptions of stress, feelings of uncontrollability, alienation and loneliness, intrusive or ruminative thinking, depression, anxiety and hostility [44, 45]. Social support has a buffering influence on stress perception, which, in turn, reduces neuroendocrine and CVR and enhances HRV and, in general, autonomic regulation. Social support is a primary human need. It also has a positive influence on health independent of the presence of stress. In such a way social isolation can be viewed as a strong stressor.

The dimension of the social support more relevant to health seems to be emotional support, which also has reliable effects on physiological function [45]. The family sources of social support could be particularly relevant to health outcomes. Family support is more predictive of CAD than workplace support. Being around family members was associated with lower ambulatory BP.

Improved social support is associated with greater adherence to medical recommendations and other health-promoting behaviours. Some prospective intervention studies, which provided opportunities for increased social interactions, have obtained reductions in systolic and diastolic BP and a positive reliable long-term affect on BP regulation [45]. In health interventions, those who dropped out of treatment could be characterised as having less social support; less perceived espousal approval and a lower level of perceived access to supportive resources. Emotional support had a significant association with successful smoking cessation. Overall, social support is associated to health-related behaviours and better health practices [45].

On the contrary, disruption of social relationships and the negative aspects of social interactions are independent (from positive aspects of support) predictors of physiological functioning [50]. The negative aspects of interpersonal relationships such as abuse or hostility could be more influential than positive aspects such as feelings of belongingness [46]. Finally, not all support are health promoting, the negative aspects of social relationships and the support that decreases competence or autonomy may be negative.

As physiological mediating mechanism, autonomic nervous system and hypothalamic pituitary adrenal axis dysregulation may link social support to CHD. Low social support has been linked to increased sympathetic and CVR and decreased HRV, vagal tone and cardiovascular recovery to stress [45, 46]. Based on suggestive data in monkeys, Knox and Uvnäs-Moberg [51] have suggested that social support triggers a specific physiological mechanism – secretion of oxytocin – which has a protective effect on the cardiovascular system. This substance is involved both in the establishment and bonding attachment relations and in cardiovascular regulation. Oxytocin lower catecholamine levels, BP, cardiac output and enhances vagal activity. In such a way, social support, mediated by oxytocin secretion, may buffer against endothelial lesion development.

Obesity and Diet

Obesity is becoming a global epidemic in both children and adults. It is associated with several co-morbidities, reduced life expectancy and is an established independent risk factor for CVD. Through its impact on the cardiovascular system, obesity predisposes to CHD, heart failure and sudden cardiac death [52].

The actual increase of obesity in children is cause for great concern. Children with a family history of cardiovascular diseases are heavier than those without family history. Very obese children are at greater risk for adult mortality from cardiovascular diseases. A body mass index (BMI) greater than the 70th percentile vs. the 25th to 50th percentiles in childhood resulted in a greater relative risk of CHD mortality in men but not in women [53].

Obesity is an important determinant of cardiovascular diseases and epidemiological studies show an inverse association between weight and risk of CHD, especially in younger age groups.

The elderly may be relatively protected from obesity-related consequences [53]. With each unit increase in BMI, the risk of ischemic stroke and hemorrhagic stroke increases 4 and 6%, respectively. These effects may be predicted by the prothrombotic/proinflamatory state that often accompanies obesity. Post-mortem examination from a young individual (15-34 years) who died from accidental causes shows that atherosclerosis was associated with obesity and size of the abdominal panniculus. Men have more fatty streaks than women and black subjects more than white [52]. Women have a lag of 10 to 20 years in the intensity of this process.

Elevated BMI predisposes to congestive heart failure. The prevalence of this disorder is of 5 (men) and 7 (women) times increase per unit increase in BMI. Stable obese subjects have an increased risk of arrhythmias and sudden cardiac death, even in the absence of cardiac dysfunction. Specifically in severely obese men, a six- and 12-fold excess mortality rate was reported in the age groups of 35-44 and 25-34 years, respectively.

Important factors are weight change over time and the distribution of body fat, especially visceral or intra-abdominal fat. Weight gain during young adult life may be one of the most important determinants of cardiovascular risk [53]. Increased intra-abdominal fat (waist circumference) is most predictive of cardiovascular diseases than BMI and the most strongly associated to hypertension, insulin resistance syndrome and levels of fibrinogen and inflammatory marker such as CRP [54]. Specifically, the presence of abdominal obesity doubled the risk of acute MI [54]. Consequences of obesity and weight loss are related to gender. Men are more affected by the negative effects of obesity and abdominal obesity is more characteristic of men. As women's educational level rises, obesity decreases, whereas no clear effect of the educational level was observed in men. Also, weight loss in women is also accompanied by bone loss [53].

Obesity is strongly associated to hypertension [52, 55]. Population studies suggest that about 75% of hypertension cases can be directly attributed to obesity. The BP increases with weight gain and decreases with weight loss. The incidence of hypertension among the obese approaches 50% and a large proportion of hypertensives tend to be obese. Obese adults are nearly twice as likely to be hypertensive as similarly aged non-obese persons. Obesity also has a strong effect on lipoprotein metabolism. Increased weight elevates levels of triglycerides, low density lipoprotein (LDL) and decreases HDL. Lipid accumulation within the myocardium, pedal edema, venous insufficiency, venous thromboembolism, pulmonary embolus, displacement of the heart, ventricular hypertrophy etc., are all consequences of obesity and all these alterations may predispose to heart failure [52].

There is a strong link between obesity and a generalised metabolic disorder, the insulin resistance syndrome [55]. Weight can account for about 50% of the variance in insulin sensitivity. Insulin resistance is associated with a constellation of metabolic abnormalities, including diabetes mellitus, hyperlipidemia, hyperglycemia, dyslipoproteinemia, hypertension, a prothrombotic state, atherosclerosis, hyperuricemia, renal dysfunction etc. Dyslipidemia is a consistent feature of the insulin metabolic syndrome. There is a positive association between insulin and triglycerides and a negative one between insulin and HDL. Increases in inflammatory markers are now also accepted as a part of the insulin resistance syndrome. In this sense, the adipocytes secrete IL-6 and TNF-α [56].

The insulin resistance syndrome is an important factor that can mediate the effect of other classical risk factors, such as hypertension, diet, obesity, sedentary life style, dyslipidemia etc. Insulin causes a dose-related increase in sympathetic nervous system (SNS) activity and norepinephrine levels. SNS activity is an important factor in the production of free fatty acids. Reciprocally, SNS activity can increase insulin resistance by stimulating lypolisis, free fatty acids production and vasoconstriction, which negatively impact glucose extraction in skeletal muscles. Insulin also reduces sodium excretion by the kidneys, increasing blood volume and pressure. Finally, insulin stimulated vascular smooth muscle hypertrophy and altered the exchanger of ions in the arteriolar smooth muscle cells, sensitising it to the pressor effects of norepinephrine and angiotensine II [55].

Insulin is closely related to diets factors. Ingestion of large quantities of alcohol can lead to increases in BP, plasma catecholamines and hypertension. The prevalence of hypertension is 50% greater in people consuming three to five drinks daily and 100% greater in those who have more than six drinks daily [55]. This increase in hypertension risk is independent of weight gain and is related to plasma catecholamine levels. Overfeeding of carbohydrates and fats activates sympathetic activity and this effect is mediated by insulin production. Although levels of circulation lipids and lipoproteins are determined to a large extent by genetic and homeostatic mechanisms, dietary habits such as consumption of saturated fats and alcohol play a significant role in the variability level of these substances. An excess intake of saturated fats can increase cholesterol levels and a change in the lipoprotein profile to an increase in LDL and a decrease in HDL. Hypercholesterolemia, associated with lesion formation and progression, elicits endothelial dysfunction in coronary arteries and LDL could inhibit endothelium-dependent vasodilatation, an effect that can be prevented by HDL [51]. Psychological stress may interact with diet to promote coronary risk. Research in monkeys has shown that when the organism has a high-fat diet along with high stress levels it results in more pronounced atherosclerosis.

The endothelium plays a critical role in the development of atherosclerosis. The healthy endothelium is a metabolically active tissue that regulates vascular tone via release of the vasodilatador nitric oxide. Endothelial integrity reduces cell adhesion, lipid deposition and other early steps in atherosclerosis process and is a critically necessary condition to the vasodilatation response. Evidence suggests that dietary factors can alter endothelial function (as vascular resistance and reactivity) not only in the middle-long term, as previously thought, but also acutely within hours of eating certain foods. This further affirms the role of dietary factors in the prevention and progression of cardiovascular diseases. Consumption of a single high-fat meal (50-105 g of fat) impairs endothelial-mediated dilatation by 45 to 80% within 2 to 5 h after. Consumption of antioxidants (vitamin C and E, polyphenols, isoflavones), folic acid, omega-3 fatty acids from blue fish, l-arginine (especially present in dry fruit as walnuts, peanuts, soybeans) and Mediterranean diet reduce systemic vascular constriction and promote healthy endothelium-dependent dilatatation [57].

Conclusion

Several studies show that anger and hostility are strongly associated with CVR and that this may be the way through which these factors influence CHD be it within a short and/or long time. However, there are also some inconsistent results. Positive results seems to depend on the following:

(i) Controlling and combining different measures of hostility and anger coping skills
(ii) Using experimental tasks involving social conflict and/or provocation

(iii) Assessing both cardiovascular reactivity and recovery and psychological processes as worry or rumination.

There is a social gradient in the relationships between SES and cardiovascular diseases. Possible mediating mechanisms of this relation could be the differences on medical care access, nutrition, risk-related behaviours, worse living conditions etc. However, these factors can explain only about one-quarter of the SES-CAD gradient. As important as these traditional factors are psychosocial factors like social support, depression, job strain and chronic stress [35].

Epidemiological and prospective studies show that social support is negatively associated to cardiovascular morbidity and mortality while social isolation predicts it. These associations remained after controlling for classical risk factors.

Obesity is strongly associated to hypertension, elevated levels of triglycerides, LDL and reduced levels of HDL, cardiac alterations predisposing to heart failure and the insulin resistance syndrome. Abdominal obesity (i.e. waist circumference) is the most predictive of cardiovascular diseases.

By a rise in insulin levels, ingestion of large quantities of alcohol or overfeeding of carbohydrates and fats activates the SNS, increases BP, reduces sodium excretion, stimulates vascular smooth muscle hypertrophy and sensitises the arteriolar smooth muscle cells to pressure responses.

Key Points

- ❑ When psychosocial factors and the traditional factor are statistically controlled, the social gradient is eliminated. Within the SES, the educative level is negatively and independently associated with all causes of cardiovascular mortality.
- ❑ Social support is negatively associated to perceptions of stress, depression, anxiety and hostility. Social support also decreases cardiovascular and neuroendocrine reactivity to stress.
- ❑ Emotional support and family sources of social support appear to be particularly relevant to health outcomes. Obesity is an established independent risk factor for CHD and, in general, for cardiovascular disease.
- ❑ Dietary factors can impair endothelial function not only in the long-term, but within hours of eating certain foods as a single high-fat meal.

References

1. Kop, W.J., 1999, "Chronic and Acute Psychological Risk Factors for Clinical Manifestations of Coronary Artery Disease", *Psychosom. Med.*, 61, pp. 476-487.
2. Smith, T.W., Glazer, K., Ruiz, J.M. and Gallo, L.C., 2004, "Hostility, Anger, Aggressiveness and Coronary Heart Disease: An Interpersonal Perspective on Personality, Emotion and Health", *J. Per.*, 72, pp. 1217-1270.
3. Miller, S.B., Friese, M., Dolgoy, L., Sita, A., Lavoie, K. and Campbell, T., 1998, "Hostility, Sodium Consumption and Cardiovascular Response to Interpersonal Stress", *Psychosom. Med.*, 60, pp. 71-77.
4. Porter, L.S., Stone, A.A. and Schwartz, J.E., 1999, "Anger Expression and Ambulatory Blood Pressure: A Comparison of State and Trait Measures", *Psychosom. Med.*, 61, pp. 454-463.

5. Ranchor, A.V., Sanderman, R., Bouma, J., Buunk, B.P. and van den Heuvel, W.J., 1997, "An Exploration of the Relation Between Hostility and Disease", *J. Behav. Med.*, 20, pp. 223-240.
6. Shapiro, D., Goldstein, I.B. and Jamner, L.D., 1996, "Effects of Cynical Hostility, Anger Out, Anxiety, and Defensiveness on Ambulatory Blood Pressure in Black and White College Students", *Psychosom. Med.*, 58, pp. 254-264.
7. Finney, M.L., Stoney, C.M. and Engebretson, T.O., 2002, "Hostility and Anger Expression in African American and European American Men is Associated with Cardiovascular and Lipid Reactivity", *Psychophysiology*, 39, pp. 340-349.
8. Burns, J.W., Evon, D. and Strain-Saloum, C., 1999, "Repressed Anger and Patterns of Cardiovascular, Self-report and Behavioral Responses: Effects of Harassment", *J. Psychosom. Res.*, 47, pp. 569-581.
9. Gendolla, G.H.E. and Krüsken, J., 2001, "The Joint Impact of Mood State and Task Difficulty on Cardiovascular and Electrodermal Reactivity in Active Coping", *Psychophysiology*, 38, pp. 548-556.
10. Gendolla, G.H.E. and Richter, M., 2005, "Ego Involvement and Effort: Cardiovascular, Electrodermal and Performance Effects", *Psychophysiology*, 42, pp. 595-603.
11. García-León, A., Reyes del Paso, G.A., Robles, H. and Vila, J., 2003, "Relative Effects of Harassment, Frustration, and Task Characteristics on Cardiovascular Reactivity", *Int. J. Psychophysiol.*, 47, pp. 159-173.
12. Harrison, L.K., Denning, S., Easton, H.L., Hall, J.C., Burns, V.E., Ring, C. and Carroll, D., 2001, "The Effects of Competition and Competitiveness on Cardiovascular Activity", *Psychophysiology*, 38, pp. 601-606.
13. Kamarck, T.W. and Lovallo, W.R., 2003, "Cardiovascular Reactivity to Psychological Challenge: Conceptual and Measurement Considerations", *Psychosom. Med.*, 65, pp. 9-21.
14. Davis, M.C., Matthews, K.A. and McGrath, C.E., 2002, "Hostile Attitudes Predict Elevated Vascular Resistance During Interpersonal Stress in Men and Women", In *Foundations in Social Neuroscience*, J.T. Cacioppo et al. (Eds.), The MIT Press, Cambridge.
15. Berkowitz, L., 1988, "Frustration, Apparisals and Aversively Stimulated Aggression", *Aggresive Behav.*, 14, pp. 3-11.
16. Brondolo, E., Rieppi, R., Erickson, S.A., Bagiella, E., Shapiro, P.A., McKinley, P. and Sloan, R.P., 2003, "Hostility, Interpersonal Interactions and Ambulatory Blood Pressure", *Psychosom. Med.*, 65, pp. 1003-1011.
17. Felsten, G., 1995, "Cynical Hostility Influences Anger, but not Cardiovascular Reactivity During Competition with Harassment", *Int. J. Psychophysiol.*, 19, pp. 223-231.
18. Demaree, H.A. and Everhart, D.E., 2004, "Healthy High-hostiles: Reduced Parasympathetic Activity and Decreased Sympathovagal Flexibility During Negative Emotional Processing", *Pers. Individ. Differ.*, 36, pp. 457-469.
19. Lawler, K.A., Harralson, T.L. and Armstead, C.A., 1993, "Gender and Cardiovascular Responses: What is the Role of Hostility?" *J. Psychosom. Res.*, 37, pp. 603-613.
20. Suarez, E.C., Kuhn, C.M., Schanberg, S.M., Williams, R.B. and Zimmermann, E.A., 1998, "Neuroendocrine, Cardiovascular and Emotional Responses of Hostile Men: The Role of Interpersonal Challenge", *Psychosom. Med.*, 60, pp. 78-88.
21. Gallo, L.C., Smith, T.W. and Kircher, J.C., 2000, "Cardiovascular and Electrodermal Responses to Support and Provocation: Interpersonal Methods in the Study of Psychophysiological Reactivity", *Psychophysiology*, 37, pp. 289-301.
22. Suarez, E.C., Saab, P.G., Llabre, M.M., Kuhn, C.M. and Zimmerman, E., 2004, "Ethnicity, Gender and Age Effects on Adrenoceptors and Physiological Responses to Emotional Stress", *Psychophysiology*, 41, pp. 450-460.

23. Brosschot, J.F. and Thayer, J.F., 1998, "Anger Inhibition, Cardiovascular Recovery and Vagal Function: A Model of the Link Between Hostility and Cardiovascular Disease", *Ann. Behav. Med.*, 20, pp. 326-332.
24. Brosschot, J.F. and Thayer, J.F., 2004, "Worry, Perseverative Thinking and Health", In *Emotional Expression and Health: Advances in Theory, Assessment and Clinical Applications*, Nyklícek, I., Temoshok, L. and Vingerhoets, A. (Eds.), Brunner-Routledge, Hove.
25. Gerin, W., Davidson, K.W., Christenfeld, N.J.S., Goyal, T. and Schwartz, J.E., 2006, "The Role of Angry Rumination and Distraction in Blood Pressure Recovery from Emotional Arousal", *Psychosom. Med.*, 68, pp. 64-72.
26. Brosschot, J.F., Gerin, W. and Thayer, J.F., 2006, "The Perseverative Cognition Hypothesis: A Review of Worry, Prolonged Stress-related Physiological Activation and Health", *J. Psychosom. Res.*, 60, pp. 113-124.
27. Glynn, L.M., Christenfeld, N. and Gerin, W., 2002, "The Role of Rumination in Recovery from Reactivity: Cardiovascular Consequences of Emotional States", *Psychosom. Med.*, 64, pp. 714-726.
28. Suchday, S., Carter, M.M., Ewart, C.K., Larkin, K.T. and Desiderato, O., 2004, "Anger Cognitions and Cardiovascular Recovery Following Provocation", *J. Behav. Med.*, 27, pp. 319-341.
29. Schwartz, A.R., Gerin, W., Davidson, K.W., Pickering, T.G., Brosschot, J.F., Thayer, J.F., Christenfeld, N. and Linden, W., 2003, "Toward a Causal Model of Cardiovascular Responses to Stress and the Development of Cardiovascular Disease", *Psychosom. Med.*, 65, pp. 22-35.
30. Neumann, S.A., Waldstein, S.F., Sollers, J.J., Thayer, J.F. and Sorkin, J.D., 2004, "Hostility and Distraction Have Differential Influences on Cardiovascular Recovery from Anger Recall in Women", *Health Psychol.*, 23, pp. 631-640.
31. Anderson, J.C., Linden, W. and Habra, M.E., 2005, "The Importance of Examining Blood Pressure Reactivity and Recovery in Anger Provocation Research", *Int. J. Psychophysiol.*, 57, pp. 159-163.
32. Adler, N.E. and Ostrove, J.M., 1999, "ESE and Health: What We Know and What We Don't", *Ann. New York Acad Sci.*, 896, pp. 3-15.
33. Marmot, M. and Feeney, A., 1996, "Socioeconomic Factors in CHD Prevention", In *Behavioral Medicine Approaches to Cardiovascular Disease Prevention*, Orth-Gomér, K. and Schneiderman, N. (Eds.), Lawrence Erlbaum Associates, New Jersey.
34. Alter, D.A., Chong, A. et al., 2006, "Socioeconomic Status and Mortality After Acute Myocardial Infarction", *Ann. Intern. Med.*, SESAMI Study Group, 144, pp. 82-93.
35. Krantz, D.S. and McCeney, M.K., 2002, "Effects of Psychological and Social Factors on Organic Disease: A Critical Assessment of Research on Coronary Heart Disease", *Annu. Rev. Psychol.*, 53, pp. 341-369.
36. Rosengren, A., Hawken, S. et al. (for the INTERHEART investigators), 2004, "Association of Psychosocial Risk Factors with Risk of Acute Myocardial Infarction in 11,119 Cases and 13,648 Controls from 52 Countries (The INTERHEART Study): A Case-control Study", *Lancet*, 364, pp. 953-962.
37. Kristenson, M., Kucinskienë, Z., Bergdahl, B. et al. (for the LiVicordia Investigators), 1998, "Increased Psychological Strain in Lithuanian vs. Swedish Men: The ViVicordia Study", *Psychosom. Med.*, 60, pp. 277-282.
38. Brunner, E.J., Marmot, M.G. et al. (for the Whitehall II Investigators), 1993, "Gender and Employment Grade Differences in Blood Cholesterol, Apolipoproteins and Haemostatic Factors in the Whitehall II Study", *Atherosclerosis*, 102, pp. 195-207.
39. Koster, A., Bosma, H., Penninx, B., Newman, A.B. et al. (for the Health ABC Study), 2006, "Association of Inflammatory Markers with Socioeconomic Status", *J. Gerontol. Series A: Biological Sciences and Medical Sciences*, 61, pp. 284-290.

40. Rasmussen, J.N., Rasmussen, S., Gislason, G.H., Buch, P., Abildstrom, S.Z. et al., 2006, "Mortality After Acute Myocardial Infarction According to Income and Education", *J. Epidemiol. Commun. H.*, 60, pp. 351-356.
41. Yan, L.L., Liu, K., Daviglus, M.L. et al. (for the CARDIA Investigators), 2006, "Education, 15-year Risk Factor Progression and Coronary Artery Calcium in Young Adulthood and Early Middle Age", *JAMA*, 295, pp. 1793-1800.
42. Ruberman, W., Weinblatt, E., Goldberg, J.D. and Chaudhary, B.S., 1984, "Psychosocial Influences on Mortality After Myocardial Infarction", *New Engl. J. Med.*, 311, pp. 552-559.
43. Loucks, E.B., Sullivan, L.M., Hayes, L.J., D´Agostino, R.B., Larson, M.G. et al., 2006, "Association of Educational Level with Inflammatory Markers in the Framingham Offspring Study", *Am. J. Epidemiol.*, 163, pp. 622-628.
44. Berkman, L.F. and Orth-Gomér, K., 1996, "Prevention of Cardiovascular Morbidity and Mortality: Role of Social Relations", In *Behavioral Medicine Approaches to Cardiovascular Disease Prevention*, Orth-Gomér, K. and Schneiderman, N. (Eds.), Lawrence Erlbaum Associates, New Jersey.
45. Uchino, B.N., Cacioppo, J.T. and Kiecolt-Glaser, J.K., 1996, "The Relationship Between Social Ssupport and Physiological Process: A Review with Emphasis on Underlying Mechanisms and Implications for Health", *Psychol. Bull.*, 119, pp. 488-531.
46. Let, H.S., Blumenthal, J.A., Babyak, M.A., Strauman, T.J., Robins, C. and Sherwood, A., 2005, "Social Support and Coronary Heart Disease: Epidemiologic Evidence and Implications for Treatment", *Psychosom. Med.*, 67, pp. 869-878.
47. Glynn, L.M., Christenfeld, N. and Gerin, W., 1999, "Gender, Social Support, and Cardiovascular Responses to Stress", *Psychosom. Med.*, 61, pp. 234-242.
48. Allen, K., Shykoff, B.E. and Izzo, J.L., 2001, "Pet Ownership, but not ACE Inhibitor Therapy, Blunts Home Blood Pressure Responses to Mental Stress", *Hypertension*, 38, pp. 815-820.
49. Kiecolt-Glaser, J.K., McGuire, L., Robles, T.F. and Glaser, R., 2002, "Emotions, Morbidity, and Mortality: New Perspectives from Psychoneuroimmunology", *Annu. Rev. Psychol.*, 53, pp. 83-107.
50. Lepore, S.J., 1995, "Cynicism, Social Support and Cardiovascular Reactivity", *Health Psychol.*, 14, pp. 210-216.
51. Knox, S.S. and Uvnäs-Moberg, K., 1998, "Social Isolation and Cardiovascular Disease: An Atherosclerotic Pathway?" *Psychoneuroendocrino*, 23, pp. 877-890.
52. Poirier, P., Giles, T.D., Bray, G.A., Hong, Y., Stern, J.S. et al., 2006, "Obesity and Cardiovascular Disease: Pathophysiology, Evaluation and Effect of Weight Loss", *Am. Heart Ass.*, 26, pp. 968-976.
53. Krauss, R.M., Winston, M., Fletcher, B.J. and Grundy, S.M., 1998, "Obesity: Impact on Cardiovascular Disease", *Circulation*, 98, pp. 1472-1476.
54. Yusuf, S., Hawken, S., Ôunpuu, S., Bautista, L., Franzosi, M.G. et al. (for the INTERHEART Investigators), 2005, "Obesity and the Risk of Myocardial Infarction in 27,000 Participants from 52 Countries: A Case-control Study", *Lancet*, 366, pp. 1640-1649.
55. Schneiderman, N. and Skyler, J.S., 1996, "Insulin Metabolism, Sympathetic Nervous System Regulation, and Coronary Heart Disease Prevention", In *Behavioral Medicine Approaches to Cardiovascular Disease Prevention*, Orth-Gomér, K. and Schneiderman, N. (Eds.), Lawrence Erlbaum Associates, New Jersey.
56. Matsuzawa, Y., 2006, "The Metabolic Syndrome and Adipocytokines", *FEBS Lett.*, 580, pp. 2917-2921.
57. West, S.G., 2001, "Effect of Diet on Vascular Reactivity: An Emerging Marker for Vascular Risk", *Curr. Ather. Rep.*, 3, pp. 446-455.

The AHA-Syndrome and Cardiovascular Diseases
Editors: Swati Y. Bhave and Sunil Saini
Copyright © 2010 Anamaya Publishers, New Delhi, India

17. Two Hearts and the Path to Heartful Living

Donald Moss
Saybrook Graduate School and Research Center, San Francisco, California, USA

Abstract: The present chapter describes two hearts, viz. the bio-electric pump of anatomy and the human heart of poetry and philosophy. This latter heart is the centre of the soul, the abode of love, caring and emotion. The chapter introduces phenomenology as an approach aiming to illuminate the individual's immediate experience of the body of life, and of health and illness. It describes the inter-twining of the scientific heart and the human heart in emotion and in illness. The human lives are swept in immediate emotion and feeling, and this subjective emotion impacts the medical and the poetic heart at once. Living heart-fully as a pathway toward heart health is advocated.

Keywords: Heart, Phenomenology, Emotion, Cardiac rhythms, Heartfulness.

"It is only with the heart that one can see rightly. What is essential is invisible to the eye."
The Little Prince, Antoine De Saint-Exupery

The Two Hearts in the Human Body

From the standpoint of clinical medicine, the heart is a bio-electric pump, defined by its anatomical structures and its electro-physiological operation:

> *"The heart is the muscle that pumps blood filled with oxygen and nutrients through the blood vessels to the body tissues. It is made up of four chambers... that receive blood from the body and pump out blood to it... Blood vessels, which compose a network of arteries and veins that carry blood throughout the body... Four valves to prevent backward flow of blood."*
> Ohio State University Medical Centre [1]

From the medical perspective, the image of pumps and pipes is central, the vital flow of blood maintained by the heart, which beats about 80 times a minute, 115,000 times a day or 42 million times a year. When physicians attempt to explain the heart to a child whose own heart is impaired, the heart is first of all depicted as a pump:

> *"It's true, your heart really is a pump and it is about as big as your fist. It's made out of a strong muscle that squeezes together to make your heart beat. Here is how it works."*
> University of Michigan Cardiovascular Centre [2]

The average human being shares this perspective of anatomy and worries at any hint that this biological pump is endangered.

There is another everyday perspective, however, equally cherished, that knows the heart as the centre of the soul, as the place in which one feels love and compassion for the beloved. We know what it means to "speak from the heart" or to be "wounded in the heart". James Barrie, the author of *Peter Pan*, wrote that "Only where the heart is, can the treasure be found". Anne Morrow Lindbergh wrote that "There is no harvest for the heart alone. The seed of love must be eternally re-sown".

This is not a new perspective. Aristotle (384-322 BC) believed that the heart was the centre of the human body, the seat of the soul and emotions, and a primary sense organ of the body. For example, he defined anger as a seething heat in the region of the heart. The 'cardiocentric' theory was widespread in the ancient world and included an assumption that the heart was the seat of mental processes including thinking and memory. This view was, in part, simply a matter of ignorance, since dissection had not yet disclosed the nervous system and the nervous pathways between brain and body [3].

Today, however, the cardiocentric view is undergoing a kind of limited revival. The research of John and Beatrice Lacey [4], for example, showed that there is a "two-way communication between the heart and the brain". The heart seems to send messages to the brain and the brain responds to those messages, in ways affecting human behaviour. Armour [5] expanded this recognition into the new field of neurocardiology, which studies the intrinsic nervous system in the heart, which has afferent pathways of its own [6]. Research has also shown that the heart produces at least two hormones, atrial natriuretic factor and oxytocin (the hormone associated with more intense emotional bonding).

The heart may be an organ of connectedness between human beings. New research is showing the hearts of some intimately connected persons synchronising with one another, even when they are separated from one another without sensory connection in sealed laboratory settings [7]. The implications of these discoveries have not yet been fully tested or explored, yet they suggest a possible bridge with the poetic attribution of a more central role to the heart, especially in emotion and human bonding.

The Phenomenology of Illness

Phenomenology is the disciplined effort, within philosophy, medicine and psychology, to unfold the moment of experience as it is lived; not to dissect or explain it, but to illuminate it. Phenomenological research brings us closer to the immediate perspective of the human being who is swept up, mid-stream in an unfolding life. From the phenomenological perspective, health and disease are not simple physiological facts, rather each involves qualitative differences in the individual's relationship to the physical environment, in personal temporality and spatiality, in relationships to the family and social world, and in the struggle for identity [8, 9].

As the Dutch phenomenological psychiatrist van den Berg showed, a sick individual – whether mentally or physically ill – lives a different existence and inhabits a perceptually and experientially different world [10, 11]. Illness and suffering turn a person back upon himself/herself. The world seems less inviting, loses its appeal, while at the same time one senses that life goes on for others without one.

For example, a woman with chronic fatigue syndrome wrote that "The destination and map I had used to navigate before were no longer useful". She continued by declaring her need to "think differently and construct new perceptions of my relationship to the world" [12]. Understanding the patient's objective medical condition, as measured through a complete blood count, magnetic resonance imaging (MRI) and other measures, without empathy for the "world of the sickbed", misses this human dimension in illness. The physician is ill-equipped to assist the ill in discovering a new destination and map or in constructing new perceptions of one's relationship with the world [13]. And yet this human dimension is often critical for any real hope of wellness or recovery.

Kingdom of the Sick

"Illness is the night-side of life, a more onerous citizenship. Everyone who is born holds dual citizenship, in the kingdom of the well and in the kingdom of the sick. Although we all prefer to use only the good passport, sooner or later each of us is obliged, at least for a spell, to identify ourselves as citizens of that other place."

Sontag [14]

Susan Sontag described the human being stricken with illness as entering the "kingdom of the sick". Becoming ill or disabled dramatically changes the patient's experience of the world. The longer an illness or disability lingers, the more radically the patient's world is transformed. If a health professional wishes to understand the patient's perspective, it is crucial to come to understand the flavour and texture of the world of illness.

Initially, patients often experience illness or injury as a 'violation' that breaks into their life uninvited. The entrance may be abrupt, in a violent injury or heart attack, or may be more gradual. One day an individual feels too ill to go to the office or to play tennis as expected. Unless the onset of illness is violent, most patients cling to the expectation of acute illness. The patient may take a few vitamins, get some extra sleep or take a medication left over from a previous illness. There is a momentary retreat from life in order to recover, but the expectation remains that, in a few hours or days, one will resume life and get back to normal life priorities.

When illness worsens or lingers, patients turn to their health professional, usually the family practice physician. Patients in mainstream cultures in the United States are typically thoroughly acculturated in the acute medicine model. They visit the physician, looking for a specific diagnostic process leading to medication and recovery. The typical primary care visit will not produce a conclusive diagnosis, but the patient remains oriented to a process of brief treatment of symptoms and a return to life as usual in short order.

As illness lingers or progresses, patients often become more emotionally invested in the process of diagnosis and a search for a cure. If the diagnostic process is prolonged, uncertainty grows and all too often primitive fears that one is not cared about. The common assumption that one is entitled to treatment and a quick cure slowly breaks down. Emergence of chronicity challenges much favoured beliefs about self and life.

Modern public hygiene and medical progress have dramatically reduced the incidence of the infectious diseases such as cholera and malaria that were the scourge of the early 20th century. The acute care medical model, which occupies the larger part of current medical school training, is enormously successful, in diagnosing and treating acute injuries and infectious conditions. Increasingly, however, the primary care clinic is congested with the care of the chronically ill. Patients with chronic illness now account for between 46 and 75% of healthcare costs. This includes such diverse conditions as diabetes mellitus, arthritis, hypertension and chronic heart disease. Little in current medical training adequately equips the physician to cope with patients who linger but will not get well.

Perhaps it is time – in this era of functional symptoms, lifestyle-based diseases and chronic illnesses – that medical thought must turn once again, to consider not only the pipes and the pumps, but how the individual will live from the heart.

Emotional Tuning of the Heart

Friedman and Rosenman [15] opened up the study of how lifestyle and emotion affect the heart. Their pioneering research followed 3,000 men for nine years and showed that "Type A behaviour" doubled the risk for heart disease. The Type A phenomenon included a variety of inter-related behaviours and traits. Type A individuals show time-urgency, competitiveness and hostility. They are hyper-aware of time and engage in multi-tasking (balancing multiple tasks simultaneously). In general, Type A individuals create their own tension by high expectations of self and others.

Later, Dembroski et al. [16] and MacDougall et al. [17] extended the research on Type A behaviour. They studied 12,000 men and isolated the toxic core of Type A hostility and anger. Angry doctors and lawyers, for example, are five times more likely to die of heart disease than their non-angry peers. It is anger and hostility, which kills, more so than all of the associated factors of competitiveness, time urgency and the like.

A number of basic research studies confirm the destructive effects of anger. Ironson et al. [18] asked research subjects to recall moments of anger and found that their ejection fraction lowered during the moments of anger. The heart does not pump as effectively when the individual is angry. Similarly, Boltwood et al. [19] studied individuals with atherosclerosis, partially clogged arteries and showed that recalling angry situations produced spasm of the arteries.

Anger and negative emotion are the enemies of the healthy heart. The cultivation of positive emotion is a pathway to health [20].

The Lonely Heart

Without loving companionship, human beings are more vulnerable to cardiovascular and other illness. Research supporting this conclusion comes from many directions. An early Israeli study of 10,000 married men with heart disease found that one simple questionnaire item had a dramatic moderating effect, even in the presence of high cholesterol, electrocardiogram (ECG) abnormalities and high anxiety [21]. Among those men who said 'Yes' to the question, "Does your wife show you her love?" only 52% developed angina. Among the group who said 'No' to the same question, 93% developed angina!

Similarly, James Lynch [22], in his book *The Broken Heart: The Medical Consequences of Loneliness* showed that the sudden loss of a partner and chronic isolation are significant contributors to cardiovascular illness and sudden death. Conversely, Lynch showed that human touch lowered heart rate and blood pressure. Dean Ornish [23] also garnered an impressive array of evidence that good relationships support cardiovascular health.

Rhythms of the Heart

The human heart beats in ever changing rhythms. Exertion increases heart rate, as does anxiety. Human touch often lowers heart rate. Healthy young hearts show high variability in heart rate. A young athlete's heart will oscillate between peak and lowest heart rates, with a difference between the two often exceeding 20 or 30 beats/min. With aging and with sedentary life style, the heart loses its variability. A sedentary 55-year-old often shows swings of only three to five beats from peak to lowest heart rates.

The level of variability is also a marker of physiological resilience, and heart rate variability (HRV) has come to be regarded as a useful prognostic index or marker for morbidity and mortality. The medical index for how much variability there is in heart rate is called the SDNN – the standard deviation of the time interval between heart beats. A higher SDNN (above 100 milliseconds (ms)) is an indicator of optimum health and a lower SDNN (below 50 ms) is an indicator of impaired health. Lower HRV predicts a greater risk for further cardiac symptoms and death after a heart attack [24]. Lowered HRV is a predictor of mortality from all causes, especially sudden death.

Negative emotion also affects HRV. Clinical depression lowers HRV and increases risk for coronary artery disease [25]. McCraty et al. [20] have identified 'coherence' as another quality of HRV. When the human being is absorbed in positive emotional states, as in a moment of closeness with a loved one, heart rate changes are smooth and well-ordered, resembling a mathematical sine curve – called 'coherence' by McCraty. When emotions are negative, the heart rate signal is ragged, irregular and low in coherence. Figure 1 shows two line graphs of moment to moment heart rate changes, contrasting the high coherence during moments of appreciation to the low coherence during frustration [20].

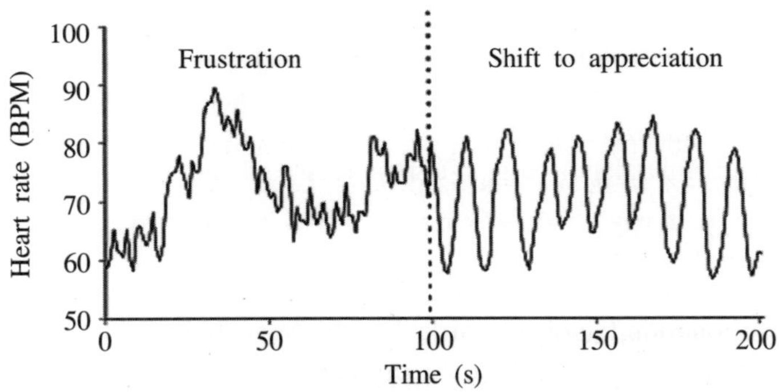

Fig. 1. Linegraphs depict the coherent variation of the heart in a state of appreciation and jagged, irregular variation in frustration.

Childre and McCraty's [26] description is as follows:

"... sustained positive emotions, such as appreciation, love, or compassion, are associated with a highly ordered or coherent pattern in the heart rhythms, reflecting greater synchronisation between the two branches of the autonomic nervous system."

> "... *during the experience of negative emotions such as anger, frustration, or anxiety, heart rhythms become more erratic or disordered, indicating less synchronisation in the reciprocal action that ensues between the parasympathetic and sympathetic branches of the autonomic nervous system.*"

Modern computer technology allows both researchers and clinicians to analyse the raw heart rate signal into component waves of varying frequency. Heart rate changes are driven by several biological governors, each producing changes in specific time frames. The Fast Fourier Transform (FFT) separates out changes in heart rate in high frequency, low frequency and very low frequency ranges. The Task Force of the European Society of Cardiology and the North American Society of Pacing and Electrophysiology [27] established a standard for categorising these frequency ranges.

Today, biofeedback practitioners are teaching individuals to gain control over their heart rhythms, increasing the coherence of the heart rate changes, consciously directing HRV into specific frequency ranges and increasing overall variability [28, 29]. During HRV biofeedback, patients learn to relax and release negative emotions, cultivate positive emotional states and develop a smooth, even mindful breathing, all of which contribute to increased coherence in heart rate changes, and increased overall HRV.

Del Pozo et al. [30] provided HRV biofeedback to patients with coronary artery disease and demonstrated a significant increase in the patient's HRV (as measured by the SDNN index). This result is preliminary evidence that HRV biofeedback is a promising tool for improving survival rates in coronary artery disease.

Living Heartfully

What does it mean to "live heartfully"? Clearly it involves learning the following lessons:

Transduce Harsh Negative Emotion into Gentler Positive Emotions

Anger is the toxic enemy of heart health and living heartfully must highlight a pathway past anger. Bhat, a cardiologist in California, asks his patients to imagine that they are cuddling a baby, petting a puppy or caring for someone who is ill [31]. Bhat calls this the *Mother Theresa effect* and sees it as a direct pathway to dissolving negative emotion. When the patient cultivates positive emotion, the result is optimal HRV.

Welcome Loving Connections with Others

MacLean [32] emphasises what he calls "open-heartedness", which involves the capacity to be emotionally available to experience the initial stages of connection with another and the capacity to stand outside of one's ego long enough to emotionally touch and be touched by another. Open-heartedness means a personal transformation, in which the heart guides one's daily life more than mental calculations and self-interest.

> "*Where ego strategises, love embraces. Where ego closes in on, love opens to. Where ego feels fear, love feels fearlessness. Where ego finds reasons to run, love knows the value in staying.*"
>
> MacLean [32]

Master the Stress of Everyday Life

A study by Blumenthal et al. [33] of patients with cardiac ischemia shocked many, when it showed that stress management had a greater effect in reducing cardiovascular effects than standard medical care or exercise. Of all the patients with standard medical care 30% suffered new cardiovascular symptoms. The addition of exercise dropped that number to only 21% and stress management dropped the number to 10%. A meta-analysis of 37 research investigations on the effects of stress management programs for patients with coronary artery disease, showed a 34% reduction in cardiac mortality and a 29% reduction in myocardial infarction.

Cultivate Mindful Breathing

The calming effects of slow, full breathing have long been recognised in schools of meditation and yoga. Traditional Chinese medicine long ago observed the reciprocal relationship between regular breathing and the subject's mental state:

> "*... the tranquility of the mind regulates the breathing naturally and in turn, regulated breathing brings on concentration of the mind naturally.*"
>
> "*... the mind and breathing are interdependent and regular respiration produces a serene mind.*"
>
> *Questions and Answers of Meisha* by Yue Yanggui, Qing Dynasty, cited by Xiangcai [34]

Regulated breathing is a powerful tool to optimise heart rate variability and improve cardiovascular health.

Cultivate Spiritual Disciplines

The pathway to heartful living is the domain of the spirit and spiritual leaders in each tradition have provided insights into healing the heart. Buddhism, for example, has a special school known as *Metta*, which focusses on the cultivation of loving-kindness, a sense of connectedness with all living beings. The *Metta Sutra* is a Buddhist spiritual text which describes this pursuit of compassionate loving-kindness towards all living beings. It describes the love of a mother who will readily risk her own life to protect her child, as the image to guide those who would develop more compassion. *Metta* prescribes specific meditations to develop a deeper compassion for others [35]. Similarly, Christian teachings guide the individual to cultivate that perfect love which casts out fear (1 John 4:18). Compassion and love can salve the corrosive effects of negative emotions.

Conclusion: The Healthy Heart

There are two hearts in the human being:

(i) The anatomical bio-electric pump, which modern medicine has so exhaustively studied
(ii) The heart as the seat of one's own soul and the abode of compassion

When we seek to heal the heart with mechanical and pharmaceutical means alone, we ignore the existential roots of many heart conditions. The manner in which the human being lives his/her life and the manner in which this person connects with others, has significance for cardiac morbidity and mortality.

The two hearts are not the same, yet also not separate. The compassionate heart, the heart of compassion for others, may also be the biological heart which secretes the hormone of bonding – oxytocin. The human being torn with anger also has a bio-electric pump whose pumping is impaired, and whose vessels are in spasm.

The human being empty of love is a human being more vulnerable to illness. Cultivating a network of supporting relationships, and opening oneself to feeling connected within relationships will optimise wellness.

It is time to make room in health care for the "lessons of the heart", along with the anatomy of pumps and pipes.

Key Points

- ❑ Two hearts are meaningful for each human being – the anatomical heart and the heart of compassion and connection.
- ❑ Phenomenology illuminates the human being's immediate experience of the living body and impact of illness on his/her relationship with the world.
- ❑ Health care professionals must become more familiar with the kingdom of the sick – the life transformed in chronic and life-threatening illness.
- ❑ Anger and negative emotions corrode the cardiovascular system, while positive emotions heal the heart.
- ❑ Loneliness and loss leave an individual vulnerable to cardiovascular illness. Human touch and human companionship support heart health and survival.
- ❑ Lowered heart rate variability is a risk factor for cardiovascular illness and death. Cultivating higher variability enhances health and wellness.
- ❑ Living heartfully involves developing positive emotions, opening one's heart to others, managing stress, learning mindful breathing and cultivating spiritual disciplines as a pathway to compassion.

References

1. Ohio State University Medical Center, 2006, "Anatomy of the Heart", Accessed on 24 November 2006, *http://medicalcenter.osu.edu/patientcare/healthinformation/diseasesandconditions/heartdisease/about/anatomy.cfm*
2. University of Michigan Cardiovascular Center, 2006, "My Heart is a Pump", Accessed on 24 January 2006, *www.med.umich.edu/cvc/mchc/kidpump.htm*
3. McCraty, R., Atkinson, M. and Tomasino, D., 2001, *Science of the Heart: Exploring the Role of the Heart in Human Performance*, Institute of Heart Math, Boulder Creek, California.
4. Lacey, J.I. and Lacey, B.C., 1978, Two-way Communication Between the Heart and the Brain: Significance of Time Within the Cardiac Cycle", *American Psychologist*, 33(2), pp. 99-113.
5. Armour, J.A., 1991, "Anatomy and Function of the Intrathoracic Neurons Regulating the Mammalian Heart", In *Reflex Control of the Circulation*, I.H. Zucker and J.P. Gilmore (Eds.), CRC Press, Boca Raton, Florida, pp. 1-37.

6. Armour, J.A. and Ardell, J. (Eds.), 1994, *Neurocardiology*, Oxford University Press, New York.
7. Mandel, D. and Kozac, L., 2007, "Resonant Hearts and Human Connectedness: Electroencephalograph, Heart Rate and Heart Rate Variability Indications of Non-local Connectedness in Intimate Pairs", *Symposium at Annual Meeting of the Association for Applied Psychophysiology and Biofeedback*, Monterey, California.
8. Moss, D., 1992, "Obesity, Objectification and Identity: The Encounter with the Body as an Object in Obesity", In *The Body in Medical Thought and Practice*, D. Leder (Ed.), Kluwer Academic Publishers, The Netherlands.
9. Moss, D., 2003b, "Phenomenology, Applied Psychophysiology and Behavioral Medicine", In *Textbook of Neurofeedback, EEG Biofeedback, QEEG and Brain Regulation*, R. Kall and J. Kamiya (Eds.), Digital Book, Futurehealth, Philadelphia, *www.futurehealth.org/book.htm*
10. van den Berg, J.H., 1966, *The Psychology of the Sick Bed*, Duquesne University Press, Pittsburgh.
11. van den Berg, J.H., 1972, *A Different Existence*, Duquesne University Press, Pittsburgh.
12. Frank, A.W., 1995, *The Wounded Storyteller: Body, Illness and Ethics*", University of Chicago Press, Chicago.
13. Moss, D., 2003a, "Existential and Spiritual Dimensions of Primary Care: Healing the Wounded Soul", *Handbook of Mind-body Medicine for Primary Care*, Sage Publications, Thousand Oaks, California.
14. Sontag, S., 1977, *Illness as Metaphor*, Farrar, Straus and Gioux, New York.
15. Friedman, M. and Rosenman, R.H., 1974, *Type A Behavior and Your Heart*, Knopf, New York.
16. Dembroski, T.M., MacDougall, J.M., Williams, R.B., Haney, T.L. and Blumenthal, J.A., 1985, "Components of Type A, Hostility and Anger-in: Relationships to Angiographic Findings", *Psychosomatic Medicine*, 47(3), pp. 219-233.
17. MacDougall, J.M., Dembroski, T.M., Dimsdale, J.E. and Hackett, T.P., 1985, "Components of Type A, Hostility and Anger-in: Further Relationships to Angiographic Findings", *Health Psychology*, 4(2), pp. 137-152.
18. Ironson, G., Taylor, C.B., Boltwood, M., Bartzokis, T., Dennis, C., Chesney, M., Spitzer, S. and Segall, G.M., 1992, "Effects of Anger on Left Ventricular Ejection Fraction in Coronary Artery Disease", *American Journal of Cardiology*, 70(3), pp. 281-285.
19. Boltwood, M.D., Taylor, C.B., Burke, M.B., Grogin, H. and Giacomini, J., 1993, "Anger Report Predicts Coronary Artery Vasomotor Response to Mental Stress in Atherosclerotic Segments", *American Journal of Cardiology*, 72(18), pp. 1361-1365.
20. McCraty, R., Atkinson, M., Tomasino, D. and Bradley, R.T., 2006, *The Coherent Heart: Heart-brain Interactions, Psychophysiological Coherence and the Emergence of a System-wide Order*, Institute of Heart Math, Boulder Creek, California.
21. Medalie, J. and Gouldbourt, U., 1976, "Angina Pectoris Among 10,000 Men", *American Journal of Medicine*, 60(6), pp. 910-921.
22. Lynch, J.J., 1979, *The Broken Heart: The Medical Consequences of Loneliness*, Basic Books, Inc., New York.
23. Ornish, D., 1998, *Love and Survival*, HarperCollins Publishers, New York.
24. Kleiger, R.E., Miller, J.P., Bigger, J.T. et al. and the Multicenter Post-Infarction Research Group, 1987, "Decreased Heart Rate Variability and Its Association with Increased Mortality After Acute Myocardial Infarction", *American Journal of Cardiology*, 59, pp. 256-262.
25. Carney, R.M., Blumenthal, J.A., Stein, P.K., Watkins, L., Catellier, D., Berkman, L.F., Czajkowski, S.M., O'Connor, C., Stone, P.H. and Freedland, K.E., 2001, "Depression, Heart Rate Variability and Acute Myocardial Infarction", *Circulation*, 104(17), pp. 2024-2028.
26. Childre, D. and McCraty, R., 2001, "Psychophysiological Correlates of Spiritual Experience", *Biofeedback*, 29(4), pp. 13-17.

27. Task Force of the European Society of Cardiology and The North American Society of Pacing and Electrophysiology, 1996, "Heart Rate Variability: Standards of Measurement, Physiological Interpretation and Clinical Use", *European Heart Journal*, 17, pp. 354-381.
28. Moss, D., 2004, "Heart Rate Variability and Biofeedback", *Psychophysiology Today: The Magazine for Mind-Body Medicine*, 1, pp. 4-11.
29. Gevirtz, R.N., 2003, "The Promise of HRV Biofeedback: Some Preliminary Results and Speculations", *Biofeedback*, 31(3), pp. 18-19.
30. Del Pozo, J.M., Gevirtz, R.N., Scher, B. and Guarneria, E., 2004, "Biofeedback Treatment Increases Heart Rate Variability in Patients with Known Coronary Artery Disease", *American Heart Journal*, 147(3), pp. G1-G6.
31. Bhat, N. and Bhat, K., 1999, "Anger Control Using Biofeedback: A Clinical Model for Heart Patients", *Biofeedback*, 29(4), pp. 15-17.
32. MacLean, B., 2004, "The Heart and the Breath of Love", *Biofeedback*, 32(4), pp. 21-25.
33. Blumenthal, J.A., Jiang, W., Babyak, M.A., Krantz, D.S., Frid, D.J., Coleman, R.E., Waugh, R., Hanson, M., Applebaum, M., O'Connor, C. and Morris, J.J., 1997, "Stress Management and Exercise Training in Cardiac Patients with Myocardial Ischaemia: Effects on Prognosis and Evaluation of Mechanisms", *Archives of Internal Medicine*, 157(19), pp. 2213-2223.
34. Xiangcai, X., 2000, *Qigong for Treating Common Ailments: The Essential Guide to Self-healing*, YMAA Publication Center, Boston, Massachusetts.
35. Nagabodhi (Ed.), 2000, *Metta: The Practice of Loving Kindness*, Windhorse Publications, Birmingham, UK.

The AHA-Syndrome and Cardiovascular Diseases
Editors: Swati Y. Bhave and Sunil Saini
Copyright © 2010 Anamaya Publishers, New Delhi, India

18. Coronary Artery Disease and Depression

Jay P. Shastri
Asha Sadan, Maharashtra State Women's Council, Mumbai; Smt. Motibai Thakcersey Institute of Research in the Field of Mental Retardation; Developmental Psychology, M.I.N.D.'s College of Special Education, Mumbai; Dr. Shastri's Clinic, 3/3, Vivina Cooperative Housing Society S.V. Road, Andheri (West), Mumbai - 400 058, India

Abstract: Depression and coronary artery disease (CAD) are diseases of the 21st century. Both lead to a significant decrease in quality of life for the patient and impose a significant economic burden on society. There is a growing body of evidence suggesting that depression is an independent risk factor for development of this disease with worst outcome in patients with established CAD. There are various behavioural factors like stress and lifestyle risk factors along with pathophysiological factors like abnormal platelet function, inflammation, drugs, autonomic dysregulation and endothelial dysfunction that seem to link depression with CAD. Management of depression in patients with this disease starts with establishment of its presence. Selective serotonin re-uptake inhibitors (SSRIs) are the first choice for treatment of depression in this group of patients. Due to their better tolerability and absence of significant cardiovascular side effects SSRIs, as a group of anti-depressant, are preferred more as compared to any other anti-depressant medication. Treatment of depression in patients with CAD improves their quality of life by better adherence to risk factor modifications, prescribed medications and rehabilitation programmes. Patients with known CAD and evidence of depression should, therefore, be evaluated for anti-depressive therapy, such as cognitive behavioural therapy, complex cardiac rehabilitation programmes and pharmacologic treatment.

Keywords: Coronary artery disease, Depression, Diagnosis, Pharmacotherapy, Psychotherapy.

Introduction

Depression is currently the fourth leading cause of disability worldwide, as per World Health Organization (WHO) and the World Bank reports and its incidence is increasing rapidly. For people living in developed countries the incidence of depression is very high and up to one-third of the population have had an episode of depression at some point in their lives. Certain studies have documented incidence of people diagnosed with chronic depression as high as 15 to 20%. By the year 2020 depression will be the second leading cause of mortality and morbidity. The only disease category which is more dreading as compared to depression is cardiovascular disease. According to WHO and World Bank reports, cardiovascular disorder is projected to become the primary cause of mortality by 2020. Thus, since both the conditions are very common, there will be many patients with both the diseases. Also, there appears to be an interaction between the two diseases that augments their respective importance when they are combined.

Although a clear understanding about co-existence of depression and coronary artery disease (CAD) has become known in the recent past, it has been talked about since mid 19th century in the literature, such as "nervous and sympathetic palpitations of heart". In 1910, Sir William Osler described his typical patient with angina pectoris as "a man whose engine is always set full speed ahead" and called his patients with cardiac disease 'worriers'.

Research in the field of psychosomatic medicine over the last 30 years has emphasised the effects of psychological, social and behavioural factors on cardiovascular disease. Concurrence of depression in patients with cardiovascular diseases is a known entity and it negatively affects its outcome. The risk of depression in terms of mortality and morbidity among cardiovascular diseases is at par with any other medical risk factor. Patients suffering from depression preserve their heart disease status, which affects their quality of life adversely. They are more likely to report coronary disease symptom burden, physical limitations, diminished quality of life and fair-to-poor health. Recognising and treating depression in this special group is a challenge in itself [1].

Epidemiology

Depression appears to be the most common psychiatric disorder in patients with CAD. Various studies have recorded the concurrence rate of depression and CAD as high as 45% [1]. Around 50% of these depressed patients suffer from major depression and the rest reported having minor depression [2]. Studies have also shown that severity of depression is directly proportional to the mortality and morbidity associated with CAD. An increased risk for CAD was not only described in patients suffering from major depression, but also in patients suffering from minor depression or dysphoria. A four year follow-up study of individuals from ages 55 to 85 years showed that major depression tripled the risk of cardiac mortality in persons without heart disease and quadrupled in those who did have cardiac aliments [3].

The prevalence of major depression in patients with CAD is much higher, especially after myocardial infraction (MI) as compared to the general population [4]. Major depression is a significant predictor of mortality at six and 18 months after an acute MI, which is equal to the effects of predictors such as history of MI or indexes of cardiac functions [5]. In one study by Lesperance et al. [6] it was noted that patients hospitalised for unstable angina and having depression were four times more likely to have MI or die the following year than those without depression. One study has shown that clinical depression even after several decades of its appearance remains an independent risk factor for CAD [7]. Depression of severe variety was present in almost 25% of the patients immediately following acute myocardial event [8]. Around 27 to 65% of the patients showed symptoms of major to minor depression following MI. In one-year follow-up studies in post-MI patients, depression was found to be associated not only with mortality and morbidity risks, but it was also seen to increase the healthcare costs [5].

Prevalence of depression was seen to be around 18% following diagnostic angiography procedure even in the absence of MI or unstable angina [6]. A one year follow-up study after diagnostic angiography has shown continuation of major depression in all the patients having it at the onset. Minor depression was also found to have become major depression. Point prevalence of depression was reported to be in the range of 20 to 30% in patients who had undergone coronary artery bypass surgery. Depression was found to be an independent risk factor for cardiac event following the surgery and was also related to higher hospital re-admission rates [9-11].

Ethiopathology

There is enough support in the literature for depression and CAD to be biologically related. The link can be considered controversial, however, as patients with depression often have more risk factors for CAD as compared with those who are not depressed and may be less attentive to modifying those risk factors. In other words, it may be that depression does not cause CAD; depression causes the behaviours that lead to CAD. Depression also results in non-compliant attitude and behaviour leading to exaggerated effects of various risk factors multiplying the morbidity and mortality associated with CAD.

Depression as a Consequence

Various psychological reactions are expected in patients who were previously normal and later developed CAD. Reactions can range from increasing concerns about dependency, autonomy, control and ability to provide for others to inciting fears about vitality, sexuality and morality. It is most difficult to maintain denial after suffering from a cardiac event. Denial can further help the patients minimise their illness or attribute symptoms to non-cardiac sources. Excessive denial can lead to either delay or non-compliance to treatment. The possibility that CAD patients with depression are in worse cardiovascular shape than those without depression cannot be ruled out. In other words, it is possible that these patients are depressed simply because they have more severe cardiovascular disease. Subjective nature of the psychological symptoms makes it more difficult for the observing clinician to recognise this with ease. In addition, the matching of cardiac anatomy and function can never be done completely. Further studies consolidating the hypothesis of co-existence of depression and CAD is the need of the hour, since all the evidence available till now while studying patients with MI or unstable angina are not conclusive.

Cardiotoxic Antidepressants vs. Cardiac Drugs Causing Depression

Whenever there is use of tricyclic anti-depressant (TCA) medications for treatment of depression the frequency of cardiac events is enhanced. Specifically, it is possible that TCAs are associated with the occurrence of cardiac arrhythmias, perhaps severe enough to result in sudden arrhythmic cardiac death in arrhythmia-prone patients. Due to their adrenergic stimulating property TCA medication can influence the release of catecholamines or cause the membrane effects that are similar to effects caused by class 1C anti-arrhythmic drugs [12]. These are the postulated mechanisms resulting in the production of arrhythmias. Newer anti-depressive agents that inhibit re-uptake of serotonin, known as selective serotonin re-uptake inhibitors (SSRIs), do not manifest these same effects and are equally effective and safe in cardiac patients [13]. Since the association of depression and CAD was known much prior to the widespread use of TCAs, their effect on cardiac morbidity and mortality cannot be established.

There are few cardiac medications that have psychiatric side effects. Medications like digoxin, α-blockers, methyldopa, reserpine, clonidine and, rarely, ACE inhibitors are associated with the development of depression.

Lifestyle Risk Factors

The most widely studied risk factors are cigarette smoking, obesity and alcohol consumption, all of which affect the development, perpetuation and exacerbation of CAD. Cigarette smoking remains the single most important modifiable risk factor for CAD and the greatest single cause of preventable premature deaths. Psychological factors affect initiation, continuation, withdrawal from and relapse into smoking. Overall, people with mental illnesses like depression are likely to smoke more as compared to those without any disturbance. After cigarette smoking obesity is the second most studied risk factor. Evidence suggests that psychological factors, such as depression and stress contribute to behaviours like overeating in some individuals, thus, leading to development of obesity. Several neuronal and hormonal inputs to the hypothalamus modulate the release of neuropeptides known to affect food intake and energy expenditure [14, 15].

Other lifestyle risk factors that are closely associated with and studied as having some relationship with depression and CAD are alcohol consumption, sedentary lifestyle, high-risk behaviours and psychoactive substance use/abuse.

Depression can also lead to non-compliant behaviour towards various aspects of disease management and prevention. Studies have shown that depressed patients show various behaviours like poor compliance to prescribed medications, missing appointments, non-adherence to dietary and exercise regimen etc. This lack of involvement in behaviours of healthy living may play a role in explaining why depressed patients have increased morbidity and mortality after acute cardiovascular events [6, 16]. Finally, although unproven, it may be that depressed patients recognise and respond to symptoms less rapidly, thus, reducing the impact of aggressive therapies on their cardiovascular disease [17].

Catecholamines

Heart disease patients show high levels of circulating catecholamines levels such as adrenaline, epinephrine or norepinephrine. When associated with poor left ventricular function these endogenous neuroactive transmitters can be a trigger for malignant cardiac arrhythmias. Depression too is associated with high levels of norepinephrine spillover. Their combination can work synergistically, leading to increased frequency of sudden cardiac deaths. A higher prevalence of ventricular tachycardia during 24 h Holter monitoring among patients with CAD and depression than among CAD patients without depression has been noted, which may contribute to the explanation of increased risk for cardiac mortality in depressed patients with CAD.

Autonomic Dysfunction

Patients with depressive disorders show reduced heart rate variability (HRV). Reduced HRV becomes an important prognostic indicator as it is associated with sudden cardiac death. This HRV is referred to as autonomic dysfunction. Patients with both acute MI and depression have substantially worse HRV, even when other factors are taken into account. Abnormal HRV is known to presage an adverse prognosis in post-MI patients. Even in healthy subjects, depressed mood was related to the magnitude of decrease in parasympathetic cardiac control during stressors. Treatment of depression in patients with CAD leads to better parasympathetic tone, which is thought to be cardioprotective [18].

Platelets

Platelets play a key role in the pathogenesis of acute coronary syndromes and anti-platelet agents are now a mainstay of therapy. Increased platelet reactivity to orthostatic challenge and heightened circulating levels of β-thromboglobulin and platelet factor 4 – markers for platelet activation – are seen in patients suffering from depression. This finding leads to the hypothesis that depressed patients have increased likelihood of thrombus formation in response to thrombogenic stimuli. Serotonin, which is stored in platelets, plays an important role in platelet aggregation and thrombus formation. Also, preliminary data suggest that treatment with SSRIs reduces the level of platelet activation, further reducing the risk of MI to that of normal controls [19]. This is primarily mediated through their action to reduce capacity of platelets to store serotonin and further reducing the capacity to initiate thrombus formation.

Stress

There are many forms of stress. Many studies have demonstrated the adverse effects of stress on patients with pre-existing heart disease. Ischemia and malignant arrhythmias induced as a response to stress in also a known fact. Psychological stress can result in lowering of the threshold of life-threatening ventricular arrhythmias. The stress response may be modified in patients with depression [20]. This "stress response" usually evokes α-adrenergic stimulation, which results in vasoconstriction, thus, raising blood pressure (BP). Normally, coronary arteries dilate in response to increase in BP, while vasoconstriction is induced in patients with CAD. Many studies have shown that experimentally induced mental stress can lead to asymptomatic or silent ischemia in patients with pre-existing heart aliment [21]. Patients having such experimental stress induced asymptomatic ischemia are twice more likely to have fatal or non-fatal cardiac event. Mental tension, frustration and sadness double the risk of ischemia in CAD [22]. Natural disasters and extreme stressful situations can lead to substantial increase in sudden cardiac death and MI. In fact, using modern imaging techniques, it has been shown that stressful activities are actually capable of inducing ischemia [23, 24].

Inflammation

Inflammation has only recently been widely recognised as another process in the development of arthrosclerosis and MI. CAD patients show elevated levels of inflammatory cytokines. Progression of CAD can be predicted by extent of elevation of certain specific markers like interleukin (IL)-6, tumor necrosis factor (TNF)-α and C reactive protein. Depression too is associated with increases in markers of inflammation such as white blood cells, C-reactive protein, IL-6 and TNF-α, as well as shifts in the relative distribution of B and T cells. Enhanced inflammatory response associated with depression or chronic stress is believed to have some role in the development of CAD. "Sickness behaviour", a condition that mimics depression, can be seen in certain individuals with subchronic inflammation, which is thought to be a core feature of CAD. Thus, depression may turn out to be either a cause or an effect of inflammatory processes that are also involved in CAD.

It has also been hypothesised that hypercortisolemia and elevated levels of corticotropin-releasing factor may be as relevant as additional pathophysiologic mechanisms of depression linked to CAD as well as Ω-3 fatty acid deficiency and elevated homocysteine levels. Furthermore, endothelial dysfunction has been reported in depressed patients. Major depression in the absence of other conventional risk factors is associated with abnormal peripheral artery endothelial function [25].

Thus, abnormal platelet function, endothelial dysfunction, inflammation and reduced HRV along with stress and various lifestyle risk factors have been identified as possible links between depression and CAD. However, more research in large-scale clinical trials is needed to confirm these interrelationships and to assess their changes after anti-depressant treatment.

Diagnosis

Depression, among all the mental health issues, is most prevalent. It is a highly disabling disorder that is under diagnosed and under treated. It is a disorder characterised by multiple disabilities and relapses. Although treatment is possible and has excellent prognosis, its diagnosis becomes a bigger challenge initially. Especially when depression is associated with CAD, clinicians have to make extra effort and show enough sensitivity to diagnose it. Many studies indicate the failure to diagnose and treat depression in patients with CAD. Many of the symptoms overlap like loss of interest, fatigue and sleep disturbances. These are often regarded as an aftermath of surgery, MI or other CAD related event and not signs of depression. Unless a clear cause for symptoms of depression, such as insomnia due to sleep apnea syndrome or fatigue due to thyroid disorders is known, presence of such symptoms in patients with CAD should be regarded as signs of underlying depression.

Depression is diagnosed by the presence of one of the/both cardinal symptoms of depression – either loss of interest in various activities or depressed mood. In addition, presence of various other symptoms is also necessary to constitute the change as depression. These other symptoms are significant weight loss or gain, an increase or decrease in appetite, insomnia or hypersomnia, psychomotor agitation or retardation, fatigue or loss of energy, feelings of worthlessness, or excessive or inappropriate guilt, diminished ability to think or to concentrate, or indecisiveness, recurrent thoughts of death, recurrent suicidal ideation without a specific plan, a suicide attempt or a specific plan for committing suicide. Presence of total five or more of these symptoms along with at least one of the cardinal symptoms constitutes a depressive episode. To diagnose a major depressive episode, the symptoms must be present for most of the day, every day, for at least two weeks, preferably longer and they must result in impairment of daily activities [26]. Key elements that should alert the clinician, beyond the usual chronic sadness and loss of interest, include statements from the patient that life is "out of control", descriptions of anxiety (feeling strained by daily minor stresses, hypervigilance, multiple somatic complaints), signs of irritability (sudden bursts of anger and hostility, frequent negative and unpleasant comments to others, hypersensitivity to noise), and reports of chronic tiredness. Making the patients aware about the presence of depression in CAD and related problems can make them more aware about the change happening within them and promote help seeking behaviours.

Depression can reliably be diagnosed by psychometric scales and standardised clinical interviews. Various well-structured questionnaires have been used and validated in the screening process, such as the Hamilton Rating Scale for depression, the recent life change questionnaire, Montgomery Asberg Depression Rating Scale and the Beck Depression Inventory. In addition, short forms of questionnaires are available which screen for depression and other psychiatric disorders including mood, anxiety, alcohol, eating and somatoform disorders. It is important to utilise these simple validated questionnaires to diagnose depression in primary care settings. Certain differential diagnosis like vascular or atherosclerotic depression, especially following cerebrovascular event, alcoholism, sleep apnea syndrome, personality disorders, drugs induced (especially beta blockers) and hypothyroidism should be kept in mind.

Management

For managing depression associated with CAD it is important to understand the following four possible ways and the relations between them:

(i) Depression when biologically caused by CAD
(ii) An individual who carries a genetic vulnerability to depression manifests the onset of depression, triggered by CAD
(iii) Depression is psychologically caused by the presence of CAD
(iv) No casual relationship exists between CAD and depression

Cases (i) and (ii) warrant initial treatment directed at the management of CAD. Treatment for depression is advocated when depression persists in spite of recovery from CAD. When depression is the psychological reaction to CAD, specific treatment for CAD is optimised; education and anti-depressant medication along with appropriate psychotherapy is warranted to treat depression. In Case (iv), wherein the two conditions are not etiologically related, appropriate treatment for both of them is advised. The decision to treat depression also relies on the factors like the severity and duration of the current episode, severity and the number of past episodes, level of impairment, foreseeable level of stresses, comorbid psychiatric disorders and the level of social support.

Cases of severe major depression require immediate attention. Although criterion for diagnosis of depression requires presence of symptom pathology for at least two weeks, symptoms of such a short duration do not always warrant treatment initiation, especially when presented with CAD. A large number of depressed patients having recent MI show spontaneous recovery from their depressive symptoms following improvement in cardiac status. All the interventions should involve liaison work with physicians and psychiatrists, especially when patients are voicing suicidal thoughts [27].

Pharmacotherapy

Pharmacotherapy of depression is generally divided into two phases. The acute phase of management handles depressive symptoms and improves day-to-day functioning. This phase can last for 6 to 12 weeks. Once the patient has achieved remission, the maintenance phase starts where the objective is to prevent the relapse of depression. The duration of maintenance therapy is either 12 months or the duration of depressive episode, whichever is longer.

Anti-depressants

Anti-depressant medications remain the mainline of pharmacological management of depression associated with CAD. Due to lack of many randomised control trials for anti-depressant drugs in the management of depression with CAD one has to rely on data collected from patients with depression only. All anti-depressant medications are effective in treating depression of various severities. The goal of pharmacotherapy is to achieve remission with lesser or no side-effects and prevent relapse.

Cyclic Anti-depressants

Before the introduction of newer and cardiac friendly anti-depressant medications, cyclic anti-depressants like imipramine, amitryptyline, nortryotyline, desipramine and doxepine were the mainstay in treatment of depression with stable patients of CAD. TCAs have effects similar to quinidine on cardiac conduction and, thus, they are referred to as type 1A anti-arrhythmic agents. TCAs influence the adrenergic tone. Thus, although these agents have anti-arrhythmic properties, they can also be pro-arrhythmic. They have also been known to cause postural hypotension. Furthermore, TCAs have anti-cholinergic effects and a high potential for drug interaction. TCAs should be reserved for those patients who do not respond to other anti-depressant classes. Otherwise, generally, they should be avoided in the case of depressed patients with CAD [12, 28].

Selective Serotonin Re-uptake Inhibitors (SSRIs)

SSRIs – the newer class of anti-depressant medications – act by inhibiting the re-uptake of serotonin from the synaptic cleft. SSRIs have little to no cardiac side-effects in healthy subjects. The most common cardiac side-effect seen with SSRIs is the slowing of heart rate, generally, by a clinical significant one-two beats per minute. Potential benefits of SSRIs in decreasing cardiac mortality might be achieved by the increase of HRV. However, patients who are also taking warfarin need more frequent monitoring of their international normalised ratio (INR) [12].

Several studies have noted the effect of SSRIs on cardiac functions in patients with pre-existing heart disease. One study using fluoxetine and paroxetine in patients with pre-existing ventricular dysfunction showed improvement in ejection fraction to a small extent. In a study comparing paroxetine and nortrityline in treatment of depression following a cardiac event, both the medications were effective but paroxetine was better tolerated and less likely to produce cardiovascular side-effects [13]. Efficacy and tolerability of sertraline has been extensively studied in the treatment of depression following a MI. Around 400 patients participated in the study, which showed that sertraline was cardiac friendly and had excellent results in treating depression, especially in patients having prior history of depression. In the case of patient experiencing their first depressive episode, it was as efficacious as placebo [19].

Other Anti-depressants

The cardiovascular effects of other anti-depressants are studied less extensively, especially in patients with cardiac disease. Buproprion appears to have fewer cardiovascular side-effects, but may cause hypertension in some patients. The serotonin and norepinephrine re-uptake inhibitor (SNRI) group of medications like venlafaxine act as a SSRI at a low dose [29]. Their main cardiovascular side-effect is in the form of hypertension, which is dose dependent and usually seen beyond 150 mg per day. There are certain ongoing trials to ascertain whether anti-depressant treatment of post-MI depression, preferably with mirtazapine, can improve cardiac prognosis.

Side-effects of various anti-depressant medications can range from nervousness to fatigue to gastrointestinal discomfort leading to drop out rates of 15 to 25%. In order to minimise the side-effects the treatment should be started at a low dose and then gradually titrated upwards. Frequent visits during the initial phase of treatment can help monitor drugs efficacy and side-effects. At the same time, change in diet and the timing of medications also helps.

Other Psychotropic Medications

Anxiolytics

With no specific cardiac effects associated with its use benzodiazepines are used to treat certain mixed anxiety depression states. Reduction anxiety tends to reduce sympathetic tone and, therefore, slows heart rate, reduces myocardial work as well as myocardial irritability.

Stimulants

Stimulants are often useful for treating medically ill patients suffering from depression, particularly those with pronounced apathy, fatigue or psychomotor slowing. Methylphenidate, generally, at doses of 5-30 mg is well tolerated by patients with heart disease, including patients with cardiac arrhythmias and angina [30].

Cardiac and Psychiatry Drug Interactions

A few drug interactions between cardiac and psychotropic drugs are worth noting. Psychotropic drugs that lower the BP should be used with caution with drugs like anti-hypertensives, diuretics and vasodilators. TCAs, which prolongs QT interval, can interact with anti-arrhythmic agents like quinidine, procainamide and moricizine, resulting in further QT prolongation [31]. Anti-depressant agents that inhibit the cytochrome P450 liver isoenzyme system (e.g. paroxetine, fluoxetine and, probably, sertraline) should not be prescribed for patients taking class 1C anti-arrhythmic agents (e.g. encainide, flecainide, mexiletine and propafenone). In addition, these anti-depressants should be used cautiously in patients taking β-blockers, since they may augment β-blockade. Other inhibitors of the cytochrome P450 system, such as nefazodone and fluvoxamine, can interfere with the metabolism of calcium-channel blockers, some statins, some anti-arrhythmics and cyclosporine.

Psychotherapy

Patients who have suffered CAD experience various psychological reactions like feeling of anxiety and sadness, concern about one's survival, associated disabilities and effects on various other aspects of life. Denial as a reaction leads to abnormal illness behaviour, unnecessary disability and impaired quality of life. Making patients aware about the changes that they are going through and enabling them to handle various stressors constitutes an important area in management of depression associated with CAD.

Psychotherapeutic approach becomes an integral part of management, and various techniques like cognitive behavioural therapy, interpersonal therapy, insight oriented therapy and group therapy can be used to handle various issues. Cognitive behavioural therapy helps patient correct certain thought processes and perceptions. This, in turn, helps them to modify behaviour processes and handle stressors. Interpersonal therapy evaluates a patient's interactions with his/her environment with the aim to help the patient re-adjust to his/her interpersonal relationships and help create an environment where his/her emotional and behavioural needs are looked after. Insight oriented therapy and group therapy are focussed on creating more awareness among the patients and also giving them methods to handle their stress.

A large number of studies have demonstrated that stress management and health education programmes have beneficial effect on cardiac outcomes in cardiac rehabilitation setting [21, 27]. This also helps in improving biological risk factors like social isolation and smoking by providing emotional support and improving the quality of life. This finding was consistent across all ages and both genders. In patients with CAD, several small clinical trials suggest that cognitive-behavioural therapy successfully reduced anxiety and depression and, thus, facilitated the modification of cardiac risk factors.

Smoking is the most difficult of risk factors when it comes to intervention. This is principally due to the psychological and physiological dependence that an individual develops on nicotine after its long term consumption. Better quitting rates are achieved when both psychological and pharmacological treatment are used as compared to when both methods are used individually.

Behavioural treatments for obesity have shown results in mild to moderate cases, especially when the emphasis is on maintenance of behavioural change [15]. When combined with strategies like dieting, exercise and longitudinal measuring of various changes during the treatment period, such treatments have shown positive results.

Conclusion

Both CAD and depression are highly prevalent disorders. Depression serves as a marker of and, perhaps, as a contributor to an adverse cardiovascular prognosis. The clearest evidence of the link between CAD and depression, however, is found in the reverse situation, when the presence of CAD has already been established. Understanding and treating the patient who suffers from both CAD and depression is a challenge. CAD is associated with acute consequences, which is life threatening and it is the presenting complaint most of the times. Most of the times both patients and physicians tend to ignore the presence of depression, rating it as a part of cardiac morbidity. Ignorance to treat depression can lead to more complications and increased cardiac morbidity and mortality. The goal is to recognise the underlying depression and treat it. Both psychotherapy and pharmacotherapy are used in combination to treat depression in patients with cardiac disorders. Clearly, the most effective approach is to forge collaboration among cardiologists, psychiatrists, psychologists and internists, all of whom can work together in lifting depression in patients with cardiac disease.

Key Points

- ❑ Depression as a co-morbid condition in patients with CAD as a known entity.
- ❑ Depression can exist as a psychological reaction to, or can biologically affect, the development of CAD.
- ❑ Treatment of depression not only improves the quality of life but also improves cardiac prognosis of such patients.

- Pharmacotherapy, psychotherapy and cardiac rehabilitation form an important part of managing both depression and CAD.

References

1. Anda, R., Williamson, D., Jones, D. et al., 1993, "Depressed Affect, Hopelessness and the Risk of Ischemic Heart Disease in a Cohort of US Adults", *Epidemiology*, 4, pp. 285-294.
2. Barefoot, J. and Schroll, M., 1996, "Symptoms of Depression, Acute Myocardial Infraction and Total Mortality in a Community Sample", *Circulation*, 93, pp. 1976-1980.
3. Barefoot, J.C., Helms, M.J., Mark, D.B. et al., 1996, "Depression and Long-term Mortality Risk in Patients with Coronary Artery Disease", *Am. J. Cardiol.*, 78, pp. 613-617.
4. Carney, R.M., Blumenthal, J.A., Catellier, D. et al., 2003, "Depression as a Risk Factor for Mortality After Acute Myocardial Infraction", *Am. J. Cardiol.*, 92, pp. 1277-1281.
5. Frasure-Smith, N., Lesperance, F. and Talajic, M., 1995, "Depression and 18 Month Prognosis After Myocardial Infraction", *Circulation*, 91, pp. 999-1005.
6. Lesperance, F., Frasure-Smith, N., Juneau, M. et al., 2000, "Depression and One-year Prognosis in Unstable Angina", *Arch. Intern. Med.*, 160, pp. 1354-1360.
7. Glassman, A.H. and Sharpio, P.A., 1998, "Depression and the Course of Coronary Artery Disease", *Am. J. Psychiatry*, 155, pp. 4-11.
8. Frasure-Smith, N., Lesperance, F. and Talajic, M., 1993, "Depression Following Myocardial Infraction: Impact on 6 Month Survival", *JAMA*, 270, pp. 1819-1825.
9. Blumenthal, J.A., Lett, H.S., Babyak, M.A. et al., 2003, "Depression as a Risk Factor for Mortality After Coronary Artery Bypass Surgery", *Lancet*, 362, pp. 604-609.
10. Connerney, I., Sharpio, P.A., McLaughlin, J.S. et al., 2001, "Relation Between Depression After Coronary Artery Bypass Surgery and 12 Month Outcome: A Prospective Study", *Lancet*, 358, pp. 1766-1771.
11. Sharpio, P.A., DePena, M., Lidagoster, L. et al., 1998, "Depression After Coronary Artery Bypass Graft Surgery", *Psychosom. Med.*, 60, p. 108.
12. Roose, S.P., Glassman, A.H., Attia, E. et al., 1994, "Comparative Efficacy of Selective Serotonin Reuptake Inhibitors and Tricyclic in the Treatment of Melancholia", *Am. J. Psychiatry*, 151, pp. 1735-1739.
13. Sheline, Y.I., Freeland, K.E. and Carney, R.M., 1997, "How Safe are Serotonin Reuptake Inhibitors for Depression in Patients with Coronary Heart Disease?" *Am. J. Med.*, 102, pp. 54-59.
14. Power, C. and Parsons, T., 2000, "Nutritional and Other Influences in Childhood as Predictors of Adult Obesity", *Proc. Nutr. Soc.*, 59, pp. 267-272.
15. Rosenbaum, M., Leibel, R.L. and Hirsch, J., 1997, "Obesity", *N. Engl. J. Med.*, 337, pp. 396-406.
16. Faris, R., Purcell, H., Henein, M.Y. et al., 2002, "Clinical Depression is Common and Significantly Associated with Reduced Survival in Patients with Non-ischemic Heart Failure", *Eur. J. Heart Failure.*, 4, pp. 541-551.
17. Luutonen, S., Holm, H., Salminen, J.K. et al., 2002, "Inadequate Treatment of Depression After Myocardial Infraction", *Acta Psychiatr. Scand.*, 106, pp. 434-439.
18. Carney, R.M., Blumenthal, J.A., Stein, P.K. et al., 2001, "Depression, Heart Rate Variability and Acute Myocardial Infraction", *Circulation*, 104, pp. 2024-2028.
19. Glass, A.H., O'Connor, C.M., Califf, R.M. et al., 2002, "Sertraline Treatment of Major Depression in Patients with Acute MI or Unstable Angina", *JAMA*, 288, pp. 701-709.
20. Gullette, E.C.D., Blumenthal, J.A., Babyak, M. et al., 1997, "Effects of Mental Stress on Myocardial Infraction During Daily Life", *JAMA*, 277, pp. 1521-1525.

21. Krantz, D.S., Sheps, D.S., Carney, R.M. et al., 2000, "Effects of Mental Stress in Patients with Coronary Artery Disease: Evidence and Clinical Implications", *JAMA*, 283, pp. 1800-1802.
22. Leor, J., Poole, W.K. and Kloner, R.A., 1996, "Sudden Cardiac Death Triggered by an Earthquake", *N. Engl. J. Med.*, 334, pp. 413-419.
23. Orth-Gomer, K., Wamala, S.P., Horsten, M. et al., 2000, "Marital Stress Worsens Prognosis in Women with Coronary Artery Disease: The Stockholm Female Coronary Risk Study", *JAMA*, 284, pp. 3008-3014.
24. Jiang, W., Babyak, M., Krantz, D.S. et al., 1996, "Mental Stress-induced Myocardial Ischemia and Cardiac Event", *JAMA*, 275, pp. 1651-1656.
25. Cesari, M., Penninx, B.W.J.H., Newman, A.B. et al., 2003, "Inflammatory Markers and Onset of Cardiovascular Events: Results from the Health ABC Study", *Circulation*, 108, pp. 2317-2322.
26. American Psychiatric Association, 1994, *Diagnostic and Statistical Manual of Mental Disorders*, 4th Edn., American Psychiatric Association, Washington, D.C.
27. Penninx, B.W.J.H., Beekman, A.T.F., Honig, A. et al., 2001, "Depression and Cardiac Mortality", *Arch. Gen. Psychiatry*, 58, pp. 221-227.
28. Roose, S.P., Glassman, A.H. and Dalack, G.W., 1989, "Depression, Heart Disease and Tricyclin Antidepressants", *J. Clin. Psychiatry*, 50, pp. 12-16.
29. Roose, S.P., Dalack, G.W., Glassman, A.H. et al., 1991, "Cardiovascular Effects of Bupropion in Depressed Patients with Heart Disease", *Am. J. Psychiatry*, 148, pp. 512-516.
30. Masand, P.S. and Tesar, G.E., 1996, "Use of Stimulants in the Medically Ill", *Psychiar. Clin. North Am.*, 19, pp. 515-548.
31. Morganroth, J. and Goin, J.E., 1991, "Quinidine Related Mortality in the Short to Medium Term Treatment of Ventricular Arrhythmias", *Circulation*, 84, pp. 1977-1983.

The AHA-Syndrome and Cardiovascular Diseases
Editors: Swati Y. Bhave and Sunil Saini
Copyright © 2010 Anamaya Publishers, New Delhi, India

19. Understanding Non-violence as an Alternative to Violence

Manisha Sen
Department of Applied Psychology, University of Mumbai, Mumbai - 400 032, India

Abstract: The history of India and the world is strife with increasing violence. There is evidence of accounts of rivalry and war. There are celebrations of lives of war heroes, attempts made to recall national victories and sense of pride in violence and the ability to defeat others. Thus, we are living in a paradox. Man is at the crossroads with an ever-increasing capacity to comprehend as well as ascend the universe and, yet, in view of nuclear developments, there is an imminent threat of total annihilation. Attention needs to be directed to these negative consequences of war and look for preserving behaviours rather than destructive ones. For most people absence of war is peace. Both these concepts have far reaching implications for individuals and societies. The primary concepts to be understood in this context are: aggression, violence and non-violence as an alternative to violence.

Keywords: Aggression, Violence, Non-violence, Health.

Definition of Aggression, Violence and Non-violence

Buss [1] explained aggression in terms of behaviour that results in harm or hurt to others. This view is limited in its approach as it ignores the 'intention' of the person who performs the act. Dollard et al. [2] referred to intention to include the aspect of goal response. The goal of an aggressive act or behaviour would be to inflict injury or harm on another object or person. Aggression was defined as "the delivery of noxious stimulus to another with the intent of harming that person and in the expectation that the aversive stimulation will reach its destination" [3]. Thus, aggression can be understood as harm or injury – physical or psychological – to another. Besides, aggression occurs only when the victim is motivated to avoid such treatment.

Buss [1] has classified various types of aggression across three dimensions, viz. physical/verbal, active/passive and direct/indirect. Examples of these kinds of aggressive acts can be seen in behaviours like stabbing another person, having an assassin to kill an enemy, a sit in demonstration, refusing to perform necessary tasks, insulting another person, spreading malicious rumours, refusing to answer questions, failing to speak up in another person's defence when the latter is being unfairly criticised.

It is generally thought that control of aggression is the best way of dealing with pressure. Lorenz [4] in his theory of aggression expressed the view that aggression can be prevented from accumulating to dangerous levels by indulging in minor non-injurious aggressive actions. Providing an angry individual with an opportunity to 'blow off steam' in some safe and non-injurious manner was assumed to cause them to feel better and weaken their tendency to engage in overt and potentially dangerous acts of aggression. This was termed as the *catharsis hypothesis*. The concept of catharsis is a part of the hydraulic model of personality, which is based on the analogy to a liquid held under pressure in a container or reservoir. Each increase in the liquid increases the pressure for release. Now, each time there is drainage, there is a decrease in pressure for release. The pressure is similar to aggressive impulses. The walls of the reservoir stand for inhibitions against the expression of aggressive impulses. The draining of the reservoir is the expression of aggression. Pressure is determined by the amount of remains in the reservoir. Thus, the less the remains in the reservoir, the less pressure is exerted by the impulse seeking release. This expression of aggression is called catharsis, and a diminution in the tendency to aggress as a consequence of this expression of aggression is called the cathartic effect.

Aggression may be perceived as a continuum with violence and non-violence as its two extreme manifestations. Violence occurs when the act engenders direct, acute insults to the psychological or physical well-being of individuals or groups and they erupt periodically as events or episodes. Violence may be direct or indirect. Bondurant [5] defined violence as "the wilful application of force in such a way that it is intentionally injurious to the person or group against whom it is applied". This definition includes physical as well as psychological harm. Bond [6] defined violence as "the use of physical force against another's body, against that person's will, and that is expected to inflict physical injury or death upon that person".

Uzma Mazhar [7] discussed the concept of *hate violence* and *hate crimes*. She conceptualised hate violence as any act of intimidation, harassment, physical force or threat of physical force directed against any person, or family, or their property or advocate. Such acts are motivated either in whole or in part by hostility to their real or perceived race, ethnic background, religious belief, sex, age, disability, or sexual orientation, with the intention of causing fear or intimidation, or to deter the free exercise or enjoyment of any rights or privileges secured by the law. Hate violence punishable under a criminal statute was termed as hate crime by her.

While the attempt to curb violence is a curative step, emphasis on the preventive aspect is required. This leads to attention being given to the concept of *peace building*.

Violence reflects instinctual, self-centred and immature approach to life that humans can have. But the progress and peace of humanity lies in cooperation, selflessness and other directedness. Individuals respond to violence in many ways. While some would rather avoid or ignore it, others are likely to rationalise its occurrence.

Mohandas Karamchand Gandhi put forth a different method of dealing with violence. He suggested the use of *non-violence* to combat violence. Non-violence may be active or passive. Active non-violence implies cultivation of a positive form of social action or a system of values. Passive non-violence involves negation or avoidance of certain actions like killing, hurting, revengefulness etc. It can also be understood in terms of principled and pragmatic non-violence. Sharp [8] defined non-violence as "noninjury in thought, word and deed to all forms of life". This views non-violence as a way of life. Thus, in the face of violence such individuals are likely to react with compassion, sacrifice, anti-punitiveness and forbearance. This value is seen in great persons like Gandhi, Nelson Mandela and Martin Luther King. But most of us cannot be like them. It is suggested to begin with using non-violence as a technique. Thus, an individual uses it as a way of dealing with differences or conflict through various forms of behaviour like non-cooperation, protests, self-punishment etc.

While the catharsis hypothesis is one explanation for reduction of aggression, there are various other theories of aggression, which emphasise factors like guilt [9] as explanation for reduction in aggression. Sen [10] contended that various theories appear to create a controversial scenario like the cathartic effect vis-à-vis the guilt mechanisms as explanations for reduction of aggression. In order to understand the role of these explanations it is pertinent to place emphasis on the type of people who may differ in their manifestation of aggression. Individuals may deal with conflict in violent or non-violent manner.

Violent and Non-violent Individuals: Genesis in Terms of Personality

The lack of conclusiveness in the theories on the reduction of aggression is the main problem. These varied criticisms arise, probably, due to the fact that no emphasis has been placed on the type of people who aggress. Although a lot of work has been done in the field of aggression to study its negative aspects, e.g. effects of instigation, annoyance, arousal etc., there has been little work done on its control and reduction.

Hence, it is absolutely necessary to analyse the personality system and behaviour patterns of those individuals who are committed to non-violence and, yet, show aggressive behaviour of their own type. For example, in India there are a number of followers of Gandhi who preach and practice non-violence and keep their aggression passively verbal and self-oriented (e.g. fasting or other self punishment methods).

Sen [10, 11] sketched a conceptual portrait of the non-violent personality that emphasises four dimensions of moral and ethical development. The prototypical non-violent individual is strongly empathic, thoroughly capable of envisioning the other's perspective, passionately committed to high moral and ethical principles, and highly pro-social and altruistic. Furthermore, the proponent of non-violence is committed to action when confronted with injustice. Finally, the non-violent person is strongly inhibited about harming others. In these cases the usual definition of aggression, that it involves delivery of noxious stimuli to the other person, does not really hold good. But then obstruction, resistance, modelling, defiance of law, hunger strike etc., are examples that show direct or indirect, passive or active ways in which 'noxious stimuli' are delivered to the other person or to oneself. Objections may be raised to the use of the term 'noxious stimuli' in the case of aggression of the non-violent person because his/her aim is to purify the other person without any intention to harm him/her. But then, a violent individual can also claim the same motive with emphasis differing only on the degree of noxious stimuli delivered.

A number of other contrasting features between these two types of people can be reified. While the non-violent individual does not show increase in aggression upon instigation and maintains an organised and controlled form, the violent individual's aggression flares up with instigation and annoyance. The latter's aggression is of a swift type with immediacy as its essence. The non-violent is more passive. The violent individual aggresses to show his/her power and to achieve the reinforcer, while the non-violent shows aggression to share the reinforcer or part away with it in goodwill. Thus, the non-violent individual's aggression has instrumentality. The violent individual is more arbitrary and indiscriminate in his/her behaviour pattern, while this is not so with the non-violent type who is more rational in his/her approach.

Factors Underlying Violence, their relation to Health and Psychological Consequences like Depression or Suicide

At the basis of violence are factors like fear, labelling others as 'bad' and reacting negatively towards them. In times of insecurity and fear, it does not take much for a stressed person to think that "others are bad because they are different from me" and "others have caused all my problems, and I am going to do something about it", thus, looking for a scapegoat. Some negative emotions involved are anger, resentment, depression (at times), sadness etc. Such an individual is preoccupied with the desire to take revenge and be non-forgiving. While violence has an element of coercion, non-violence involves persuasion. Richard Gregg [12] in his classic book *The Power of Non-violence* points out that when an individual responds to violence with violence, in essence, he/she justifies the violent act of the attacker. If the response is non-violent, then the individual would have created a kind of moral jiu-jitsu, a situation in which the lack of physical opposition by the user of psychic jiu-jitsu causes the attacker to lose his/her moral balance.

Robert Ginsberg [13] asserted that non-violence must be understood as resistance to violence. It is an active engagement in defeating violence by winning over hearts. The non-violent individual is able to win the conquest within, which releases considerable energy as a positive gain for active living. Thus, non-violence is not mere negation or neutralising, but it is dynamic and activating.

Variables Having a Correlation with Non-violence and Health

Selye [14] related stress to constitutional weaknesses and Oetgen [15] related it to immunological weaknesses. A relationship between stress resistance and health practices like paced respiration has also been established [16]. But psychologists have observed that if a negative event is appraised in a manner that changes the perceived degree of stressfulness of that event, with action promoted to facing it, the consequences are likely to be healthy.

Kobasa [17] proposed the concept of *hardiness* which includes a "constellation of personality characteristics that function as a resistance resource in the encounter with stressful events". Such an individual is more likely to be physically and mentally healthy. These individuals reflect commitment, control and challenge in their disposition.

Hardiness is an important variable to be considered. Ganellen and Blaney [18] reported that alienation from self, a component of commitment, was related to depression. Composite Hardiness Score was observed to predict depression where individuals high on hardiness score showed less depression. Maddi et al. [19] observed that alienation measured by commitment was positively related to optimism. Rhodewalt and Agustsdottir [20] reported that hardy individuals have a high tendency to perceive events as positive.

The relationship between hardiness and physical health was studied by Kobasa et al. [21, 22]. A significant relationship between hardiness and later illness was observed by Weibe and McCallum [23]. However, Schmeid and Lawler [24] found no significant relationship between these two variables. In the study by Weibe [25], results suggested that hardiness has a moderating effect on stress. This effect occurs because of adaptive stress appraisal processes. In addition, Contrada [26] has reported that Type-B individuals, high on hardiness score, have a low diastolic blood pressure and also demonstrate least anger.

An interactive relationship between stress, hardiness and psychosomatic illness was demonstrated by Shepperd and Kashani [27]. They observed that individuals who experience high stress but have high control and commitment show less psychosomatic symptoms than individuals with high stress and low control and commitment. Glass and Singer [28] demonstrated that subjects who had greater perceived control also showed a greater tolerance of frustration. Seligman [29] postulated that individuals exhibiting control over their actions will not exhibit learned helplessness.

Other important variable is *resilience*. Resilience has a relationship with productivity and non-violence. This theory was postulated by Joseph [30] who asserted that hardiness is a component of resilience. The theoretical model is presented below:

What goes in to resilience		What comes out of resilience
Hardiness	R	Productivity
	E	
Other orientedness	S	
	I	
Self-efficacy and inner control	L	Stress resistance
	I	
Coherence	E	
	N	
Positive disposition	C	
Channel negative feelings in positive ways	E	Non-violence

Source: Joseph [30].

Joseph suggested that encouraging cooperative behaviour as against competitive behaviour, promoting social sensitivity to the needs of others, teaching effective problem solving skills and training in taking responsibility, is likely to bring about increase in interpersonal understanding, tolerance and self and social efficacy. These are essential ingredients for a non-violent personality.

In a study by Chandra and Sen [31], hardiness predicted non-violent predisposition, explaining the variance of nearly 4%, which was significant at the 0.001 level. These results implied that individuals with a hardy personality are likely to be non-violent. Kobasa [17] conceptualised hardiness as having three components, viz. challenge, commitment and inner locus of control. The component of challenge envisages an individual as accepting change and novelty as a normal phenomenon in life. The component of commitment describes hardiness as "an ability to believe in truth, importance and interest values of what one is doing, and the willingness to exercise influence or control in the personal and social situations in which one is involved" [32]. Therefore, it can be concluded that a hardy individual, when faced with a stressful situation, is likely to take charge of the situation, interpret stress as a challenge and work toward resolving the stress in a manner that would help to achieve his/her goals. Such individuals are likely to have an increased tolerance of frustration and, hence, do not exhibit hostile behaviour. These findings imply that an individual with a hardy personality, committed to his/her goals and who takes responsibility even in adverse circumstances is likely to be non-violent.

The study by Apter et al. [33] attempted to identify variables having a correlation to the risk of suicide. Two patient groups that differed mainly in their level of expressed aggression were included in this study. Results revealed that in the non-violent patient group there was a high correlation between risk of suicide and sadness. However, among the violent patients there was no correlation between these variables. The low correlation between sadness and risk of suicide in the violent patients, and the low prevalence of affective disorder diagnoses in these patients compared to other patients, suggested that suicidal risk should be managed differently in highly violent patients as compared to others.

The analysis of correlations in the violent group showed that lack of impulse control, anger, fear, instability, suspiciousness, rebelliousness, and state and trait anxiety were positively correlated to risk of suicide, whereas, calmness was negatively correlated to risk of suicide. In the non-violent group a similar pattern existed. There were, however, two striking differences in the pattern of correlations between the groups after risk of violence was partialed out. In the forensic patients (with history of violence), but not the municipal hospital patients (without history of violence), there was a highly significant correlation between anger and risk of suicide ($r = 0.71$, $p < 0.001$). There was a significant correlation between sadness and suicide risk in the non-violent patients ($r = 0.52$, $p < 0.01$) but not in the violent patients. In addition, happiness correlated negatively and significantly to suicide risk in the non-violent patients ($r = -0.57$, $p < 0.01$) but not in the violent patients.

Apter et al. [33] explained the low correlation between sadness and suicide risk in the violent patients in terms of an ego defect in such patients that inhibits the expression of depressive symptoms. This hypothesis is supported by their finding of a significant correlation between anger and suicide risk in violent patients but not in non-violent patients. These findings can be explained in terms of Sen's portrayal of the violent personality vis-à-vis non-violent personality. It supports the conceptual framework comparing the two personalities. She explains that while the non-violent person does not show increase in aggression upon the instigation, the violent individual flares up and is affected by the degree of self-arousal in him/her. This strongly implies that the dynamics underlying aggression of the violent and non-violent individuals is different.

There are studies, which have reported the relation between personality attributes and medical conditions like cancer and heart pathology. A predictive relationship between some personality attributes and cancer and heart disease has been documented by Ronald Grossarth-Maticek et al. [34]. They claimed that disease-prone personality types are those wherein emotions are repressed and it is accompanied with a feeling of hopelessness, resulting in cancer. Also, their findings that hostility and aggression cause heart problems fit in very well with the other findings that have shown the health-personality connection. He claimed that personality type predicts a death from cancer six times better than smoking does. Research done at the Johns Hopkins School of Medicine demonstrates that people who go through life behaving passively, like doormats, appear to get more than their share of cancer. A number of animal studies have shown that certain strains of rats living in a stressful environment are very prone to the disease. Grossarth-Maticek and Eysenck [35, 36] reported strong evidence for the role of psychotherapy in preventing cancer and heart problems. Other studies have shown that human hostility and cynicism are two hallmarks of the notorious Type-A behaviour pattern that leads to heart trouble.

However, Joshua Fischman [37] held the view that the classic Type-As, showing harried and hostile behaviour, may not always suffer from heart trouble. The predisposing factor may be the high frequency of situations with interpersonal conflicts and a cynical worldview. These situations when followed by an extreme bodily reaction to stress, including increased heart rate, blood pressure and blood flow to the muscles (part of the "flight or fight" response to a threat) may be the most relevant factors causing heart damage.

Edward Suarez, a psychologist at Duke University Medical Center, and his colleagues [38, 39] have found a link between high hostility and bodily responses. They asked a group of students to solve word puzzles. Suarez then added an element of harassment to the experiment and got strikingly different results. Under these circumstances they found that "high hostiles do tend to react with greater increases in blood pressure and blood flow". High hostiles also reported feeling a lot more angry, with their blood pressure remaining high for about 15 minutes after they completed the puzzles. The results were interpreted to imply that high hostiles tended to view other people's actions and motives very cynically. They thought the researchers were "out to get them", felt threatened and reacted, while low hostiles did not perceive the researchers actions as such a personal attack.

Attribution

Ross [40] has presented A Model of the Psychological Causes of Oppositional Political Terrorism which consists of five etiological factors: the development of facilitating traits, frustration or narcissism-aggression, associational drives, learning opportunities, and cost-benefit calculations.

Gutmann [41] examined the view that specific personality characteristics predispose certain people to engage individually in terrorism, join terrorist organisations, and/or commit this type of political violence on behalf of the group. A few of the more prominent characteristics are, from least to the most reported: fear, hostility, depression, guilt, anti-authoritarianism, perceived lack of manliness, self-centredness, extreme extroversion, need for high risks or stress, and alienation.

Although periodically discredited [42], some researchers have expressed the view that terrorism is caused by frustration manifested in aggression. This frustration may arise from the accumulation of grievances. The psychological injury, caused by blows to their ego leads to aggression, if an individual encounters an appropriate target. Terrorism can be labelled as a form of collective violence. In keeping with Sutherland's [43] concept of differential association, a reason for joining terrorist organisations for some individuals is a conscious or unconscious attempt to affiliate with others who share similar personalities, can provide benefits and fulfill their individual goals adding a sense of belonging. In particular, Post [44] suggested that viewing the group as all good and society as all bad is central to the group's ideology and is the rationale for committing acts of violence against the established authorities. Thus, it reflects an either/or pattern of attribution in keeping with Baumgardner's findings [45].

Terrorism can also be explained in terms of learning theories involving processes like positive reinforcements and punishments [46, 47]. The decision to engage in a terrorist action is also a function of a conscious or unconscious cost-benefit analysis [48, 49].

An individual's reaction to any situation is determined by attribution of the intent behind another person's behaviour. Attributions are critical mediators to the social world. The behaviour of one individual towards another frequently depends upon interpretations made of the world in terms of causal attributions made for specific events.

Sources of Misperception

There is a distinction between errors that are now usually called *motivated errors* and those that are called *cognitive* or *unmotivated*. Motivated errors are those that seem to serve a definable human need, such as the need to think well of oneself or to clear oneself of guilt. Cognitive or unmotivated errors can be defined simply as those in which no specific psychological need is evident. Another cognitive error is premature cognitive closure, which leads to inadequately considered decisions. A third cognitive error, underlying the second, is a lazy tendency to avoid the complicated kinds of thinking (cognitive complexity) that realism requires: making necessary distinctions, seeing alternative explanations, and considering adequately alterative courses of action.

Processes of Misperceptions

Selective Inattention

What is not said is often more significant than what is said. 'Sins' of omission are often more frequent and potent in producing misperception than sins of commission.

Slanted Interpretation

This occurs when in an ambiguous situation, the mind prefers the explanation that best suits the purpose of rationalisation or projection.

Studies have brought out the role of factors like perception and attribution. There is a link between the attributions an individual makes of an event and the effect it will have on his/her behaviour. Abramson et al. [50] formulated that in situations where the person attributes a cause of uncontrollable events to internal factors as opposed to external factors, stable factors as opposed to unstable factors and global factors as opposed to specific factors, helplessness and depression is likely to occur.

It is important to note that even for Gandhi, non-violence was not a simple or absolute rejection of violent action. In fact, violence was preferable to cowardice in the face of injustice. Justice and non-violence are central and coexisting values. Ideally, justice is sought through non-violent means. The study by Steve R. Baumgardner [45] tried to identify violent and non-violent individuals, as defined by the Non-violent Test [51] and to investigate the differences between violent and non-violent individuals in judgments of cause, responsibility and blame for rape. Results indicated that judgments for the rapist and the victims are at opposite ends of the scale for the violent group, and much less so for the non-violent group. Responsibility and blame for the victim are especially distinct between the two groups, with non-violent individuals assigning more responsibility and blame for the victim than violent individuals.

While violent individuals' attributions reflected an either/or judgment pattern, the non-violent individuals' attribution did not reveal this pattern. The latter held both, the rapist and the victim, as responsible. It was also observed that non-violent persons attributed more causality, responsibility and blame to rape victims, when the victims responded violently or did nothing (inaction). Less blame was attributed when the victim was verbally aggressive or tried to humanise the rapist. It was observed that violent individuals tended to make attributions according to a "cost/accounting just world view".

Research has suggested that biases in children's social perception may act as mediators of deviant interpersonal aggressive behaviour. According to Dodge [52], aggressive boys are more likely to attribute hostility to peers in ambiguous situations than non-aggressive boys. Dodge and Newman [53] stipulated that aggressive boys responded more quickly and with less attention to available social cues as compared to non-aggressive boys. They suggested that aggressive boys could be trained to respond after paying attention to social cues. This is likely to lead to reduction of aggressive behaviour. Weiner et al. [54], have provided empirical evidence linking specific causal attributions to anger and arousal. According to them, anger is experienced when an individual holds another person responsible for the negative or harmful consequences of social transactions. Fondacaro and Heller [55] also established that attributing blame to others in personally threatening situations serves to externalise the negative affect. Thus, studies have revealed that cognitive distortions play an important part in promoting aggressive behaviour. Hence, it would be important to understand these attributions and re-style them to help reduce aggression.

Seligman [29] observed that individuals with a non-violent predisposition have an attributional style for negative events, which is different from that of violent individuals. Kool [56], and Kool and Sen [51] have measured non-violent behaviour. In a study by Chandra and Sen [31], it was observed that non-violent individuals attribute internal and controllable causes to negative events demonstrating a specific attributional style. In view of this research finding the pertinence of attribution therapy becomes evident. If the belief structure of the cause of an event is changed, it would result in phenomenologically changing the perception of the event. It is pertinent, therefore, to take a proactive approach in reducing aggression in society through appropriate intervention.

Research with adults and children has shown that both adults and children on experiencing catastrophic events show a wide range of reactions such as fear, depression, withdrawal or anger, which can occur immediately or some time after the tragic event [57, 58]. March et al. [59] postulated that the more direct the exposure to the traumatic event, the higher the risk for emotional harm. Children and adolescents experience loss of trust in adults, fear of events occurring again [60-63], show regressive behaviour, suicidal thoughts, depression and anxiety. These kinds of consequences are greater for those who have been victims of earlier incidents of trauma [64-67] and who lack family support [68].

Research has indicated a link between affect and cognition, which then impacts behaviour. Sen [69] conducted an interventional study that emphasised the importance of:

(i) Identification of the nature of attribution along three dimensions, viz. causality in terms of internal/external locus of control, controllability and stability.
(ii) The use of cognitive restructuring for changing the attributions where required.

Research has revealed that cognitive distortions play an important part in promoting aggressive behaviour. The attributions made by an individual for negative events determine the emotional response. In view of this, the proposed intervention programme on attribution restyling would help in reducing aggressive behaviour in society. The results of this research will have far reaching implications. It would help in the following ways:

(i) Help orient individuals to identify the role of attribution in determining their aggressive behaviour.
(ii) Replication with other target groups.
(iii) Training of trainers to help implement such an intervention programme.

Conclusion

The present chapter has attempted to present the relevance of non-violence as an alternative to violence. It is important to understand that violence has negative consequences for all those involved. Since it impacts the emotional framework of a person, hence, it has both physical and psychological consequences for the individual and society at large. Here, the author has attempted to bring out the relation between non-violence and its positive health consequences. Interventions in keeping with research on non-violence have been brought out to convey that non-violence is not inaction but action. If we follow the rule "an eye for an eye", it would end up making the whole world blind. The only alternative is non-violence. The late Mrs. Indira Gandhi [70] said that "Development, independence, disarmament and peace are closely related. Can there be peace alongside nuclear weapons? Without peace all our dreams of development will turn to ashes. No Peace today – No life tomorrow".

Key Points

- With increasing violence in the society, there is an imminent threat of total annihilation.
- There is a great need to understand the concepts of aggression, violence and non-violence.
- Non-violence is an important alternative to violence and there is a positive relationship with physical and psychological consequences for the individual and society at large.

References

1. Buss, A.H., 1961, *The Psychology of Aggression*, Widen, New York.
2. Dollard, J., Doob, L., Miller, N., Mowrer, O.H. and Sears, R.R., 1939, *Frustration and Aggression*, Yale University Press, New Haven, Connecticut.
3. Geen, R.G., 1990, *Human Aggression*, Brook/Cole, Pacific Grove, California, p. 28.
4. Lorenz, K., 1996, *On Aggression*, Harcourt, Brace and World, New York.
5. Bondurant, J.V., 1988, *Conquest of Violence: The Gandhian Philosophy of Conflict*, New Revised Edn., Princeton University Press, Princeton, New Jersey, p. 9.
6. Bond, D., 1994, "Nonviolent Direct Action and the Diffusion of Power", In *Justice Without Violence*, W. Paul, H. Burgess and G. Burgess (Eds.), Lynne Rienner Publishers, London, p. 9.
7. Mazhar, U., "Hate Violence and Hate Crimes", *www.crescentlife.com*
8. Sharp, G., 1979, *Gandhi as a Political Strategist*, Allen and Unwin, Boston, Massachusetts, p. 134.
9. Berkowitz, L., 1974, "Some Determinants of Impulsive Aggression: The Role of Mediated Associations with Reinforcements for Aggression", *Psychological Review*, 81, pp. 165-176.
10. Sen, M., 1996, *Reducing Aggression*, Famous Publishers, New Delhi, India.
11. Sen, M., 1993, "Non-violence: An Empirical Study in India", In *Non-violence: Social and Psychological Issues*, V.K. Kool (Ed.), University Press of America, Inc., pp. 157-166.
12. Gregg, R., 1938, *The Power of Non-violence,* Navajivan Press, Ahmedabad.

13. Ginsberg, R., 1993, "The Paradoxes of Violence, Moral Violence and Non-violence", In *Nonviolence: Social and Psychological Issues*, V.K. Kool (Ed.), University Press of America, Inc., pp. 161-167.
14. Selye, H., 1956, *The Stress of Life*, McGraw-Hill, New York.
15. Oetgen, H.T., 1977, "Immunotherapy of Cancer", *New England Journal of Medicine*, 297, pp. 484-491.
16. McCaul, K.D., Solomon, S. and Holmes, D.S., 1979, "Effects of Paced Respiration and Expectations on Physiological and Psychological Responses to Threat", *Journal of Personality and Social Psychology*, 37, pp. 564-571.
17. Kobasa, S.C., 1979, "Stressful Life Events, Trait Situations", *Journal of Consulting and Clinical Psychology*, 46, pp. 280-287.
18. Ganellen, R.J. and Blaney, P.H., 1984, "Hardiness and Social Support as Moderators of the Effects of Life Stress", *Journal of Personality and Social Psychology*, 47, pp. 156-163.
19. Maddi, S.R., Kobasa, S.C. and Hoover, M., 1979, "An Alienation Test", *Journal of Humanistic Psychology,* 19, pp. 73-76.
20. Rhodewalt, F. and Agustsdottir, S., 1984, "On the Relationship of Hardiness to the Type A Behaviour Pattern: Perception of Life Events vs. Coping with Life Events", *Journal of Research in Personality*, 18, pp. 212-223.
21. Kobasa, S.C., Maddi, S.R. and Courington, S., 1981, "Personality and Constitution as Mediators in the Stress Illness Relationship", *Journal of Health and Social Behaviour*, 22, pp. 368-378.
22. Kobasa, S.C., Maddi, S.R. and Kahn, S., 1982, "Hardiness and Health: A Prospective Inquiry", *Journal of Personality and Social Psychology*, 42, pp. 168-177.
23. Weibe, D.J. and McCallum, D.M., 1986, "Health Practices and Hardiness as Mediators in the Stress-illness Relationship", *Health Psychology*, 5, pp. 425-438.
24. Schmeid, L.A. and Lawler, K.A., 1986, "Hardiness, Type A Behaviour and the Stress-illness Relationship in Working Women", *Journal of Personality and Social Psychology*, 51, pp. 1218-1223.
25. Weibe, D.J., 1991, "Hardiness and Stress Moderation: A Test Proposed Mechanism", *Journal of Personality and Social Psychology*, 60, pp. 89-99.
26. Contrada, R.J., 1989, "Type-A Behaviour, Personality Hardiness and Cardiovascular Responses to Stress", *Journal of Personality and Social Psychology*, 57, pp. 895-903.
27. Shepperd, J.A. and Kashani, J.H., 1991, "The Relationship of Hardiness, Gender and Stress to Health Outcomes in Adolescents", *Journal of Personality*, 59, pp. 747-768.
28. Glass, D.C. and Singer, J.E., 1972, *Urban Stress*, Academic Press, New York.
29. Seligman, M.E.P., 1975, *Helplessness: On Depression, Development and Death*, Freeman, San Francisco.
30. Joseph, J.M., 1993, "Resiliency and its Relationship to Productivity and Non-violence", In *Non-violence: Social and Psychological Issues*, V.K. Kool (Ed.), University Press of America, Inc., pp. 138-139.
31. Chandra, L. and Sen, M., 2001, "An Empirical Study of Correlates of Nonviolent Behaviour", Unpublished, Mumbai.
32. Kobasa, S.C. 1982, "The Hardy Personality: Toward a Social Psychology of Stress and Health", In *Social Psychology of Health and Illness*, G.S. Sanders and J. Suls (Eds.), Erlbaum, New Jersey, pp. 3-32.
33. Apter, A., Kotler, M., Sevy, S., Plutchik, R., Brown, S., Foster, H., Hilibrand, M., Korn, M. and Praag, H., 1991, "Correlates of Risk of Suicide in Violent and Nonviolent Psychiatric Patients", *American Journal of Psychiatry*, 148, pp. 883-887.
34. Grossarth-Maticek, R., Siegrist, J. and Vetter, H., 1982, "Interpersonal Repression as a Predictor of Cancer", *Social Science and Medicine*, 16, pp. 493-498.

35. Grossarth-Maticek, R. and Eysenck, H.J., 1995, "Self-Regulation and Mortality from Cancer, Coronary Heart Disease and Other Causes: A Prospective Study", *Personality and Individual Differences*, 19(6), pp. 781-795; *Research and Therapy* 1994, 16, pp. 167-215.
36. Grossarth-Maticek, R. and Eysenck, H.J., 1991, "Creative Novation Behavioral Therapy as a Prophylactic Treatment for Cancer and Coronary Heart Disease: Part I – Description of Treatment", *Behavioral Research and Therapy*, 29(1), pp. 1-16; Part II, pp. 17-32.
37. Fischman, J., 1988, "The Character of Controversy: Fighting Cancer and Heart Disease", *Psychology Today*, p. 22.
38. Suarez, E.C. and Williams, R.B., 1989, "Situational Determinants of Cardiovascular and Emotional Responses in High and Low Hostile Men", *Psychosomatic Medicine*, 51, pp. 404-418.
39. Suarez, E.C. and Williams, R.B., 1990, "The Relationships between Dimensions of Hostility and Cardiovascular Reactivity as a Function of Task Characteristics", *Psychosomatic Medicine*, 52, pp. 558-570.
40. Ross, J.I.A., 1996, "Model of the Psychological Causes of Oppositional Political Terrorism", *Journal of Peace and Psychology*, 2(2), p. 129.
41. Gutmann, D., 1979, "Killers and Consumers: The Terrorist and His Audience", *Social Research*, 46, pp. 516-526.
42. Friedland, N., 1992, "Becoming a Terrorist: Social Individual Antecedents", In *Terrorism: Roots, Impact, Responses*, L. Howard (Ed.), Praeger, New York, pp. 81-93.
43. Sutherland, E.H., 1947, *Principles of Criminology*, 4th Ed., Lippincott, Philadelphia.
44. Post, J.M., 1986, "Hostilite, Conformite, Fraternite: The Group Dynamics of Terrorist Behaviour", *International Journal of Group Psychotherapy*, 36(2), pp. 211-214.
45. Baumgardner, S.R., 1993, "Attribution of Cause, Responsibility, and Blame Among Violent and Nonviolent Individuals", In *Non-violence: Social and Psychological Issues*, V.K. Kool (Ed.), University Press of America, Inc., pp. 54-64.
46. Skinner, B.F., 1938, *The Behaviour of Organisms: An Experimental Analysis*, Appleton-Century-Crofts, New York.
47. Bandura, A., 1973, *Aggression: A Social Learning Analysis*, Prentice Hall, Englewood Cliffs, New Jersey.
48. Crenshaw, M., 1990a, "The Logic of Terrorism: Terrorist Behaviour as a Product of Strategic Choice", In *Origins of Terrorism*, W. Reich (Ed.), Cambridge University Press, pp. 7-24.
49. Corrado, R.R., 1981, "A Critique of the Mental Disorder Perspective of Political Terrorism", *International Journal of Law and Psychiatry*, 4, pp. 1-17.
50. Abramson, L., Seligman, M.E.P. and Teasdale, J., 1978, "Learned Helplessness in Humans", *Journal of Abnormal Psychology*, 87, pp. 49-74.
51. Kool, V.K. and Sen, M., 1984, "The Non-violence Test", In *Second Handbook of Psychological and Social Instruments*, D.M. Pestonjee (Ed.), Indian Institute of Management, Ahmedabad, India, pp. 48-54.
52. Dodge, K.A., 1980, "Social Cognition and Children's Aggressive Behaviour", *Child Development,* 51, pp. 162-170.
53. Dodge, K.A. and Newman, J.P., 1981, "Biased Decision-making Processes in Aggressive Boys", *Journal of Abnormal Psychology*, 90, pp. 375-379.
54. Weiner, B., Graham, S. and Chandler, C., 1982, "Pity, Anger and Guilt: An Attributional Analysis", *Personality and Social Psychology Bulletin*, 8, pp. 226-232.
55. Fondacaro, M.R. and Heller, K., 1990, "Attributional Style in Aggressive Adolescent Boys", *Journal of Abnormal Child Psychology*, 18, pp. 75-89.
56. Kool, V.K., 1993, "Toward a Theory of the Psychology of Non-violence", In *Non-violence: Social and Psychological Issues*, V.K. Kool (Ed.), University Press of America, Inc., pp. 1-24.

57. Smith, E.M. and North, C.S., 1993, "Post-traumatic Stress Disorder in Natural Disasters and Technological Accidents", In *International Handbook of Traumatic Stress Syndromes*, J.P. Wilson and B. Raphael (Eds.), Plenum Press, New York, pp. 405-419.
58. Yehuda, R., McFarlane, A.C. and Shalev, A.Y., 1998, "Predicting the Development of Post-traumatic Stress Disorder from the Acute Response to a Traumatic Event", *Biological Psychiatry*, 44(12), pp. 1305-1313.
59. March, J.S., Amaya-Jackson, L., Terry, R. and Costanzo, P., 1997, "Post-traumatic Symptomatology in Children and Adolescents After an Industrial Fire", *Journal of the American Academy of Child and Adolescent Psychiatry*, 36(8), pp. 1080-1088.
60. Osofsky, J.D., 1995, "The Effects of Exposure to Violence on Young Children", *American Psychologist*, 50(9), pp. 782-788.
61. Pynoos, R.S., Steinberg, A.M. and Goenjian, A.K., 1996, "Traumatic Stress in Childhood and Adolescence: Recent Developments and Current Controversies", In *Traumatic Stress: The Effects of Overwhelming Experience on Mind, Body and Society*, B.A. Van der Kolk, A.C. McFarlane and L. Weisaeth (Eds.), Guilford Press, New York, pp. 331-358.
62. Marans, S. and Adelman, A., 1997, "Experiencing Violence in a Developmental Context", In *Children in a Violent Society*, J.D. Osofsky et al. (Eds.), Guilford Press, New York, pp. 202-222.
63. Vogel, J.M. and Vernberg, E.M., 1993, "Psychological Responses of Children to Natural and Human-made Disasters: I, Children's Psychological Responses to Disasters", *Journal of Clinical Child Psychology*, 22(4), pp. 464-484.
64. Garbarino, J., Kostelny, K. and Dubrow, N., 1991, "What Children Can Tell Us About Living in Danger", *American Psychologist*, 46(4), pp. 376-383.
65. Duncan, R.D., Saunders, B.E., Kilpatrick, D.G., Hanson, R.F. and Resnick, H.S., 1996, "Childhood Physical Assault as a Risk Factor for PTSD, Depression and Substance Abuse: Findings from a National Survey", *American Journal of Orthopsychiatry*, 66(3), pp. 437-448.
66. Boney-McCoy, S. and Finkelhor, D., 1995, "Prior Victimization: A Risk Factor for Child Sexual Abuse and for PTSD-related Symptomatology Among Sexually Abused Youth", *Child Abuse and Neglect*, 19(12), pp. 1401-1421.
67. Roth, S.H., Newman, E., Pelcovitz, D., Van der Kolk, B.A. and Mandel, F.S., 1997, "Complex PTSD in Victims Exposed to Sexual and Physical Abuse: Results from the DSM-IV Field Trial for Post-traumatic Stress Disorder", *Journal of Traumatic Stress*, 10(4), pp. 539-555.
68. Morrison, J.A., 2000, "Protective Factors Associated with Children's Emotional Responses to Chronic Community Violence Exposure", *Trauma, Violence and Abuse: A Review Journal*, 1(4), pp. 299-320.
69. Sen, M., 2007, "An Intervention Program for Reduction of Aggression in Adolescence through Attributional Style Therapy", Research Project, Unpublished, University of Mumbai, India.
70. Gandhi, I., 1983, *Disarmament and Development*, Speech at the Seventh Conference of Heads of State or Government of Non-aligned Countries, New Delhi.

The AHA-Syndrome and Cardiovascular Diseases
Editors: Swati Y. Bhave and Sunil Saini
Copyright © 2010 Anamaya Publishers, New Delhi, India

20. Lifestyle Disease Prevention by Early Intervention

Swati Y. Bhave
Indraprastha Apollo Hospital, Sarita Vihar, New Delhi - 110 076, India

Abstract: The major risk factors for developing coronary heart disease (CHD) are obesity, hyperlipidemia, hypertension, diabetes and stress, all of which can be tracked from childhood to adolescence to adulthood and, therefore, are called lifestyle diseases. All these diseases are preventable if a good and healthy lifestyle is adopted as early as possible, in fact right from childhood. Obesity is the end result of a variety of factors. However, the major cause is unhealthy lifestyle that involves reduced physical activity and unhealthy food habits and, hence, is very much preventable. Obesity will predispose to development of hyperlipidemia, hypertension, diabetes and cardiovascular disease. The present chapter focusses on prevention of the major risk factors that cause cardiovascular disease. Indians, like many Asians, are at a higher risk [1] for CHD even if they are born or staying outside the country or the continent as they are genetically more prone to a syndrome called metabolic syndrome. This syndrome and its prevention will also be discussed in detail.

Keywords: Lifestyle diseases, Metabolic syndrome, Obesity, Early intervention.

Introduction

Lifestyle risk factors developed during childhood or adolescence (unhealthy food habits, alcohol intake, smoking, poor physical activity, drugs etc.) get carried into adult life as well. By adopting a healthy lifestyle from childhood, especially adolescence, it is possible to prevent these diseases [2]. The risk of having coronary heart disease (CHD) is increased if a person has obesity. Obesity leads to many metabolic abnormalities like hyperlipidemia, Type II diabetes mellitus (DM) and hypertension. The prevention for CHD, thus, should ideally begin in childhood when parents should be sensitised to adopting a healthy lifestyle for themselves and for their children. Adolescents should be given preventive counselling for problems related to high risk behaviours like substance abuse, consumption of junk food and lack of exercise.

CHD has a higher incidence in the Indian population and Asians, in general, as they are at risk for metabolic syndrome, also called insulin resistance syndrome or syndrome X.

Metabolic Syndrome/Insulin Resistance Syndrome/Syndrome X

This is associated with increased risk of obesity, insulin resistance, Type II DM and cardiovascular disease [3]. As per the 2005 International Diabetes Federation definition [4], the criteria for the diagnosis of the metabolic syndrome are as follows:

(a) Central obesity (waist circumference > 90 cm for males and > 80 cm for females)
(b) Any two of the following four factors:

   (i) Raised serum triglycerides ≥ 150 mg/dl
   (ii) Reduced serum HDL cholesterol < 45 mg/dl
   (iii) Raised blood pressure (BP) systolic > 130 and diastolic > 85 mm Hg
   (iv) Raised fasting blood sugar level > 100 mg/dl

Additional features associated with metabolic syndrome are:

(a) Insulin resistance (fasting insulin, HOMA IR)
(b) Dyslipidemia (in addition to above, increased small dense LDL)
(c) Hypercoagulability of blood (increased plasminogen activator inhibitor)
(d) Vascular dysregulation (beyond elevated BP) endothelial dysfunction-microalbuminuria
(e) Inflammatory state: Raised high sensitive C-reactive protein, TNC-α and IL
(f) Polycystic ovarian disease (PCOS)
(g) Acanthosis nigricans

All the above factors (i)-(iv) and (a)-(g) increase the risk of a person developing CHD.

Why Does Metabolic Syndrome Occur in India and Other Countries in the Asian Region?

This can be explained by the Barker's Hypothesis [5] for fetal origin of adult onset disease (FOAD) 1986. There have been rapid epidemiological transitions, especially nutritional and socio-economic, in Asian countries. In all parts of India we see a complex picture of under nutrition and overweight occurring simultaneously. Indian mothers are chronically malnourished (stunted) and Indian babies are the smallest in the world with low birth weight (LBW) accounting for more than 25% of all "normal births". With this background, India is now witnessing plentiful problems, such as obesity with its attendant risks [3].

Predictive Adaptive Responses (PARS) [6, 7]

The developing organism predicts its future environment. The embryo/fetus depend on the information transmitted by the mother/placenta to evaluate/predict the present and future environments. Predictive adaptive responses (PARs) are the decisions made by the developing organism to change the course of its development. PARs can be *appropriate* or *inappropriate*, depending on whether the physiological responses that the mature organism can have are adapted to the environment it is exposed to.

Appropriate PARs are those where the physiological responses that the mature organism can have are adapted to the environment it is exposed to. When this is not the case, i.e. inappropriate PARs, the risk of disease in later life is greater. PARs only happen during critical windows of development when developmental plasticity operates. The windows of potential induction differ for different organs. The key concept of the PARS model is match/mismatch PARs. If there is a *match* then the risk of disease is low; if there is *no match* then the risk of disease is higher.

The metabolic, nutrient and hormonal signals that come from the mother can be interfered with, if there is maternal or placental dysfunction. For a human baby, the information received about its nutritional environment is the feeding it receives from the mother or caretaker. The baby's size *in utero* depends on the supply of food and accommodation provided by the mother.

Undernutrition and unfavourable intra-uterine environment at critical periods in early life can cause permanent changes (in both structure and function) in the developing systems of the fetus. This is called 'programming', which may manifest as a disease over a period of time due to 'dysadaptation' with the changed environmental circumstances.

The model to explain the "developmental origins of child disease" suggests that the relationship between the predicted and actual mature environments determines disease risk. If the environments match, the risk of disease is low. If they do not match, the risk of disease is greater. The physiological settings established during the plastic and predictive phases (that occur before and after birth in the case of some organs) are not appropriate for the environment of the non-plastic mature phase [8]. For example, if the nutritional signals show poor food availability the fetus sets a physiology of *insulin resistance*, which is advantageous before and after birth in poor nutritional environments. But this insulin resistance creates a disease risk in later life depending upon the environment the child/adult will be living in. As nutritional intakes in childhood and adulthood increase rapidly in many societies, the risk of mismatch rises and the risk of diabetes increases. This knowledge changes our views about how to intervene in the epidemic 'lifestyle' disease. Interventions on lifestyle only are partially effective in those affected by inappropriate PARs.

Improving maternal and fetal health will help in dealing better with post-natal nutritional conditions. The periconceptual period is vital. Hence, it is very important that a woman should get excellent nutrition during conception and during early pregnancy.

Thrifty Phenotype Hypothesis

The fetus responds to adverse environment by making irreversible changes in its development. It reduces its growth to keep the energy for cardiac function and neurodevelopment. Nutritional deprivation signals insulin resistance and reduced vascularity in organs. If such a baby becomes obese at middle age, cardiovascular and metabolic diseases would appear.

Affluent countries have emphasised the importance of birth weight and other measures of poor fetal growth in the genesis of FOAD disorders. However, in the recent years, cohort studies from India (beginning in Pune in 1990, followed by those in Mysore, Delhi and Vellore) have highlighted the importance of subsequent overnutrition in the development of this disorder [9]. FOAD is now called developmental origins of health and disease (DOHaD).

Hypothesis for DOHaD

Multi-phasic nutritional insult = Genes + Early undernutrition + Subsequent overnutrition fetal origins or later lifestyles or both.

Studies of DOHaD in India

The Pune Cohort Study has effectively shown that there are deleterious effects of accelerated weight gain in childhood, i.e. "crossing of centiles", especially in LBW babies. Indices of insulin resistance and cardiovascular risk factors were found to be highest in those who were born 'small' but were big by eight years of age even though they were not obese in absolute terms. Accelerated growth in childhood is associated with early puberty and greater risk of obesity [10].

Maternal nutritional studies have shown convincingly that this high risk body composition is present even at birth, i.e. LBW, lower muscle mass, but relatively high fat mass and hyper insulinemia ('thin fat' phenotype). It is possible that such fat offers survival benefits to newborns, but also endangers predisposition to insulin resistance from birth itself [11]. Newborns with truncal adiposity, even though relatively small at birth (birth weight < 2.9 kg), have been reported to have greater subscapular skin fold thickness, which is shown to correlate well with truncal obesity [12]. It has also been shown that this adiposity goes up to four years of age [13].

Most FOAD related disorders can be prevented or effectively managed if detected early in life. The main prevention is through public health campaigns directed towards lifestyle changes in the family or society as a whole. The benefits of healthy eating, increased physical activity and reduction in sedentary activities have to be inculcated from early age. School-based programmes are most likely to be successful, but health authorities and media have an important role to play to spread this awareness.

Obesity

There is increasing evidence of overweight and obesity in India, especially in the children and adolescents belonging to affluent families. Many studies have shown high prevalence of the same. In a Chennai study of school children overweight/obesity was seen in 4.5% in the low socioeconomic (LSE) group, 15% in the middle socioeconomic (MSE) group, and as high as 22% in the high socioeconomic (HSE) group [14]. In urban Delhi, obesity and overweight was found in 45% females and 25% males. A Delhi study involving young adults showed that an increase of body mass index (BMI) of 1 SD from 2 to 12 years of age increased the odds ratio for disease (IGT/DM) by 1.36. Further, continuing cohort studies in Pune suggest that accelerated growth in childhood, especially in LBW is associated with early puberty and greater risk of obesity [10]. It is important to watch carefully if any child or adolescent starts crossing his/her centiles of growth and be especially alert to the 'healthy' weight gain during adolescence.

The causes of obesity are multifactorial – genes, endocrine, diet, exercise, behaviour psychology, child and adolescent lifestyle pattern. Obesity results when energy intake exceeds energy expenditure as a result of genetic or acquired changes in: feeding control, control of energy efficiency and adipogensis.

Cause of the Obesity Epidemic Around the World Today

There was a time when the food supply was very unreliable and humans had to work very hard to procure food to survive, which involved a lot of physical activity. Hence, there was no need to develop a strong physiological defence against weight gain. The gradual weight gain seen in the 21st century is a relatively new phenomenon. It is most likely due to the changed environment of this century that provides a constant food supply and with reduced needs for physical activity. Thus, in the past there was a physiological control that matched the human food intake to the individual energy requirement. Today, the affluent people have abundant food supply. They need to make very active and conscious effort to restrict energy intake in order to match a very low level of energy expenditure [15].

It is extremely difficult to resist and restrict consumption of food given the constant availability of good-tasting, low cost food or affordability of purchasing high cost food. The present day lifestyle does not have fixed food intake timings and the environment promotes eating when food is available, i.e. round the clock. Today, healthy body weight is difficult to achieve without conscious effort. Cognitive management is vital to restrict food intake and increase physical activity. This means behaviour change strategies are very important in preventing obesity and reducing weight. Most of the affluent population has been in slight positive energy balance over the past 10-15 years.

The global epidemic of obesity is driven by an environment that encourages overeating and discourages physical activity, creating a consistent bias toward positive energy balance. This small degree of sustained, positive energy balance of less than 50 kcal/day is causing weight gain at a rate of 0.5-2 kg/year as seen in the Cardia Study [16]. Prevention of this weight gain should take far less than 60-90 min/day of moderate intensity physical activity. Substantial efforts need to be directed toward modifying the environment to increase physical activity.

Current Environment Facilitates Obesity [17]

Built Environment

This includes transportation systems, architectural design, use of land, parks, and public spaces. Today's lifestyle discourages physical activity and encourages the use of automobiles and other vehicles. The residential areas are built without proper footpaths, which discourages walking. Tall buildings discourage staircases and encourage use of lifts [18].

Commercial Environment

Low cost junk food is easily available everywhere. Such food is heavily advertised, especially to children. In developed countries, many schools have vending machines with high energy dense (HED) food and fast food outlets. There is heavy promotion of activities and products that discourage physical activity. People are enjoying sedentary forms of entertainment more and more like the home entertainment systems, video and computer games etc.

Policy Environment

It is very important to bring out the following changes in various policies:

- Restrictions on 'undesirable' eating behaviour
- Removal of junk foods from schools
- Taxes or ban imposed on 'unhealthy' foods/drinks
- Regulation of advertising for undesirable foods
- Labelling of all nutritive contents
- Reduction of sugar consumption
- Discouragement of consumption of HDE/manufactured foods
- Encouragement to consumption of fruits and vegetables
- Making physical education in schools compulsory
- Setting up of physically active transportation

The Social and Cultural Environment

The technological advances of today reduce the need for physical activity. In most occupations, jobs, schools, daily living and household activities there is great competition between physical and sedentary activities via the invasion of video and computer games, internet television and movies etc.

Low level of physical activity is a well-known cause of weight gain. Today there are many components in food that promote obesity. The portion size of food is progressively increasing in hotels, restaurants, packed foods etc. The bigger the portion the more is the amount a person gets accustomed to eating. There is too much consumption of soft drinks, which contain sugar and empty calories. Most readymade and fast food have high fat and are energy dense with a high Glycemic Index. Also, junk food is made to appeal to the taste buds, is easily available and comes in a large variety. In fact, it is cheaper and easily accessible than healthy foods!

The prevention of obesity, therefore, consists of changes in lifestyle to adopting a more healthy way of living. This can be achieved by modifying physical activity and dietary intake, as well as by choosing a strategy to change one's environment and behaviour. The need of the hour is primary prevention of weight gain in those who are not obese. Secondary prevention in obese persons involves the following:

- Prevention of further weight gain
- Sustained weight loss till the desired weight is achieved
- Prevention of weight regain

It is best to begin with small changes. There are various programmes for this, e.g. America on the Move (AOM) [19], which is an American national initiative to inspire people to make two small changes to prevent further weight gain and improve lifestyle. AOM asks people to do the following:

(i) Walk an additional 2,000 steps (about 1 mile) each day (burns about 100 kcal)
(ii) Choose one eating behaviour each day that eliminates about 100 kcal

With the above two simple behaviours, most of the population, regardless of age, can prevent further weight gain. For children, these changes can reduce excessive weight gain. The US Surgeon General recommends 30-60 min of moderate exercise per day for a healthy lifestyle [20]. A lot of literature is available on information regarding healthy lifestyle [21, 22].

Prevention of Weight Gain by Modification of Diet [18]

Public support for healthier lifestyles needs to begin with children and adolescents. They need to be taught early on the importance of physical activity and healthy eating [23]. They must be provided with the knowledge and the cognitive skills to manage energy balance in the modern environment. Changing the environment is the best long-term solution, but it is a decades-long effort. In the short-term, efforts have to be put into helping people make behaviour changes to keep the problem from worsening [15].

Genes play a very important role in determining whether or not obesity will develop. For example, differences in genotype will determine to what extent body weight gain is seen within a given environment. Different individuals maintain different levels of body weight within a given environment. Some individuals are genetically resistant to weight.

The other diseases that are high risk factors for cardiovascular diseases, in addition to obesity, are Type II DM, hypertension, and stress (both acute and chronic).

Type II DM

It has an insidious onset and patients may have hyperglycemia for a number of years before diagnosis. It constitutes high risk for cardiovascular and cerebro-vascular mortality and morbidity [24]. Obesity, particularly of the central type, appears to be a direct correlate of Type II DM. Obese children are insulin resistant and have up to 40% lower glucose utilisation than non-obese children. Hypertension and other cardiovascular system (CVS) risk factors (hyperlipidemia, hypercoagulability). People who are obese are more prone to Type II diabetes, hypertension and hyperlipidemia. In turn, these also make them more susceptible to cardiovascular disease. The high incidence of mortality and morbidity due to myocardial infarctions and stroke in young adults shows that these problems start insidiously in childhood/adolescence and are asymptomatic for long periods. Indian cohort studies have suggested that high risk factors for CVS diseases are associated with both fetal origins and later lifestyles.

Hypertension or High BP

The precipitating factors for hypertension are obesity, lack of exercise, unhealthy diet and chronic stress. All these are due to bad lifestyle and are preventable. Once hypertension has already developed, only anti-hypertensive medications are never enough. A change in lifestyle via daily exercise, reduction in body weight and having a healthy diet are equally important for the control of hypertension.

Daily Exercise and Obesity

Lack of exercise and obesity are both important factors that can lead to hypertension. This can be prevented by daily exercise of 30-60 min. If a person is overweight or obese then a weight reduction regime should be started. It is well documented that each 1 kg increase in body weight increases the BP by 1 mm Hg and vice versa.

A decrease of as less as 2-10 mm Hg in BP reduces the morbidity of heart attacks and strokes by 2%. Hence, it is extremely important to prevent BP increase. In persons who have already got high BP, exercise and weight loss helps to keep it under control.

Unhealthy Diet and Hypertension

Use of excessive sodium, low potassium and high intake of saturated fatty acids can lead to hypertension. The dietary approach to stop hypertension (DASH) eating plan is a clinical study that tested the effects of nutrients in food on BP. The results show that high BP can be reduced by a diet having fruits, vegetables, low fat dairy foods, low saturated fat, total fat and cholesterol. The DASH eating plan encourages eating whole grains, poultry, fish and nuts, as well as limits fats, red meats, sweets and sugared beverages. A second clinical study, called DASH-Sodium, looked at the effect of a reduced dietary sodium intake on BP as people followed either the DASH eating plan or a typical American diet. Results showed that reducing dietary sodium lowered BP for both the DASH eating plan and the typical American diet. The biggest BP lowering benefits were for those following the DASH eating plan at the lowest sodium level (1,500 mg/day) [25].

One must restrict intake of excess sodium right from childhood to adulthood. Use of table salt should be minimised. Herbs and spices should be used to flavour instead of salt. Processed foods should be checked for the sodium content. In addition to reduced intake of sodium, increased intake of potassium is also found to be beneficial in reduction of hypertension.

Saturated fat has adverse effects on the health of the heart and blood vessels. It is found in animal fats, e.g. fatty meats, poultry skin and whole-milk dairy products, such as butter, cheese, cream and ice cream. It is present in oils of coconut, palm kernel and palm. These oils are used in processed foods, e.g. baked goods, snacks etc. Saturated fat should be replaced by margarine and canola, sunflower and olive oil. If a person wants to lose weight, all fats have to be restricted [26].

Omega-3 Fatty Acid and High BP [27, 28]

Intake of more than 3 g of omega-3 fatty acids per day may be necessary to obtain clinically relevant effects. But, there is an increased risk of bleeding at this dose level. Other approaches are known to have greater effects on BP, such as salt reduction, weight loss, exercise, or anti-hypertensive drug therapy. Therefore, although omega-3 fatty acids do appear to have effects in this area, their role in the management of high BP is limited.

Healthy Diet and Prevention and Treatment of Cardiovascular Disease

Omega-3 Fatty Acids

Dietary sources of omega-3 fatty acids include fish oil and certain plant/nut oils. Fish oil contains both docosahexaenoic acid (DHA) and eicosapentaenoic acid (EPA). Nuts and vegetable oils (canola, soybean, olive) contain α-linolenic acid (ALA).

Intake of recommended amounts of DHA and EPA in the form of dietary fish or fish oil is very beneficial [29, 30]. Multiple mechanisms have been proposed for the beneficial effects of omega-3 fatty acids [31], which include reduced triglyceride levels [32], reduced inflammation, slightly lowered BP [33], reduced tendency of the heart to develop dangerous abnormal rhythms, and diminished buildup of atherosclerotic plaques in arteries of the heart [34]. Experiments suggest that omega-3 fatty acids may reduce platelet derived growth factor (PDGF), decrease platelet aggregation, inhibit the expression of vascular adhesion molecules that reduces blood clotting, and stimulate relaxation of endothelial cells in the walls of blood vessels [35], and reduce strokes in people with known cardiovascular disease [36-38]. They are also shown to reduce the risk of death and heart attack [30-41].

Although similar benefits are proposed for α-linolenic acid, scientific evidence is less compelling, and beneficial effects may be less pronounced [42]. High doses (> 3 g/day) of omega-3 fatty acids may have harmful effects, such as an increased risk of bleeding. Hence, they should always be taken under medical supervision. Some species of fish carry a higher risk of environmental contamination, such as with methyl mercury, and should be used with caution in young children [43].

C-reactive Protein (CRP) Levels

CRP is a marker of inflammation. Persons with high CRP levels are more prone to cardiovascular disease. Weight reduction, smoking cessation, and medications like statin drugs and COX-2 inhibitors all appear to reduce CRP. The evidence regarding fish oil remains equivocal.

Primary Cardiovascular Disease Prevention [44]

Several epidemiologic studies show a significantly lower rate of death from heart disease in men and women who regularly eat fish [45]. The American Heart Association (AHA) [46], in its 2003 recommendations, suggested that all adults should eat fish at least two times per week, in particular fatty fish, e.g. mackerel, lake trout, herring, sardines, albacore tuna, and salmon. In addition, all adults should consume plant-derived sources of omega-3 fatty acids, such as tofu/soybeans, walnuts, flaxseed oil and canola oil.

Secondary Cardiovascular Disease Prevention

In people with a history of heart attack, regular consumption of oily fish (200-400 g of fish each week = 500-800 mg of daily omega-3 fatty acids) or fish oil/omega-3 supplements (containing 850-1800 mg of EPA + DHA) reduces the risk of non-fatal heart attack, fatal heart attack, sudden death, and all-cause mortality (death due to any cause) [47-50].

Most patients in these studies were also using conventional heart drugs, suggesting that the benefits of fish oils may add to the effects of other therapies. The AHA, in its 2003 recommendations, also suggested that people with known CHD should take in approximately 1 g of EPA and DHA (combined) each day. The World Health Organization (WHO) and government health agencies of several countries recommend consuming 0.3-0.5 g daily of EPA + DHA and 0.8-1.1 g daily of α-linolenic acid.

Clinicians Dealing with Children and Adolescents Can Do a Lot to Prevent Diseases Caused by Metabolic Syndrome [23]

Clinicians can help increase awareness via advocacy programmes in schools and community for children, adolescents, parents and community regarding the diseases caused by metabolic syndrome. They can use the visits by children and adolescents to check their height and weight, chart their BMI, and advise them accordingly. This data can be compared with past records. if available. They can check BP and keep an annual record. It would also be possible to take a good look at a child's or adolescent's family history for cardiovascular disease and diabetes. If found positive and/or the child or adolescent is obese, they can check for lipid profile and do a glucose tolerance test. If any features of metabolic X syndrome are detected, the child or adolescent may be subjected to additional tests to rule out associated features.

Children, adolescents, parents and community must also be informed about the need to cut down sedentary activities like watching TV, playing computer or video games etc. By citing the food pyramid, healthy diet – eating plenty of fresh fruits, vegetables, whole grains and avoiding junk food or heavy greasy, fried food – must be explained. The dangers of smoking, alcohol consumption and substance abuse need to be emphasised and the importance of physical activity for at least one hour daily highlighted.

Stress and Disease

Adolescents face conflicting demands from parents, teachers and friends, which create a lot of stress [51]. Stress is a challenge to the body homeostasis. It causes a biological and biochemical reaction that begins in the brain and causes an autonomic nervous system effect, causing hormone release and adversely affecting the immune system – the "neuro-endocrine immuno axis".

Stress can be physical, psychological and psychosocial. Stresses can manifest as *eustress*, i.e. the positive stress which motivates our everyday actions. Inability to cope up with stress means *distress*. The key to good health is learning how to turn distress into eustress. The body response to stress is called the general adaptation syndrome. Chronic stress can cause chronic health problems, as wellness cannot be maintained when a large percentage of body energy is channeled into coping with stress [52]. Stress affects the whole body; causing gastrointestinal disturbances (dyspepsia, peptic ulcer, irritable bowel syndrome), neuromuscular disorders (chronic back pain, vague aches and muscle pains, migraine), sleep disorders, inability to concentrate on performing well academically and in extracurricular activities, cardiovascular disease (hypertension, coronary disease), allergic disorders, and recurrent infections, due to depressed immunity.

Teenagers can manifest stress with a variety of psychosomatic symptoms (pertaining to any systems) and these may mislead the diagnosis to somatic illness. Hence, pediatricians treating adolescents must go deep into proper history. Teenagers can be stressed due to various factors: biological, family, peer factors, societal etc. Most teenagers turn to tranquilisers to manage stress. Hence, it is important to teach them how to manage stress without using drugs and follow a lifestyle that prevents stress related diseases. If stress is not properly managed it can result in depression, suicidal behaviour, drug or alcohol abuse, and eating disorders. It has been found that day-to-day stress is more difficult for adolescents to handle than major life events. Adolescents generally cope with stress by listening to music and watching television. They must also be helped to find a meaning in stressful experiences. The best way to deal with stress is to get into the relaxation response, which means bringing down one's heart rate by breathing exercises, relaxation techniques and by mentally deciding that the situation is not stressful.

Religion and Spirituality

These are known to give mental peace and keep a person on the right track in life. However, adolescents are used to being extremely involved and intense about the activities they undertake. Hence, care must be taken that they do not become religious fanatics or indulge in religious bigotry. Care also has to be taken that they do not come under the influence of unscrupulous people who can pose as religious leaders to exploit the innocent.

Yoga, Meditation, *Pranayama* and the Art of Living

These are known to reduce stress and induce positive thinking in life. Adolescents should be encouraged to learn and practice these arts.

Conclusion

Many diseases originate during childhood and get carried through adolescence into adulthood. Fortunately, many of them are preventable by a healthy lifestyle that includes healthy eating habits, exercise, effective stress management, and avoidance of alcohol and substance abuse. Clinicians dealing with children and adolescents should help them to understand the importance of a healthy lifestyle for prevention of disease and should clinically monitor them to detect early signs. Stress management should form an important part of daily life.

References

1. Reddy, K.S., 2002, "Cardiovascular Diseases in Developing Countries: Dimensions, Determinants, Dynamics and Directions for Public Health Action", *Pub. Hlth. Nut.*, 5, pp. 231-237.
2. WHO/NMH/NPH, 2001, "Life Course Perspectives on Coronary Heart Disease, Stroke, and Diabetes", World Health Organization, Geneva, 01 April.
3. Pandit, A.N., Bhave, S., Bavadekar, 2006, "Fetal Origin of Adult Onset Disease", In *Bhave's Textbook of Adolescent Medicine*, S.Y. Bhave (Chief Ed.), 1st Edn., Jaypee Medical Publishers, New Delhi, Chapter 3, pp. 104-108.
4. IDF, 2005, "The IDF Consensus Worldwide Definition of the Metabolic Syndrome", International Diabetes Federation, Brussels, May, *www.idf.org/webdata/docs/IDF-Metasyndrome-definition.pdf*
5. Barker, D.J.P., 1998, *Mothers, Babies and Health in Later Life*, Churchill Livingstone, Edinburgh.
6. Gluckman, 2005, "The Fetal, Neonatal and Infant Environments: The Long-term Consequences for Disease Risk", *Early Human Development*, 81, p. 51.
7. Barker, 2002, "Fetal Origins of Adult Disease: Strengths of Effects and Biological Basis", *International Journal of Epidemiology*, 31, p. 1235.
8. Extramurally Speaking, 2002, "Fetal Basis of Childhood and Adult Disease: Role of the Environment", *EHP*, 110 (6), *ehp.niehs.nih.gov/docs/2002/110-6/extram-speaking.html*
9. Yajnik, C.S., 2001, "The Insulin Resistance Epidemic in India: Fetal Origins, Later Lifestyle, or Both? Fetal Origins of Adult-onset Diseases (FOAD)", *Nutr. Rev.*, 59, pp. 1-9.
10. Bavdekar, A., Yajnik, C.S., Caroline, H.D., Bapat, S., Pandit, A., Deshpande, V. et al., 1999, "Insulin Resistance Syndrome in 8-year-old Indian Children: Small at Birth, Big at 8 years, or Both?" *Diabetes*, 48, pp. 2422-2429.
11. Yajnik, C.S., Fall, C.H.D., Koyaji, K.J., Hirve, S.S., Rao, S., Barker, D.J.P. et al., 2003, "Neonatal Anthropometry: The Thin-fat Indian Baby – The Pune Maternal Nutrition Study", *Int. J. Obes.*, 27, pp. 173-180.
12. Krishnaveni, G.V., Hill, J.C., Veena, S.R. and Fall, C.H.D., 2005, "Truncal Obesity is Present at Birth and in Early Childhood in South Indian Children", *Indian Pediatr.*, 42, pp. 527-538.
13. Agarwal, K.N., Saxena, A., Bansal, A.K. and Agarwal, D.K., 2001, "Physical Growth Assessment in Adolescence", *Indian Pediatr.*, p. 38.
14. Ramachandran, A., Snehalatha, C., Vinitha, R., Thayyil, M., Sathish Kumar, C.K., Sheeba, L. et al., 2002, "Prevalence of Overweight in Urban Indian Adolescent School Children", *Diabetes Res. Clin. Pract.*, 57, pp. 185-190.
15. Hill, J.O., Wyatt, H.R., Reed, G.W. and Peters, J.C., 2003, "Obesity and the Environment: Where do We Go from Here?" *Science*, 299, pp. 853-855.
16. CARDIA, *www.dopm.uab.edu/cardia/*
17. Booth, S.L., Sallis, J.F. et al., 2001, "Environmental and Societal Factors Affect Food Choice and Physical Activity: Rationale, Influences and Leverage Points", *Nutrition Reviews*, 9(3), pp. S21-S39.
18. *http://ceq.eh.doe.gov/nepa/nepanet.htm*
19. *americaonthemove.org*
20. *www.surgeongeneral.gov/topics/obesity*
21. US Department of Health and Human Services, *healthfinder.gov*

22. National Heart Lung and Blood Institute, *www.nhlbi.nih.gov*
23. Greydanus, D.E. and Bhave, S.Y., 2004, "Editorial: Obesity and Adolescents: Time for Increased Activity", *Indian Pediatr.*, 41(6).
24. Ramachandran, A., Snehalatha, C., Kapur, A., Vijay, V., Mohan, V., Das, A.K. et al., 2001, "High Prevalence of Diabetes and Impaired Glucose Tolerance in India: National Urban Diabetes Survey", *Diabetologia*, 9, pp. 1094-1111.
25. *www.nhlbi.nih.gov/hbp/prevent/h_eating/h_eating.htm*
26. *www.nhlbi.nih.gov/hbp/prevent/h_eating/fats.htm*
27. Knapp, H.R. and Fitzgerald, G.A., 1989, "The Antihypertensive Effects of Fish Oil: A Controlled Study of Polyunsaturated Fatty Acid Supplements in Essential Hypertension", *N. Engl. J. Med.*, 320(16), pp. 1037-1043.
28. Bonaa, K.H., Bjerve, K.S., Straume, B. et al., 1990, "Effect of Eicosapentaenoic and Docosahexaenoic Acids on Blood Pressure in Hypertension: A Population-based Intervention Trial from the Tromso Study", *N. Engl. J. Med.*, 322(12), pp. 795-801.
29. Hooper, L., Thompson, R., Harrison, R. et al., 2004, "Omega 3 Fatty Acids for Prevention and Treatment of Cardiovascular Disease", *Cochrane Database Syst. Rev.*, 4, CD003177.
30. Bucher, H.C., Hengstler, P., Schindler, C. et al., 2002, "N-3 Polyunsaturated Fatty Acids in Coronary Heart Disease: A Meta-analysis of Randomized Controlled Trials", *Am. J. Med.*, 112(4), pp. 298-304.
31. Dolecek, T.A., 1992, "Epidemiological Evidence of Relationships Between Dietary Polyunsaturated Fatty Acids and Mortality in the Multiple Risk Factor Intervention Trial", *Proc. Soc. Exp. Biol. Med.*, 200(2), pp. 177-182.
32. Harris, W.S., Dujovne, C.A., Zucker, M. et al., 1988, "Effects of a Low Saturated Fat, Low Cholesterol Fish Oil Supplement in Hypertriglyceridemic Patients: A Placebo-controlled Trial", *Ann. Intern. Med.*, 109(6), pp. 465-470.
33. Howe, P.R., 1997, "Dietary Fats and Hypertension: Focus on Fish Oil", *Ann. N.Y. Acad. Sci.*, 827, pp. 339-352.
34. Erkkila, A.T., Lichtenstein, A.H., Mozaffarian, D. et al., 2004, "Fish Intake is Associated with a Reduced Progression of Coronary Artery Atherosclerosis in Postmenopausal Women with Coronary Artery Disease", *Am. J. Clin. Nutr.*, 80(3), pp. 626-632.
35. Mori, T.A., Watts, G.F., Burke, V. et al., 2000, "Differential Effects of Eicosapentaenoic Acid and Docosahexaenoic Acid on Vascular Reactivity of the Forearm Microcirculation in Hyperlipidemic, Overweight Men", *Circulation*, 102(11), pp. 1264-1269.
36. Simon, J.A., Fong, J., Bernert, J.T. Jr. et al., 1995, "Serum Fatty Acids and the Risk of Stroke", *Stroke*, 26(5), pp. 778-782.
37. Iso, H., Rexrode, K.M., Stampfer, M.J. et al., 2001, "Intake of Fish and Omega-3 fatty Acids and Risk of Stroke in Women", *JAMA*, 285(3), pp. 304-312.
38. Orencia, A.J., Daviglus, M.L., Dyer, A.R. et al., 1996, "Fish Consumption and Stroke in Men: 30-year Findings of the Chicago Western Electric Study", *Stroke*, 27(2), pp. 204-209.
39. Stone, N.J., 1996, "Fish Consumption, Fish Oil, Lipids and Coronary Heart Disease", *Circulation*, 94(9), pp. 2337-2340.
40. Ascherio, A., Rimm, E.B., Giovannucci, E.L. et al., 1996, "Dietary Fat and Risk of Coronary Heart Disease in Men: Cohort Follow Up Study in the United States", *BMJ*, 313(7049), pp. 84-90.
41. Daviglus, M.L., Stamler, J., Orencia, A.J. et al., 1997, "Fish Consumption and the 30-year Risk of Fatal Myocardial Infarction", *N. Engl. J. Med.*, 336(15), pp. 1046-1053.
42. Oomen, C.M., Ocke, M.C., Feskens, E.J. et al., 2001, "Alpha-Linolenic Acid Intake is Not Beneficially Associated with 10-year Risk of Coronary Artery Disease Incidence: The Zutphen Elderly Study", *Am. J. Clin. Nutr.*, 74(4), pp. 457-463.

43. *www.naturalstandard.com*
44. Kris-Etherton, P.M., Harris, W.S. and Appel, L.J., 2003, "Fish Consumption, Fish Oil, Omega-3 fatty Acids and Cardiovascular Disease", *Arterioscler. Thromb. Vasc. Biol.*, 23(2), pp. e20-e30.
45. Hu, F.B., Bronner, L., Willett, W.C. et al., 2002, "Fish and Omega-3 Fatty Acid Intake and Risk of Coronary Heart Disease in Women", *JAMA*, 287(14), pp. 1815-1821.
46. American Heart Association, *www.americanheart.com*
47. Djousse, L., Pankow, J.S., Eckfeldt, J.H. et al., 2001, "Relation Between Dietary Linolenic Acid and Coronary Artery Disease in the National Heart, Lung, and Blood Institute Family Heart Study", *Am. J. Clin. Nutr.*, 74(5), pp. 612-619.
48. Kromhout, D., Menotti, A., Bloemberg, B. et al., 1995, "Dietary Saturated and Trans Fatty Acids and Cholesterol and 25-year Mortality from Coronary Heart Disease: The Seven Countries Study", *Prev. Med.*, pp. 308-315.
49. Burr, M.L., Fehily, A.M., Gilbert, J.F. et al., 1989, "Effects of Changes in Fat, Fish, and Fibre Intakes on Death and Myocardial Reinfarction: Diet and Reinfarction Trial (DART)", *Lancet*, 2(8666), pp. 757-761.
50. Singh, R.B., Niaz, M.A., Sharma, J.P. et al., 1997, "Randomized, Double-blind, Placebo-controlled Trial of Fish Oil and Mustard Oil in Patients with Suspected Acute Myocardial Infarction: The Indian Experiment of Infarct Survival 4", *Cardiovasc. Drugs Ther.*, 11(3), pp. 485-491.
51. Bansal, C.P. and Bhave, S.Y., 2006, "Stress in Adolescents", *Textbook of Adolescent Medicine*, 1st Edn., Chapter 24, Jaypee Brothers, New Delhi, pp. 844-853.
52. Asterita, M.F., 1985, *The Physiology of Stress*, New York Human Sciences Press, pp. 4-5.
53. *www.aacap.org/publications/factsfam/66.htm*, Helping Teenagers with Stress.

The AHA-Syndrome and Cardiovascular Diseases
Editors: Swati Y. Bhave and Sunil Saini
Copyright © 2010 Anamaya Publishers, New Delhi, India

21. Nutrition, Food Habits and Cardiovascular Diseases

Alka Sharma,[1] Diwakar Prakash Sharma[2] and Neeraj Dilbaghi[3]
[1]Department of Food Technology, Guru Jambheshwar University of Science and Technology
Hisar - 125 001, India
[2]Department of Animal Products Technology, Chaudhary Charan Singh Haryana Agricultural University
Hisar - 125 004, India
[3]Department of Bio and Nano Technology, Guru Jambheshwar University of Science and Technology
Hisar - 125 001, India

Abstract: Various factors associated with increased risk of coronary heart disease (CHD) are discussed in this chapter. Some of them cannot be altered and others are potentially reversible. Emphasis is laid on discussing dietary factors, mainly lipids and related constituents, that are thought to be contributing towards development of CHD. Various other dietary factors including vitamins and minerals are also suitably discussed.

Keywords: Coronary heart disease, Atherosclerosis, Thrombosis, Hypertension.

Introduction

Coronary heart disease (CHD), the common cause of heart attack, is one of the most frequent causes of death in the developed and developing countries [1]. Several inherited and lifestyle factors affect the risk of heart diseases [2, 3]. Lifestyle factors, particularly diet, account for substantial proportion of variations in CHD risk. In the past, health oriented dietary approaches were reduced salt, sugar and saturated fats in the diet. Nowadays, more attention is being given to specific nutrients that can reduce the risk of CHD [4]. Dietary fibre, *n*-3 fatty acids, vitamin C, vitamin E and plant sterols are of particular interest as many studies have pointed out their potential in reducing the risk of CHD.

The primary cause of coronary artery disease is atherosclerosis of the coronary arteries. Atherosclerosis is a quiet disease and significant symptoms appear only when the process has advanced to a stage where blood flow to the heart has been greatly reduced. Atherosclerosis is the major disease and underlying pathologic process in CHD. The reasons are atheromas, which are raised fibrous plaques appearing on the interior surface of blood vessels around the unaffected surrounding area [5]. They contain fatty materials such as lipoproteins, which are carriers of cholesterol in the blood. The fatty degeneration and thickening constricts the lumen of blood vessels. Ultimately, the blood flow is cut-off in the affected artery, leading to oxygen and nutrient unavailability. This process is called *ischemia* and it leads to death of an area of the heart called myocardial infarction.

Another event is thrombosis, which is formation of a large blood clot in the vessels, sometimes as a result of the rupture of an atherosclerotic plaque. It stops the blood supply from reaching an area of the heart leading to heart attack. Platelet aggregation causes clotting of blood.

In recent years most of the emphasis has been on drug therapy and surgical interventions. Little attention has been paid to the nutritional approach [6]. It is a well accepted fact that lifestyle factors, particularly diet, account for substantial proportion of variation in CHD risk. Earlier, dietary approaches included reduction in salt, refined sugar and saturated fats in the diet. But, in recent years, more attention has been focussed on the consumption of specific nutrients that are present in natural food sources [4].

Risk Factors for CHD

A large number of factors are associated with increased risk of CHD but some of them cannot be altered, e.g. masculine gender, increasing age, genetic traits and body build. Other risk factors are related to behaviour and lifestyle (e.g. cigarette smoking, dislipidemia, centrally distributed obesity, hypertension, physical inactivity, and hyperglycemia) and are potentially reversible. Control of these risk factors is particularly important for those people who have non-modifiable risk factors, such as a family history of heart disease. The risk factors interact with each other and their effect is cumulative. Besides these, stressful situations, cold weather and soft drinking water have also been indicated to contribute towards development of CHD [7]. Some important contributors have been briefly discussed.

Genetic Factors

Genetic and environmental factors cause mutation of a single smooth muscle cell from near the side of the plaque (like a benign tumour of the artery wall). The conditions involved may be similar to that which transform cells and initiate cancers.

Injury and Blood Clot

Injury to the blood vessel wall occurs from mechanical damage or physical condition, leading to rupture of small capillary blood vessels and formation of a blood clot or thrombosis. Physical injury may result from elevated blood pressure (BP), chemical damage from cigarette smoking and resulting carbon monoxide (CO) in the blood.

Lipids and CHD

Triglycerides

A definite relationship between the amount of triglycerides in the diet and elevated blood lipid levels has been established. Dietary substitution of foods high in saturated animal fats with polyunsaturated fatty acids has produced a lowering of blood cholesterol.

Cholesterol

Increased concentration of cholesterol carrying lipoproteins, the low density lipoproteins (LDL) in the plasma have been shown repeatedly to be related to an increased risk of atherosclerosis. Cholesterol is essential for the body in small amounts. It is produced in the liver and some of it is also obtained from the diet. It is a constituent of cells, e.g. brain cells. Cholesterol is carried around the body in the blood by lipoproteins – LDL and high density lipoprotein (HDL). LDL cholesterol is the primary lipoprotein found in atherosclerotic plaque [8]. LDL oxidation is the key factor in the development of atherosclerosis [9-11]. Oxidised LDL is cytotoxic and is taken up by macrophages, which are the primary factor in plaque formation [8]. HDL is often called "good cholesterol" because it retrieves cholesterol from body tissues and helps to transfer it to the liver for disposal. The level of cholesterol in the blood depends partly on genetic factors but diet is also important. The levels of blood cholesterol are measured in millimoles/litre (mmol/l) against which the risks of heart disease are calculated, as given in Table 1 [12].

Table 1. Cholesterol levels and risk of heart disease

Cholesterol (mmol/1)	Risk factor
< 5.2	Low
5.2-6.5	Average
6.5-7.8	Moderate
> 7.8	High

Homocysteine and CHD

Homocysteine is a metabolic product of methyl group donation of amino acid methionine [13]. Hyperhomocysteinemia has been shown to be a significant risk factor for cardiovascular diseases. It arises from the lack of key enzymes or vitamins, such as methylenetetra hydropholate reductase, vitamin B6 and folate, which are involved in homocysteine metabolism [14]. Its seriousness as a risk factor for CHD has been equated to hypercholesterolemia and smoking [14]. It has been shown to produce multiple effects, such as alteration of platelet function and coagulation factors [15-17], endothelial damage and dysfunction [18, 19], encouraging the oxidation of low-density lipoprotein [20, 21], smooth muscle proliferation [22, 23], and endothelian-leukocyte interactions [24]. Homosysteine's physiological role is to assist in maintaining sulphur-amino acid homeostasis. Beyond this metabolic process, it is beginning to be recognised as a significant risk factor for cardiovascular diseases [14].

Research work is still going on the involvement of lipids, especially cholesterol in CHD, but it is established that atherosclerosis is a multiple risk factor disease process, enhanced serum cholesterol is a major contributor to CHD and saturated animal fat can affect serum cholesterol level. Hence, importance of dietary factors in control of CHD is being recognised now.

Dietary Factors and CHD

Dietary Lipids

There is now overwhelming evidence that dietary factors reflect the risk of CHD [25-27]. Three most common atherogenic dietary risk factors are saturated fats, cholesterol and obesity [26, 27].

Blood cholesterol level is affected more by the amount and type of fat in the diet than the amount of dietary cholesterol. A high intake of saturated fatty acids in diet can increase the amount of cholesterol produced in the liver and, hence, in the blood. Strong correlation has been noted between CHD and percentage of energy derived from saturated fatty acids [7]. The major sources of saturates in the diet include cooking fats and spreads (e.g. butter, margarine, lard), fatty meats and meat products, full fat milk and dairy products, chips, biscuits, cakes, pastries and confectionery. Dietary cholesterol has a weaker effect on blood cholesterol levels. Cholesterol is found only in foods of animal origin. Liver, egg yolk and shellfish are the major sources of dietary cholesterol but red meats, poultry, whole milk and cheese also contribute to the cholesterol content of the diet. In most of the cases, reducing saturated fat intake is more important than monitoring dietary cholesterol.

Fatty acids are usually in the cis configuration, which is determined by the way in which the carbon and hydrogen molecules of fat are joined together. Trans fatty acids (which contain a double bond in the trans configuration) occur seldom in nature but can be found in ruminant fats and milk being produced by fermentation in the rumen of cows, sheep and goats. Trans double bonds can be produced during the hydrogenation process whereby oils are used to make margarines. High intake of trans fatty acids appear to be associated with CHD [7]. The main dietary sources are hard margarine and foods prepared by using this type of fat.

Replacing saturates in the diet with either mononsaturated fatty acids or polyunsaturated fatty acids can lower LDL cholesterol levels. For example, monounsaturates found in olive oil, rapeseed oil and cereal products may have benefits in terms of heart disease.

Essential Fatty Acids (EFAs)

Essential fatty acids (EFAs) are necessary fats that are not synthesised in the body and must be obtained through diet. EFAs are long chain polyunsaturated fatty acids derived from oleic, linoleic and linolenic acids. There are two families of EFA: Ω-3 and Ω-6. Ω-9 is necessary yet "non-essential" because the body can manufacture a modest amount on its own, provided essential EFAs are present. The number following 'Ω-' represents the position of the first double bond, counting from the terminal methyl group on the molecule. Ω-3 fatty acids are derived from linolenic acid, Ω-6 from linoleic acid, and Ω-9 from oleic acid.

EFAs support the cardiovascular, reproductive, immune and nervous systems. The body requires EFAs for formation and repair of cell membranes. EFAs primary function is production of prostaglandins, which regulate body functions, such as heart rate, BP, blood clotting, fertility, conception, and play a role in immune function by regulating inflammation. EFA deficiency and Ω-6/Ω-3 imbalance are linked to serious health conditions, such as heart attacks, cancer, insulin resistance, asthma, lupus, schizophrenia, depression, postpartum depression, accelerated aging, stroke, obesity, diabetes, arthritis and alzheimer's disease etc. EFA deficiency is common worldwide, particularly Ω-3 deficiency. An ideal intake ratio of Ω-6 to Ω-3 fatty acids is between 1:1 to 4:1, with most people only obtaining a ratio between 10:1 and 25:1. The minimum healthy intake for both linolenic (Ω-3) and linoleic (Ω-6) acid via diet, per adult per day, is 1.5 g of each. One tablespoon of flaxseed oil can provide this amount. As high heat destroys linolenic acid, cooking in linolenic rich oils or eating cooked linolenic rich fish is unlikely to provide a sufficient amount.

Ω-3 (Linolenic Acid)

α-linolenic acid is the principal Ω-3 fatty acid, which a healthy human will convert into eicosapentaenoic acid and, later, into docosahexaenoic acid. Ω-3 fatty acids are used in the formation of cell walls, improving circulation and oxygen uptake with proper red blood cell flexibility and function. Ω-3 deficiencies are linked to increased tendency to form blood clots, increased triglycerides, increased LDL cholesterol, impaired membrane function, hypertension and irregular heart beats [5]. Ω-3 fatty acids are found in flaxseed oil, which has the highest linolenic acid content of any food. Besides these, hempseed oil, hempseeds, walnuts, pumpkin seeds, Brazil nuts, sesame seeds, avocados, some dark leafy green vegetables (kale, spinach, purslane, mustard greens, collards etc.), canola oil, soybean oil, wheat germ oil, salmon, mackerel, sardines, anchovies, albacore tuna and others are good source of this fatty acid. Ω-3 poly unsaturated fatty acid (1 g/day) has been recommended for reduction in risk of mortality by cardiac arrhythmia [28]. Flaxseed oil used for dietary supplementation should be maintained under refrigeration or freezing conditions.

Fibre

Dietary fibre is characterised on the basis of its solubility in the intestine. Fibres with high water holding capacity, such as pectins, gums and psyllium have been referred as soluble fibres. Both soluble and insoluble fibres are important for gastrointestinal health as well as cholesterol lowering benefit [29]. Wheat, rye, rice and most other grains are primarily composed of insoluble fibre [30, 31]. Oats have a greater proportion of soluble fibre than any other grain. Barley contains both, but is mainly insoluble fibre. Legumes, beans and peas are very good sources of both types of fibres. Certain fruits and vegetables are also good sources of both soluble and insoluble fibres. [29]. However, more amounts of fruits and vegetables should be consumed to equal the fibre content obtained from beans and cereal grains.

Recent research provides evidence that viscous polysaccharides act in the gastrointestinal tract to reduce blood cholesterol by decreasing absorption of cholesterol or fatty acids and decreasing absorption of biliary cholesterol [32, 33]. Fibre may also cause altered serum concentration of hormones or short-chain fatty acids that affect lipid metabolism. β-Glucan, the water soluble fibre prevalent in oats and barley, has been shown in animal models to be the active agent causing the altered cholesterol metabolism [34]. Another type of dietary fibre called resistant starch may also reduce the risk of CHD. Resistant starch is a type of starch that resists digestion to its component sugar, glucose in the small intestine and passes unchanged into the large intestine. Here, resistant starch is fermented by gut bacteria producing short-chain fatty acids, which may help reduce blood cholesterol levels. Some foods rich in resistant starch are whole or partly-milled grains and seeds, pulses and corn flakes.

Numerous studies have shown that vegetarians have lower serum cholesterol and mortality rates than non-vegetarians, but whether it is due to fibre itself or due to greater intake of complex carbohydrates and saturated fats is difficult to understand [35-37]. The mechanism by which increased fibre intake reduces serum cholesterol is still unclear. Nonetheless, benefits of diet rich in whole grains, fruits and vegetables has been amply indicated in United States Food and Drug Administration (USFDA) food guide pyramid. Food containing wheat, rice, oats and corn are at the base of the pyramid and are the foundation of health promoting diet [38].

Soy Protein

It has long been recognised that CHD rates are lower in Japan where soy consumption is more common than Western countries [39]. This beneficial effect has been suggested due to alcohol extractable isoflavones like genistein and daidzein. However, in a study on monkeys, whole soy protein was found to be causing significant improvement in LDL and HDL cholesterol levels than alcohol extractable isoflavones [39]. The potential mechanisms by which soy protein might prevent atherosclerosis include a beneficial effect on plasma lipid concentration, increased LDL receptor activity, anti-oxidant effect, anti-proliferative effect of smooth muscles, effect on thrombus formation, maintenance of normal vascular activity, and modulation of hormone which affect cholesterol metabolism [5, 39].

Plant Sterols and Stanols

Plant sterols and stanols are members of the phytosterol family of compounds, which occur naturally in a variety of plants and vegetable oils, such as soy, corn and wheat. Plant sterols resemble cholesterol but have ethyl or methyl group or unsaturation in the side chain. They lower cholesterol by inhibiting cholesterol absorption and themselves are poorly absorbed [40]. Stanols are the product of 5-α saturation of sterols, which can be achieved commercially. Earlier, sterols were shown to be effective in lowering cholesterol [41, 42]. Then interest switched over to stanols, which are found in much smaller quantities [43]. But now the line between the two has blurred and they are considered equally effective [44]. Spreads with plant sterols/stanols are commercially available and USFDA has authorised their use in food labels as health claims based upon available evidences. Both have been reported to reduced cholesterol by 20 to 30% [43, 44].

Tea

A study in the US showed that self-reported moderate and heavy consumption of tea in the year before acute myocardial infarction was associated with lower mortality after infarction [45]. Improvement in endothelial dependent dialatation have been consistently observed in randomised control trials after both acute and chronic intake of green and black tea [46, 47]. Polyphenolic fraction found in green and black tea enhances nitric oxide bioavailability, which is impaired by free radical proxidation [48, 49]. Beneficial effect of green tea has been suggested due to inhibition of human platelet aggregation by epigallocatechin-3 gallate [50] and green tea catechin [51]. However, often, there are no improvements in anti-oxidant status after tea uptake, which therefore, does not support an anti-oxidant mechanism [4]. Hence, it has been suggested that the effect of tea may be due to polymeric polyphenols or other tea components which chelate transition metals [4].

Garlic

Garlic contains many important compounds including S-allyl systeine, which may protect from atherosclerosis by various mechanisms. Consumption of garlic decreases total and LDL cholesterol, increases HDL cholesterol, reduces serum triglycerides and fibrinogen concentration, lowers BP and inhibits platelet aggregation [52]. Aged garlic extract has been reported to inhibit LDL oxidation by scavenging peroxides and by chelation of copper ions [53]. LDL oxidation has been recognised as playing an important role in the initiation and progression of atherosclerosis. Oxidised LDL promotes vascular dysfunction by cytotoxicity towards endothelial cells [54]. Garlic has been suggested to play not only preventive but curative role in atherosclerosis by slightly regressing the plaque volume [55].

Alcohol

Inverse association between CHD and the moderate consumption of alcohol has been shown. Several studies have shown that self-reported low-to-moderate alcohol consumption is associated with low mortality that arises out of cardiovascular complications following acute myocardial infarction [56, 57]. It has been suggested that red wine, which contains anti-oxidant polyphenols, may offer greater protection than other types of alcohol. Wine is predominantly consumed in groups of higher socio-economic status where diet usually consists of a variety of foods and availability of different nutrients is sufficient [58]. Thus, definitive trials are required to confirm the effect of wine consumption on clinical end point in CHD patients [4]. A high level of consumption is associated with increased mortality [59]. In terms of chronic heart disease prevention, moderate drinking is generally recommended to those who already take alcohol but evidences do not justify that alcohol should be recommended to a non-drinker for its cardio protective effect.

Minerals and CHD

Sodium

The role of high amount of sodium in increasing the arterial BP by extra cellular volume expansion has been known since long [60, 61]. High BP predisposes to CHD and patients are routinely advised to lower sodium intake through diet. Minimum daily intake of 200 mg sodium (equivalent to 0.5 g NaCl) is sufficient to maintain normal physiological balance in the human body [62]. Normal diet contains sufficient sodium and, hence, table salt should be avoided.

Chromium

Chromium is a trace metal that is vital to human health. There are growing evidences from both animal and human studies showing role of chromium in atherosclerosis. Chromium supplementation in normal adult man has been reported to increase HDL cholesterol, decreased triglycerides and total cholesterol [63]. Animal studies also indicate improvement in serum cholesterol, aortic lipids and plaque formation due to supplementation with chromium [63]. Trace amounts of chromium are present in many foods. The best dietary source is brewer's yeast, which contains chromium in the form of glucose tolerance factor. Other good sources of chromium include peanuts, legumes, and whole grains.

Calcium

The degree of hardness in drinking water is inversely related to CHD incidence in epidemiological studies. Since water hardness is partly determined by calcium content, it has been suggested that calcium has protective effect [5]. Absorption of calcium is reduced in older people due to lower sensitivity of intestines to calcitriol and less renal synthesis of calcitriol [64]. Also, synthesis of vitamin D, which is required for absorption of calcium, is lower in aged people [65]. There is few evidence that calcium reduces BP and platelet aggregation by interfering with absorption of saturated fats [64]. Hypocalcaemic cardiomyopathy responds dramatically to calcium supplementation [66-68]. Milk, sardines (with bones) and cheese are good source of calcium.

Magnesium

Lack of magnesium has been linked to an increased risk of CHD, heart attacks and improper heartbeats. Low magnesium level is common in elderly patients with atrial fibrillations, heart failure [69, 70] and ventricular fibrillations [71]. Diuretics like thiazides increase magnesium loss. Incidence of magnesium deficiency in chronic heart failure has been reported at more than 30% and is accompanied by muscular magnesium deficiency [72]. Magnesium deficiency also causes positive sodium balance and negative potassium balance [73]. Deficiency of magnesium has been linked to free radical production as ascorbic acid supplementation inhibited cardiac failure in rats with magnesium deficiency [74, 75]. Heart failure as a consequence of hypomagnesaemia has also been reported in humans and correction of magnesium levels lead to improvement [76]. Hence, intake of magnesium may have inverse association with risk of CHD [77]. Magnesium can be found in almonds, parsley and spinach.

Zinc and Copper

Zinc is an anti-oxidant that helps maintain proper immune function. High level of lipid peroxides in rat hearts has been associated with zinc deficiency [78]. Lipid peroxides are an indicator of oxidative stress in body. Hence, it is suggested that zinc acts as an anti-oxidant [79]. Lower serum and high urinary zinc levels have been found in the case of heart failure [80]. Older people generally have zinc deficiency, which may be due to reduced nutritional protein [81]. Copper is also reported to play a role in regulation of oxidative free radicals and its deficiency increases lipoprotein peroxidation [82]. It has also been suggested that its deficiency may lead to increase in plasma cholesterol [83, 84]. Copper deficient cardiomyopathy has been recognised [85]. However, a proper balance in zinc and copper is a major factor in the etiology of CHD. High zinc to copper imbalance results in hypercholesterolemia and high mortality due to CHD [86]. We get more than enough copper from cereals, barley, legumes, nuts, shellfish and meats.

Selenium

The lower level of selenium in the blood and red blood cells may be related to the risk of CHD and heart attacks. Selenium activates glutathione peroxidase, one of the most potent anti-oxidants, which prevents the free radicals from attacking LDL cholesterol and prevents its conversion into its more artery damaging, oxidised form. Pure selenium deficiency is rare but symptoms may appear on additional stress, such as vitamin E deficiency [64]. A cardiomyopathy is prevalent in China known as Keshan disease due to selenium deficiency [87]. Patients on long-term parenteral nutrion have suffered from selenium deficiency leading to cardiomyopathy [88]. Deficiency leads to lipid peroxidation and increased oxidative stress [64]. Its supplementation in diet, therefore, may protect against CHD by preventing atherosclerosis. Selenium is provided by many foods, such as barley, shrimp, whole grains, tomatoes, poultry, shellfish, garlic, meat and egg yolk.

Vitamins and CHD

β-Carotene

β-carotene is present in plants, which gets converted to vitamin A in the body. There are reports that β-carotene protects against heart diseases by inhibiting the oxidation of LDL. Epidemiological evidence exists associating low β-carotene intake with the risk of acute myocardial infarction [89]. In combination with vitamin E and selenium it has been shown to reduce mortality due to heart diseases [90]. Whether its routine supplementation should be advocated or not, is unclear. β-carotene is found in yellow fruits and vegetables.

Niacin

Niacin has been used for many years for the treatment of hyperlipidemia. It has been shown to reduce coronary death and non-fatal myocardial infarction. It reduces total cholesterol, LDL cholesterol and triglycerides, and increases HDL cholesterol [91, 92]. The major drawbacks of niacin use are its side effects like flushing, palpitation, peptic ulcers, gout and hepatitis [91]. Still, combination of niacin with bile acid sequestrant is a powerful lipid altering therapy. Niaspan (extended release niacin), at a maximum recommended dosage of 2000 mg/day, has been reported to change lipid and lipoprotein levels in the desirable direction [92].

Vitamins B6, B12 and Folate

These vitamins are discussed together as they play a role in homocysteine metabolism. B6 is a co-factor for cystathionine β-synthase which mediates the transformation of homocysteine to cystathionine and altemately urinary excretion of sulphur. Homocysteine is remethylated to methionine via step requiring folic acid and vitamin B12 [93].

Strong inverse relationship has been reported between folate consumption and homocysteine levels [94, 95]. There is epidemiological evidence of an inverse link between folate consumption and risk of CHD [96, 97]. Association of low level of folate and vitamin B12 with higher levels of homocysteine has been documented [98]. Intake of folate and vitamin B6 above the current RDA may be important in primary prevention of CHD [99]. The rich food sources of folate are dark green leafy vegetables, whole grain cereals, legumes and animal products. Table 2 [100] shows the current reference daily intake of vitamins [100]. Vitamin B6 is amply found in poultry, fish, meat, legumes, nuts, potatoes and whole grains [101]. Vitamin B12 is found in animal products only, i.e. meat, poultry, fish, egg and milk.

Table 2. Current reference daily intake of vitamins

Vitamins	Daily value
Vitamin A	1500 μg/l (5000 IU)
Vitamin C	60 mg
Vitamin D	10 μg/l (400 IU)
Vitamin E	20 mg (30 IU)
Vitamin K	80 μg/l
Vitamin B6	2 mg
Vitamin B12	6 μg/l
Folate	400 μg/l
Thiamin	1.5 mg
Riboflavin	1.7 mg
Niacin	20 mg

Vitamins C and E

Vitamins C and E are anti-oxidants and are believed to prevent oxidation of LDL, thus, reducing the risk of CHD. Vitamin C administration has been shown to increase fibrinolytic activity [102]. Supplementation with vitamin C has also been shown to be effective in lowering BP by vasodilatation [103-106]. Vitamin E prevents atherosclerosis by its anti-oxidant effects and inhibitory effect on smooth muscle proliferation [107] and platelet adhesion [108]. In a study, supplementation with vitamin E has been shown to improve the imbalance between oxidative stress and anti-oxidant status in plasma [109]. Good sources of vitamin C include citrus fruits, strawberries, sweet red pepper and *aonla*. Germinated pulses and fish oils are good source of vitamin E.

Other Dietary Factors

Bromelain

It is an extract found in pineapple, which has demonstrated anti-thrombic and fibrinolytic activity [110]. It can be administered orally, is safe and without side effects. Its therapeutic benefits include reversible inhibition of platelet aggregation and angina pectoris. In a study, oral and intravenous application of bromelain inhibited thrombus formation in rats [111]. Its acceptance as a drug for inhibition of platelet aggregation will depend upon more clinical trials.

Policosanols

These are aliphatic alcohols obtained from purified sugarcane. Policosanols have been shown to decrease risk of atheroma formation by reducing platelet aggregation [112] and endothelial damage [113]. They also lower LDL cholesterol and improve HDL cholesterol, possibly by reducing cholesterol synthesis and enhancing LDL clearance [113]. Policosanols appear to be promising in prevention and therapy of CHD.

Guggulipid

Herbal extract of guggul tree (*Commiphora mukul*) – used in ayurvedic medicines for hundreds of years in Asia for treating a variety of diseases – has been growing in popularity as a cholesterol lowering agent in the US [114]. It has been shown to be effective in decreasing serum cholesterol and triglycerides [115-117]. Its anti-hyperlipidemic effect has been suggested to be due to guggul sterones. But, a short-term trial indicated that it is ineffective and may even raise LDL cholesterol [114]. Further studies are needed before its recommendation as a cholesterol lowering agent.

Ubiquinone (Co-enzyme Q10)

It is a naturally occurring vitamin-like fat soluble substance found in high concentration in mitochondria of myocardium, liver and kidney [64]. Heart failure is associated with low intra-myocardial ATP and Q10 levels [118]. It has properties which have the potential of preventing cellular damage during myocardial ischemia [119]. Daily doses of 50 to 150 mg orally for three months have been shown to improve arrhythmia and palpitation [118].

Turmeric

Turmeric is a spice that is obtained from the root of *Curcuma longa*, a member of the ginger family, Zingaberaceae. In ayurveda, turmeric has been used for its medicinal properties for various indications and through different roots of administration, including tropically, orally and inhalation. Curcuminoids are components of turmeric, which include mainly curcumin (diferuloyl methane), demethoxycurcumin and bisdemethoxycurcumin [120]. The effect of curcumin administration in reducing the serum levels of choleseterol and lipid peroxides was studied in ten healthy human volunteers, receiving 500 mg of curcumin per day for seven days. A significant decrease in the level of serum lipid peroxides, increase in HDL cholesterol and a decrease in total serum cholesterol were noted. As curcumin reduced serum lipid peroxides and serum cholesterol, the study of curcumin as a chemopreventive substance against arterial diseases is suggested [121].

Conclusion

Nutrition and food habits play an important role in precipitating as well as in reducing cardiovascular reactivity.

Key Points

- ❑ Dietary factors play an important role in either precipitating CHD or have the potential of reducing the occurrence of CHD.
- ❑ Dietary lipids, cholesterol and LDL contribute to the development of CHD.
- ❑ In the past, health-oriented dietary approaches focussed on reduced salt, sugar and saturated fats in diet. Nowadays, more attention is being given to specific nutrients that can reduce the risk of CHD.
- ❑ Food is a complex system where nutrient's interaction with each other affects their absorption and their ultimate bioavailability. However, beneficial effect of dietary fibre, plant sterols/ stanols, Ω-3 fatty acids, tea, garlic, chromium, calcium, magnesium, zinc, selenium, vitamins B6 and B12, folate, niacin, vitamins C and E have been shown in numerous reports.
- ❑ Besides these, bromelain (pineapple), policosanols (sugarcane), guggulsterones (*Commiphora mukul*) and curcuminoids (turmeric) appear to have the potential of preventing the CHD.
- ❑ Absorption of vitamins and minerals in the intestine decreases in old age, which is generally the period of occurrence of cardiovascular diseases. Hence, dietary supplements are essential for enhancement of quality of life and prevention of CHD, even if their benefits are marginal.
- ❑ It is certain that in the near future emphasis will be more on a vegetarian pattern of diet.

References

1. AHA, 1989, *Heart Facts*, American Heart Association, Dallas.
2. Elson, C.E., 1992, "Tropical Oils: Nutritional and Scientific Issues – Critical Reviews", *Food Science and Nutrition*, 3, pp. 79-102.
3. Macnair, A.L., 1994, "Physical Activity, Not Diet, Should be the Focus of Measures for the Primary Prevention Cardiovascular Disease", *Nutritional Research and Reviews*, 7, pp. 43-65.
4. Hamer, M. and Steptoe, A., 2006, "Influence of Specific Nutrients on Progression of Atherosclerosis, Vascular Function, Haemostasis and Inflammation in Coronary Heart Disease Patients: A Systematic Review", *British Journal of Nutrition*, 95, pp. 849-859.
5. Wheatcroft, S., Noronh, B. and Kearney, M., 2005, "The Heart and Blood Vessels", In *Clinical Nutrition*, M.J. Gibney, M. Elia, O. Lungquist and J. Dowsett (Eds.), Nutrition Society Textbook Series, Blackwell Publishing, pp. 268-293.
6. de Lorgeril, M., Salen, P. and Defaye, P., 2005, "Importance of Nutrition in Chronic Heart Failure Patients", *European Heart Journal*, 26, pp. 2215-2217.
7. Mann, J., 2004, "Cardiovascular Disease", In *Public Health Nutrition*, M.J. Gibney, B.M. Margetts, J.M. Kerney and L. Arab, Blackwell Publishers, pp. 317-329.

8. Adams, A.K., Wermuth, E.O. and Mcbride, P.E., 1999, "Antioxidant Vitamins and Prevention of Coronary Heart Disease", *American Academy of Family Physicians*, 60, pp. 895-904.
9. Diaz, M.N., Frei, B., Vita, J.A. and Keaney, J.F. Jr., 1997, "Antioxidants and Atherosclerotic Heart Disease", *New England Journal of Medicine*, 337, pp. 408-416.
10. Schwartz, C.J., Valente, A.J. and Sprague, E.A., 1993, "A Modern View of Atherogenesis", *American Journal of Cardiology*, 71, pp. 9B-14B.
11. Jialal, I. and Grundy, S.M., 1992, "Influence of Antioxidant Vitamins on LDL Oxidation", *Annals of New York Academy of Science*, 669, pp. 237-248.
12. McWhirter, A. and Clasen, L., 1996, "Foods that Harm, Foods that Heal", *An A-Z Guide to Safe and Healthy Eating*, Reader's Digest Association Ltd., London, New York, Sydney, Cape Town, Montreal.
13. Haynes, W.G., 2002, "Hyperhomocysteinemia, Vascular Function and Atherosclerosis: Effects of Vitamins", *Cardiovascular Drugs and Therapy*, 16(5), pp. 391-399.
14. Fanapour, P.C., Yug, B. and Kochar, M.S., 1999, "Hyperhomocysteinemia: An Additional Cardiovascular Risk Factor", *Wisconsin Medical Journal*, 98(8), pp. 51-54.
15. Lentz, S.R. and Sadler, J.E., 1991, "Inhibition of Thrombomodulin Surface Expression and Protein C Activation by the Thrombogenic Agent Homocysteine", *Journal of Clinical Investigation*, 88, pp. 1906-1914.
16. Nappo, F., DeRosa, N., Marfella, R., DeLucia, D., Ingrosso, D., Perna, A.F., Farzati, B. and Giugliano, D., 1999, "Impairment of Endothelial Functions by Acute Hyperhomocysteinemia and Reversal by Antioxidant Vitamins", *Journal of American Medical Association*, 281, pp. 2113-2118.
17. Rodgers, G.M. and Kane, W.H., 1996, "Activation of Endogenous Factor V by a Homocysteine-induced Vascular Endothelial Cell Activator", *Journal of Clinical Investigation*, 77, pp. 1909-1916.
18. Wall, R.T., Harlan, J.M., Harker, L.A. and Striker, G.E., 1980, "Homocysteine-induced Endothelial Cell Injury *In Vitro*: A Model for the Study of Vascular Injury", *Thrombosis Research*, 18, pp. 113-121.
19. Berman, R.S. and Martin, W., 1993, "Arterial Endothelial Barrier Dysfunction: Actions of Homocysteine and the Hypoxanthine-xanthine Oxidase Free Radical Generating System", *British Journal of Pharmacology*, 108, pp. 920-926.
20. Blom, H.J., Engelen, D.P. and Boers, G.H., 1992, "Lipid Peroxidation in Homocysteinemia", *Journal of Inherited Metabolic Disease*, 15, pp. 419-422.
21. Blom, H.J., Kleinveld, H.A. and Boers, G.H., 1995, "Lipid Peroxidation and Susceptibility of Low-density Lipoprotein to *In Vitro* Oxidation in Hyperhomocysteinemia", *European Journal of Clinical Investigation*, 25, pp. 149-154.
22. Tyagi, S.C., 1998, "Homocysteine Redox Receptor and Regulation of Extracellular Matrix Components in Vascular Cells", *American Journal of Physiology*, 274, pp. C396-C405.
23. Tsai, J.C., Perella, M.A. and Yoshizumi, M., 1994, "Promotion of Vascular Smooth Muscle Cell Growth by Homocysteine: A Link to Atherosclerosis", *Proceedings of National Academy of Sciences*, USA, 91, pp. 6369-6373.
24. Dudman, N.P., Temple, S.E., Guo, X.W., Fu, W. and Perry, M.A., 1999, "Homocysteine Enhances Neutrophil-endothelial Interactions in Both Cultured Human Cells and Rats *In Vivo*", *Circulation Research*, 84, pp. 409-416.
25. National Academy of Sciences, 1989, *Diet and Health*, National Academy Press, Washington, D.C.
26. National Cholesterol Education Program, 1990, "Report of the Expert Panel on Population Strategies for Blood Cholesterol Reduction", NIH Publication, US Department of Health and Human Services, Bethesda, Maryland, 90-3046.
27. The Nutrition Committee, AHA, 1996, "Dietary Guidelines for Healthy American Adults", *Circulation*, American Heart Association, 94, pp. 1795-1800.

28. Marchioli, R., Brazi, F. and Bomba, E., 2002, "Early Protection Against Sudden Death by n-3 Polyunsaturated Fatty Acids after Myocardial Infraction: Time-course Analysis of the Results of the Grouppo Italiano per lo Studio della Sopravvivenza nell'Infarto Miocardico (GISSI)-Prevenzione", *Circulation*, 105(16), pp. 1897-1903.
29. Horn, L.V., 1997, "Fiber, Lipids and Coronary Heart Disease: A Statement for Healthcare Professionals from the Nutrition Committee, American Heart Association", *Circulation*, 95, pp. 2701-2704.
30. Englyst, H., Wiggins, H.S. and Cummings, J.H., 1982, "Determination of the Non-starch Polysaccharides in Plant Foods by Gas-liquid Chromatography of Constituent Sugars as Alditol Acetates", *Analyst*, 107, pp. 307-318.
31. Southgate, D.A., Hudson, G.J. and Englyst, H., 1978, "The Analysis of Dietary Fiber: The Choices for the Analyst", *Journal of Science of Food and Agriculture*, 29, pp. 979-998.
32. Marlett, J.A., Hosig, K.B., Vollendorf, N.W., Shinnick, F.L., Haack, V.S. and Story, J.A., 1994, "Mechanism of Serum Cholesterol Reduction by Oat Bran", *Hepatology*, 20, pp. 1450-1457.
33. Anderson, J.W., Story, L., Sieling, B., Chen, W.J., Petro, M.S. and Story, J., 1984, "Hypocholesterolemic Effects of Oat-bran or Bean Intake for Hypercholesterolemic Men", *American Journal of Clinical Nutrition*, 40, pp. 1146-1155.
34. Shinnick, F., Mathews, R. and Ink, S., 1991, "Serum Cholesterol Reduction by Oats and Other Fiber Sources", *Cereal Foods World*, 36, pp. 815-821.
35. Burslem, J., Schonfeld, G., Howald, M.A., Weidman, S.W. and Miller, J.P., 1978, "Plasmaapoprotein and Lipoprotein Lipid Levels in Vegetarians", *Metabolism*, 27, pp. 711-719.
36. Knuiman, J.T. and West, C.E., 1982, "The Concentration of Cholesterol in Serum and in Various Serum Liproproteins in Macrobiotic, Vegetarians and Non-vegetarians Men and Boys", *Atherosclerosis*, 43, pp. 71-82.
37. Sacks, F.M., Castelli, W.P., Donner, A. and Kass, E.H., 1975, "Plasma Lipids and Lipoproteins in Vegetarians and Controls", *New England Journal of Medicine*, 292, pp. 1148-1151.
38. Kahlon, T.S. and Smith, G.E., 2004, "Health Benefits of Grains, Fruits and Vegetables and the USFDA Good Guide Pyramid", *Cereal Food World*, 49, pp. 50288-50290.
39. Anthony, M.S., Clarkson, T.B. and Williams, J.K., 1998, "Effects of Soy Isoflavones on Atherosclerosis: Potential Mechanisms", *American Journal of Clinical Nutrition*, 68 (Suppl. 6), pp. 1390S-1393S.
40. Jenkins, D.J.A. and Kendall, C.W.C., 1999, "Plant Sterols, Health Claims and Strategies to Reduce Cardiovascular Disease Risk", *Journal of the American College of Nutrition*, 18(6), pp. 559-562.
41. Lees, A.M., Mok, H.Y., Lees, R.S., McClusky, M.A. and Grundy, S.M., 1977, "Plant Sterols as Cholesterol-lowering Agents: Clinical Trials in Patients with Hypercholesterolemia and Studies of Sterol Balance", *Atherosclerosis*, 28, pp. 325-338.
42. Lees, R.S. and Lees, A.M., 1976, "Effects of Sitosterol Therapy on Plasma Lipid and Lipoprotein Concentration", In *Lipoprotein Metabolism*, H. Greten, Springer-Verlag, New York.
43. Becker, M., Staab, D. and von Bergmann, K., 1993, "Treatment of Severe Familial Hypercholesterolemia in Childhood with Sitosterol and Sitostanol", *Journal of Pediatrics*, 122, pp. 292-296.
44. Westrate, J.A. and Meijer, G.W., 1998, "Plant Sterol-enriched Margarines and Reduction of Plasma Total- and LDL-cholesterol Concentrations in Normocholesterolaemic and Mildly Hypercholesterolaemic Subjects", *European Journal of Clinical Nutrition*, 52, pp. 334-343.
45. Mukamal, K.J., Maclure, M., Muller, J.E., Sherwood, J.B. and Mittleman, M.A., 2002, "Tea Consumption and Mortality After Acute Myocardial Infarction", *Circulation*, 105, pp. 2476-2481.
46. Hodgson, J.M., Burke, V. and Puddey, I.B., 2005, "Acute Effects of Tea on Fasting and Post Prandial Vascular Function and Blood Pressure in Humans", *Journal of Hypertension*, 23, pp. 47-54.
47. Widlansky, M.E., Duffy, S.J., Hamburg, N.M., Gokcy, N., Warden, B.A., Wiseman, S., Keaney, J.F. Jr., Frie, B. and Vita, J.A., 2005, "Effects of Black Tea Consumption on Plasma Catechin and

Markers of Oxidative Stress and Inflammation in Patients with Coronary Artery Disease", *Free Radical Biology and Medicine*, 38, pp. 499-506.
48. Anter, E., Thomas, S.R., Schulz, E., Shapira, O.M., Vita, J.A. and Keaney, J.F. Jr., 2004, "Activation of Endothelial Nitric Oxide Synthase by the p38 MAPK in Response to Black Tea Polyphenol", *Journal of Biological Chemistry*, 279, pp. 46637-46643.
49. Lorenz, M., Wessler, S., Follmann, E., Michaelis, W., Dusterhoft, T., Baumann, G., Stangl, K. and Stangl, V.A., 2004, "Constituent of Green Tea, Epigallocatechin-3-gallate, Activates Endothelial Nitric Oxide Synthase by a Phophatidylinositol-3-OH-kinase-,cAMP-dependent Protein Kinase- and Akt- Dependent Pathway and Leads to Endothelial-dependent Vasorelaxation", *Journal of Biological Chemistry*, 279, pp. 6190-6195.
50. Deana, R., Turetta, L., Donella-Deana, A., Dona, M., Brunati, A.M., De Michiel, L. and Garbisa, S., 2003, "Green Tea Epigallocatechin-3-gallate Inhibits Platelet Signalling Pathways Triggered by Both Proteolytic and Non-proteolytic Agonists", *Thrombosis and Haemostasis*, 89(5), pp. 866-874.
51. Kang, W.S., Chung, K.H., Chung, J.H., Lee, J.Y., Park, J.B., Zhang, Y.H., Yoo, H.S. and Yun, Y.P., 2001, "Antiplatelet Activity of Green Tea Catechins is Mediated by Inhibition of Cytoplasmic Calcium Increase", *Journal of Cardiovascular Pharmacology*, 38(6), pp. 875-884.
52. Siegel, G., Walter, A., Engel, S., Walper, A. and Michel, F., 1999, "Pleiotropic Effects of Garlic", *Wiener Medizinische Wochenschrift*, 149(8-10), pp. 217-224.
53. Dillon, S.A., Burmi, R.S., Lowe, G.M., Billington, D. and Rahman, K., 2003, "Antioxidant Properties of Aged Garlic Extract: An *In Vitro* Study Incorporating Human Low Density Lipoprotein", *Life Science*, 72(14), pp. 1583-1594.
54. Lau, B.H., 2001, "Suppression of LDL Oxidation by Garlic", *J. of Nutrition*, 131(3s), pp. 985S-988S.
55. Koscielny, J., Klussendorf, D., Latza, R., Schmitt, R., Radtke, H., Siegel, G. and Kiesewetter, H., 1999, "The Antiatherosclerotic Effect of Allium Sativum", *Atherosclerosis*, 144(1), pp. 237-249.
56. Muntwyler, J., Hennekens, C.H., Buring, J.E. and Jaziano, J.M., 1998, "Mortality and Light to Moderate Alcohol Consumption After Myocardial Infarction", *Lancet*, 352, pp. 1882-1885.
57. Mukamal, K.J., Maclure, M., Muller, J.E., Sherwood, J.B. and Mittleman, M.A., 2001, "Prior Alcohol Consumption and Mortality Following Acute Myocardial Infarction", *Journal of American Medical Association*, 285, pp. 1965-1970.
58. Nielsen, N.R., Schnohr, P., Jensen, G. and Gronbaek, M., 2004, "Is the Relationship between Type of Alcohol and Mortality Influenced by Socio-economic Status?", *Journal of International Medicine*, 255, pp. 280-288.
59. Bobak, M. and Marmot, M., 2005, "Alcohol and Coronary Heart Disease", In *Coronary Heart Disease Epidemiology: From Etiology to Public Health*, 2nd Edn., M. Marmot and P. Elliott (Eds.), Oxford University Press, pp. 261-263.
60. Sebranek, J.G., Olson, D.G., Whiting, R.C., Benedict, R.C., Rust, R.E., Kraft, A.A. and Woychik, J.H., 1983, "Physiological Role of Dietary Sodium in Human Health and Implications of Sodium Reduction in Muscle Foods", *J. Food Technol.*, 37, pp. 51-59.
61. Truswell, A.S., 1994, "The Evolution of Diets for Western Diseases", In *Food Multidisciplinary Perspective*, B. Harris-While and R. Hoffenderg (Eds.), Basil Blackwell, Oxford.
62. Gerdenswartz, M.H. and Schrier, R.W., 1982, "Renal Regulation of Sodium Excretion", In *Sodium: Its Biological Significance*, S. Papper (Ed.), CRC Press, Boca Raton, Florida, p. 19.
63. Anderson, R.A., 1986, "Trace Elements and Cardiovascular Diseases", *Acta. Pharmacol. Toxicol. (Copenh.)*, 59 (Suppl. 7), pp. 317-324.
64. Klaus, K.A., Witte, M.B., Andrew, L.C. and John, G.F., 2001, "Chronic Heart Failure and Micronutrients", *Journal of American College of Cardiology*, 37, pp. 1765-1774.
65. Maclaughlin, J. and Holick, M.F., 1985, "Aging Decreases the Capacity of Human Skin to Produce Vitamin D3", *Journal Clinical Investigation*, 76, pp. 1536-1538.

66. Brunvand, L., Haga, P., Tangsrud, S.E. and Haug, E., 1995, "Congestive Heart Failure Caused by Vitamin D Deficiency?", *Acta Paediatricia*, 84, pp. 106-108.
67. Rimailho, A., Bouchard, P., Schaison, G., Richard, C. and Auzopy, P., 1985, "Improvement of Hypocalcemic Cardiomyopathy by Correction of Serum Calcium Level", *American Heart Journal*, 109, pp. 611-613.
68. Palazzuoli, V., Martini, G., Giovani, S., Mondillo, S., Giusti, R., D'Arpino, A. and Ricci, D., 1990, "Dilated Cardiomyopathy Secondary to Idiopathic Hypoparathyroidism in Adults (Description of a Case)", *Recenti Progressi in Medicina*, 81, pp. 263-265.
69. Martin, B.J., McAlpine, J.K. and Devine, B.L., 1988, "Hypomagnesemia in Elderly Digitalized Patients", *Scottish Medical Journal*, 33, pp. 273-274.
70. DeCarli, C., Sprouse, G. and LaRosa, J.C., 1986, "Serum Magnesium Levels in Symptomatic Atrial Fibrillation and Their Relation to Rhythm Control by Intravenous Digoxin", *American Journal of Cardiology*, 57, pp. 956-959.
71. Perticone, F., Ceravolo, R., de Novara, G., Torchia, L. and Cloro, C., 1992, "New Data on the Anti-arrhythmic Value of Parenteral Magnesium Treatment: Magnesium and Ventricular Arrhythmias", *Magnesium Research*, 5, pp. 265-272.
72. Wester, P.O. and Dyckner, T., 1986, "Intracellular Electrolytes in Cardiac Failure", *Acta Medica Scandinavia*, Suppl., 707, pp. 33-36.
73. Shils, M.E., 1969, "Experimental Production of Magnesium Deficiency in Man", *Annals of New York Academy of Science*, 162, pp. 847-855.
74. Wu, F., Zou, L., Altura, B.T., Barbour, R.L. and Altura, B.M., 1992, "Low Extracellular Magnesium Results in Cardiac Failure in Isolated Perfused Rat Hearts", *Magnesium and Trace Elements*, 10, pp. 364-373.
75. Wu, F., Altura, B.T., Gao, J., Barbour, R.L. and Altura, B.M., 1994, "Ferrylmyoglobin Formation Induced by Acute Magnesium Deficiency in Perfused Rat Heart Causes Cardiac Failure", *Biochimica et Biophysica Acta*, 1225, pp. 158-164.
76. Fonseca, V. and Havard, C.W., 1985, "Electrolyte Disturbances and Cardiac Failure with Hypomagnesemia in Anorexia Nervosa", *British Medical Journal*, 291, pp. 1680-1682.
77. Al-Delaimy, W.K., Rimm, E.B., Willet, W.C., Stampfer, M.J. and Hu, F.B., 2004, "Magnesium Intake and Risk of Coronary Heart Disease Among Men", *Journal of American College of Nutrition*, 23(1), pp. 63-70.
78. Coudray, C., Charlon, V., de Leiris, J. and Favier, A., 1993, "Effect of Zinc Deficiency on Lipid Peroxidation Status and Infarct Size in Rat Hearts", *International Journal of Cardiology*, 41, pp. 109-113.
79. Kang, Y.J., 1999, "The Antioxidant Function of Metallothionein in the Heart", *Proceedings of the Society for Experimental Biology and Medicine*, 222, pp. 263-273.
80. Golik, A., Cohen, N., Ramot, Y., Maor, J., Moses, R.,Weissgarten, J., Leonov, Y. and Modai, D., 1993, "Type II Diabetes Mellitus, Congestive Cardiac Failure and Zinc Metabolism", *Biological Trace Element Research*, 39, pp. 171-175.
81. Greger, J.L., 1977, "Dietary Intake and Nutritional Status in Regard to Zinc of Institutionalized Aged", *Journal of Gerontolology*, 32, pp. 549-553.
82. Rayssiguier, Y., Gueux, E., Bussiere, L. and Mazur, A., 1993, "Copper Deficiency Increases the Susceptibility of Lipoproteins and Tissues to Peroxidation in Rats", *Journal of Nutrition*, 123, pp. 1343-1348.
83. Klevay, L.M., Inman, L., Johnson, L.K., Lawler, M., Mahalko, J.R., Milne, D.B., Lukaski, H.C., Bolonchuk, W. and Sandstead, H.H., 1984, "Increased Cholesterol in Plasma in a Young Man During Experimental Copper Depletion", *Metabolism*, 33, pp. 1112-1118.

84. Klevay, L.M., 1987, "Dietary Copper: A Powerful Determination of Cholesterolemia", *Medical Hypotheses*, 24, pp. 111-119.
85. Kopp, S.J., Klevay, L.M. and Feliksik, J.M., 1983, "Physiological and Metabolic Characterization of a Cardiomyopathy Induced by Chronic Copper Deficiency", *American Journal of Physiology*, 245, pp. H855-H866.
86. Klevay, L.M., 1975, "Coronary Heart Disease: The Zinc/copper Hypothesis", *Journal of American College of Nutrition*, 28(7), pp. 764-774.
87. Cenac, A., Simonoff, M., Moretto, P. and Djibo, A., 1992, "A Low Plasma Selenium is a Risk Factor for Peripartum Cardiomyopathy", *International Journal of Cardiology*, 36, pp. 57-59.
88. Lockitch, G., Taylor, G.P., Wong, L.T., Davidson, A.G., Dison, P.J., Riddell, D. and Massing, B., 1990, "Cardiomyopathy Associated with Nonendemic Selenium Deficiency in a Caucasian Adolescent", *American Journal of Clinical Nutrition*, 52, pp. 572-577.
89. Tavani, A., Negri, E., D'Avanzo, B. and La Vecchia, C., 1997, "Beta-carotene Intake and Risk of Non-fatal Acute Myocardial Infarction in Women", *European Journal of Epidemiology*, 13, pp. 631-637.
90. Blot, W.J., 1993, "Nutrition Intervention Trials in Vitamin/mineral Combinations, Cancer Incidence and Disease-specific Mortality in the General Population", *Journal of the National Cancer Institute*, 85, pp. 1483-1492.
91. Crouse, J.R. III., 1996, "New Developments in the Use of Niacin for Treatment of Hyperlipidemia: New Considerations in the Use of an Old Drug", *Coronart Artery Diseases*, 7(4), pp. 321-326.
92. Goldberg, A.C., 1998, "Clinical Trial Experience with Extended-release Niacin (Niaspan): Dose-escalation Study", *American Journal of Cardiology*, 82, pp. 35U-38U.
93. Wilcken, D.E. and Wilcken, B., 1998, "B Vitamins and Homocysteine in Cardiovascular Disease and Aging", *Annals of New York Academy of Science*, 854, pp. 361-370.
94. Kang, S.S., Wong, P.W. and Norusis, M., 1987, "Homocysteinemia Due to Folate Deficiency", *Metabolism*, 36, pp. 458-462.
95. Nygord, O., Refsum, H., Veland, P.M. and Vollset, S.E., 1998, "Major Life Style Determinants of Plasma Total Homocysteine Distribution: The Hordaland Homocysteine Study", *American Journal of Clinical Nutrition*, 67, pp. 263-270.
96. Panchurinti, N., Lewis, C.A. and Sauberlich, H.E., 1994, "Plasma Homocysteine, Folate and Vitamin B 12 Concentrations and Risk of Early Onset Coronary Artery Disease", *American Journal of Clinical Nutrition*, 59, pp. 940-948.
97. Morrison, H.I., Schaubel, D., Derneules, M. and Wigle, D.T., 1996, "Serum Folate and Risk of Fatal Coronary Heart Disease", *Journal of American Medical Association*, 275, pp. 1893-1896.
98. Genser, D., Prachar, H., Hauer, R., Halbmayer, W.M., Mlczoch, J. and Elmadfa, I., 2006, "Homocysteine, Folate and Vitamin B12 in Patients with Coronary Heart Diseases", *Annals of Nutritional Metabolism*, 50(5), pp. 413-419.
99. Rimm, E.B., Willet, W.C., Hu, F.B., Sampson, L., Colditz, G.A., Manson, J.E., Hennekens, C. and Stampfer, M.J., 1998, "Folate and Vitamin B6 from Diet and Supplements in Relation to Risk of Coronary Heart Disease Among Women", *Journal of American Medical Association*, 279(5), pp. 359-364.
100. Fairfield, K.M. and Fletcher, R.H., 2002, "Vitamins for Chronic Disease Prevention in Adults", *Journal of American Medical Association*, 287, pp. 3116-3126.
101. Dong, M.H., McGown, E.L., Schwenneker, B.W. and Saubrich, H.E., 1980, "Thiamin, Riboflavin and Vitamin B6 Contents of Selected Food as Served", *Journal of American Dietetic Assocociation*, 76, pp. 156-160.
102. Bordia, A.K., 1980, "The Effect of Vitamin C on Blood Lipids, Fibrinolytic Activity and Platelet Adhesiveness in Patients with Coronary Artery Disease", *Atherosclerosis*, 35(2), pp. 181-187.

103. Taddei, S., Virdis, A., Ghiadoni, L., Magagna, A. and Salvetti, A., 1998, "Vitamin C Improves Endothelium-dependent Vasodilation by Restoring Nitric Oxide Activity in Essential Hypertension", *Circulation*, 97, pp. 2222-2229.
104. Duffy, S.J., Gokce, N., Holbrook, M., Huang, A., Frei, B., Keany, J.F. Jr. and Vita, J.A., 1999, "Treatment of Hypertension with Ascorbic Acid", *Lancet*, 354, pp. 2048-2049.
105. Gokce, N., Keaney, J.F., Frei, B., Holbrook, M., Olesiak, M., Zachariah, B.J., Leeuwenburgh, C., Heinecke, J.W. and Vita, J.A., 1999, "Long-term Ascorbic Acid Administration Reverses Endothelial Vasomotor Dysfunction in Patients with Coronary Artery Disease", *Circulation*, 99, pp. 3234-3240.
106. Levine, G.N., Frei, B., Koulouris, S.N., Gerhard, M.D., Keany, J.F. Jr. and Vita, J.A., 1996, "Ascorbic Acid Reverses Endothelial Vasomotor Dysfunction in Patients with Coronary Artery Disease", *Circulation*, 93, pp. 1107-1113.
107. Boscoboinik, D., Szewczyk, A., Hensey, C. and Azzi, A., 1991, "Inhibition Cell Proliferation by Alfa Tocoferol: Role of Protein Kinase C", *Journal of Biological Chemistry*, 266, pp. 6188-6194.
108. Steiner, M., 1993, "Vitamin E More than an Antioxidant", *Clinical Cardiology*, 16, pp. 116-118.
109. Micheletta, F., Natoli, S., Misuraca, M., Sabarizia, E., Diczfalusy, U. and Iuliano, L., 2004, "Vitamin E Supplementation in Patients with Carotid Atherosclerosis: Reversal of Altered Oxidative Stress Status in Plasma But Not in Plaque", *Arteriosclerosis, Thrombosis and Vascular Biology*, 24(1), pp. 136-140.
110. Maurer, H.R., 2001, "Bromelain: Biochemistry, Pharmacology and Medical Use", *Cellular and Molecular Life Science*, 58(9), pp. 1234-1245.
111. Metzig, C., Grabowska, E., Eckert, K., Rehse, K. and Maurer, H.R., 1999, "Bromelain Proteases Reduce Human Platelet Aggregation In Vitro, Adhesion to Bovine Endothelial Cells and Thrombus Formation in Rat Vessels *In Vivo*", *In Vivo*, 13(1), pp. 7-12.
112. Arruzazabala, M.L., Valdes, S., Mas, R., Carbazol, D. and Fernandez, L., 1997, "Comparative Study of Policosanol, Aspirin and the Combination Therapy Policosanol-aspirin on Platelet Aggregation in Healthy Volunteers", *Pharmacology Research*, 36(4), pp. 293-297.
113. Varady, K.A., Wang, Y. and Jones, P.J., 2003, "Role of Policosanols in the Prevention and Treatment of Cardiovascular Disease", *Nutrition Reviews*, 61(11), pp. 376-383.
114. Szapary, P.O., Wolfe, M.L., Bloedon, L.T., Cucciara, A.J., Dermarderosian, A.H., Cirigliano, M.D. and Rader, D.J., 2003, "Guggulipid for the Treatment of Hypercholesterolemia: A Randomized Controlled Trial", *Journal of American Medical Association*, 290(6), pp. 765-772.
115. Nityanand, S., Srivastava, J.S. and Asthana, O.P., 1989, "Clinical Trials with Gugulipid: A New Hypolipidaemic Agent", *J. Assoc. Physicians India*, 37(5), pp. 323-328.
116. Urizar, N.L., Liverman, A.B., Dodds, D.N.T., Silva, F.V., Ordantlich, P., Yan, Y., Gonzalez, F.J., Heyman, R.A., Mangelsdorf, D.J. and Moore, D.D., 2002, "A Natural Product that Lowers Cholesterol as an Antagonist Ligand for FXR", *Science*, 296(5573), pp. 1703-1706.
117. Urizar, N.L. and Moore, D.D., 2003, "Goggolipid: A Natural Cholesterol-lowering Agent", *Annual Reviews in Nutrition*, 23, pp. 303-313.
118. Baggio, E., Gandini, R., Plancher, A.C., Passerie, M. and Carmosino, G., 1994, "Italian Multicenter Study on the Safety and Efficacy of Coenzyme Q10 as Adjunctive Therapy in Heart Failure: CoQ10 Drug Surveillance Investigators", *Molecular Aspects of Medicine*, 15 Suppl., pp. s287-s294.
119. Greenberg, S. and Frishman, W.H., 1990, "Co-enzyme Q10: A New Drug for Cardiovascular Disease", *Journal of Clinical Pharmacology*, 30(7), pp. 596-608.
120. Chainani-Wu, N., 2003, "Safety and Anti-inflammatory Activity of Curcumin: A Component of Tumeric (Curcuma longa)", *Journal of Alternative and Complementary Medicine*, 9(1), pp. 161-168.
121. Soni, K.B. and Kuttan, R., 1992, "Effect of Oral Curcumin Administration on Serum Peroxides and Cholesterol Levels in Human Volunteers", *Indian Journal of Physiology and Pharmacology*, 36(4), pp. 273-275.

Index